P9-APU-690

Atlas of
DRUG REACTIONS

Atlas of DRUG REACTIONS

R. Douglas Collins, M.D.

Fellow of the American College of Physicians
Formerly, Associate Clinical Professor of Medicine
University of Florida College of Medicine
Gainesville, Florida
Formerly, Director, Internal Medicine Residency Program
Pensacola Foundation for Education
and Research, Inc. (P.E.P.)
Pensacola, Florida

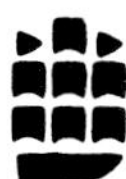

CHURCHILL LIVINGSTONE
New York, Edinburgh, London, and Melbourne 1985

Acquisitions Editor: Gene Kearn
Copy Editor: Margot Otway
Production Editor: Charlie Lebeda
Production Supervisor: Kerry Ann O'Rourke
Compositor: Progressive Typographers, Inc.
Printer/Binder: Mandarin Offset International, Ltd.

Distributed in the United States by Churchill Livingstone Inc., 1560 Broadway, New York, N.Y. 10036. Distributed in the United Kingdom by Churchill Livingstone, Robert Stevenson House, 1–3 Baxter's Place, Leith Walk, Edinburgh EH1 3AF and associated companies, branches and representatives throughout the world.

First published in 1985

Printed in Hong Kong

ISBN 0-443-08377-0

7 6 5 4 3 2 1

Library of Congress Cataloging in Publication Data

Collins, R. Douglas.
Atlas of drug reactions.

Includes indexes.
1. Drugs—Side effects. 2. Drugs—Safety measures.
3. Drug interactions. 4. Drugs—Toxicology.
I. Title, [DNLM: 1. Drug Interactions—atlases.
2. Drug Therapy—adverse effects—atlases. 3. Drugs—
adverse effects—atlases. QZ 17 C712a]
RM302.5.C65 1985 615'.704 85-11033
ISBN 0-443-08377-0

This book is dedicated to the family doctor in recognition of his many victories in the war against disease, which so often go unrecognized by anyone but himself and his patients.

Preface

Several times during the day — when prescribing an unfamiliar drug, when checking a possible drug reaction reported by a patient — it becomes necessary for most physicians to consult the standard references on drug reactions and interactions. These sources are comprehensive and therefore indispensible, but they are not designed for rapid reference.

There is a clear need for an alternative to these existing sources — for a quick reference presenting the adverse reactions to the common drugs in a simple, organized, and easily remembered fashion. This atlas was written to fulfill that need.

The text consists of individual discussions of the most important drugs in clinical use, arranged according to therapeutic category. Each discussion clearly and concisely presents adverse reactions, contraindications, precautions for use, and interactions with other drugs. The discussions are accompanied by color illustrations which graphically display the common and serious reactions to the drugs. Numerous tables compare the adverse reactions to the drugs in each therapeutic class, providing the clinician with appropriate alternatives. Finally, the book contains appendices listing drugs by trade name and generic name, which provide a quick reference to the identification of a drug and its important adverse reactions.

I wish to thank the people whose hard work made this book possible. Teri Langheld turned my miserable scribbling into a handsome typewritten manuscript. Lynn Kubasek transformed my rough sketches into beautifully finished illustrations. Gene Kearn and the staff of Churchill Livingstone turned the manuscript into a book that any author could be proud of.

I could not close this preface without mentioning how much the patience, love, and understanding of my lovely wife, Deborah, have meant to me throughout the creation of this book.

R. Douglas Collins, M.D., F.A.C.P.

Introduction

How is this book organized, and how may it be used most efficiently?

In the body of the text will be found separate discussions of drugs or groups of related drugs, organized into chapters by therapeutic category. Each discussion gives the various reactions associated with the drug or drugs, and also contraindications, precautions for use, and interactions with other drugs. If a reaction presented by a patient is not mentioned in the discussion, it is extremely unlikely to have been caused by the drug in question.

The discussions of the more common drugs and drug groups are accompanied by a color illustration displaying the more frequent or serious reactions. Although many of the less common drugs are not individually illustrated, the class of drug into which they fall usually is.

At the end of the text are two appendices which provide the physician with concise, basic information and help guide him to the relevant discussion in the text. The Generic Index lists drugs by generic name and gives their therapeutic category, under which they are discussed in the text. The Index of Drugs by Trade Name lists proprietary drugs, gives their generic ingredients, and for each ingredient gives the therapeutic category and the most significant adverse reactions. Thus a drug may be looked up by either generic or trade name.

In addition to the two appendices, there is a standard index at the back of the book which gives the pages on which a drug is discussed.

Not every drug is discussed in this book. However, for virtually any drug that is not individually discussed, the appendices will provide the therapeutic category so that a general idea of the significant reactions may be obtained.

Certain types of reactions are common to most drugs. Almost any drug ingested orally can cause a gastrointestinal reaction of some type — nausea, vomiting, diarrhea, constipation, etc. Almost any drug can cause a hypersensitivity reaction. Finally, individual patients can have a reaction of almost any sort, so the clinician must keep an open mind at all times.

Perhaps the most unique feature of this book is the **toxicity rating.** Each drug is rated low, medium, or high in toxicity according to the frequency, severity, and reversibility of its adverse reactions. Drugs such as sympathomimetics, antihistamines, and hypnotics are mostly rated low. At the other end of the spectrum are drugs such as the aminoglycosides, which cause ototoxicity and nephrotoxicity, and phenylbutazone and chloramphenicol, which cause agranulocytosis. In between are a host of drugs with a medium to high rating, which require careful consideration before they are prescribed. Some drugs have a moderate to high rating only when given parenterally.

Contents

Chapter 1

ANTACIDS

Antacids

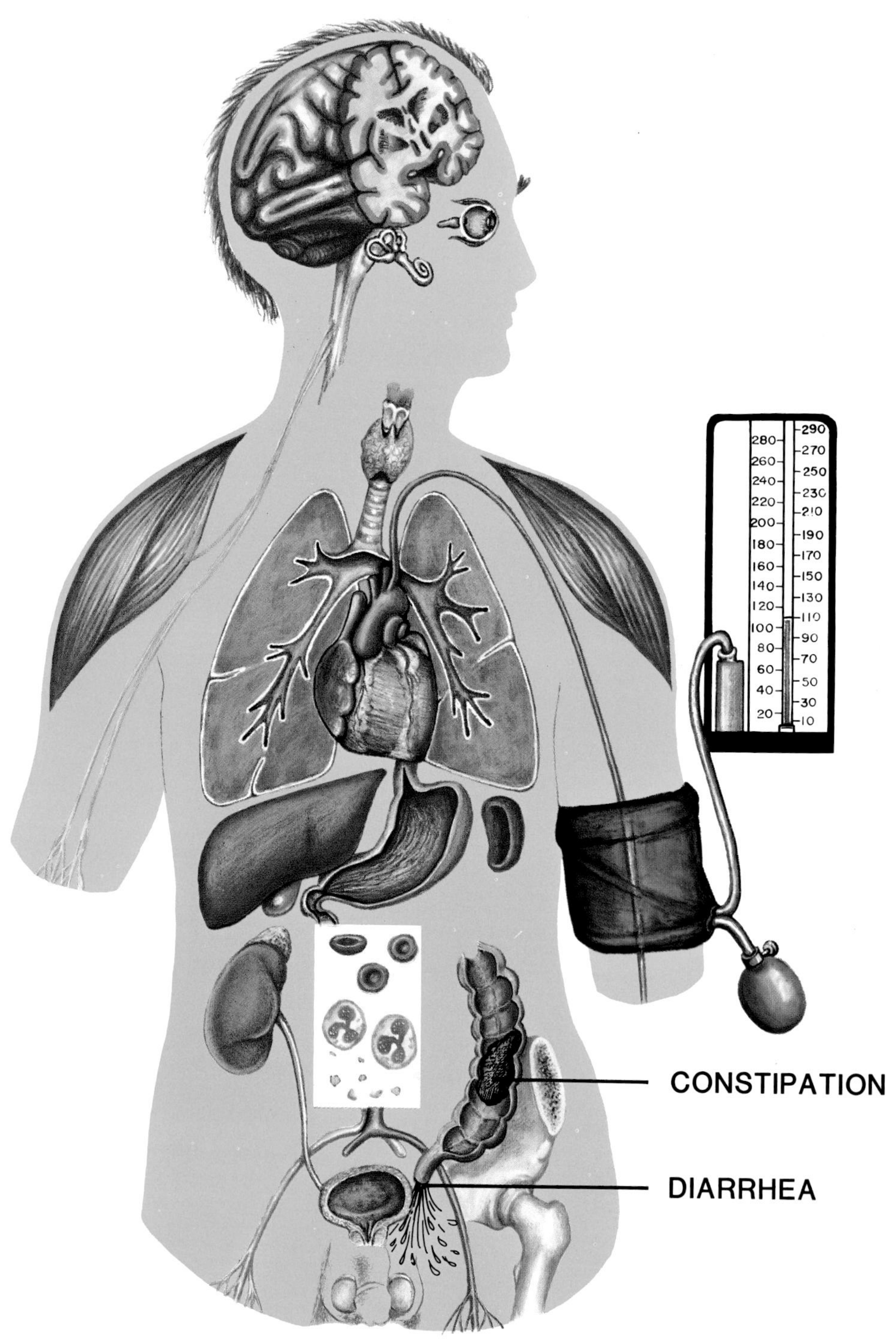

Antacids

Principal Drugs

Generic Name	Representative Trade Names
Aluminum hydroxide	Amphojel
Combination with magnesium hydroxide	Aludrox, Maalox
Combination with magnesium trisilicate	Gaviscon
Combinations with magnesium hydroxide and simethicone	Gelusil, Mylanta
Magnesium hydroxide	Milk of Magnesia
Calcium carbonate (in combination with aluminum hydroxide and magnesium hydroxide)	Camalox
Sodium bicarbonate	baking soda

Toxicity Rating: Low

Adverse Reactions

Gastrointestinal The principal side effects of all antacids are diarrhea and constipation. In general, too much magnesium hydroxide will give a patient diarrhea, whereas too much aluminum hydroxide will produce constipation. Calcium carbonate is also usually constipating.

Other Too frequent ingestion of antacids may produce hypercalcemia and the milk-alkali syndrome characterized by metabolic alkalosis, renal calculi, and nephrocalcinosis. Calcium carbonate may cause acid rebound because it stimulates gastrin production.

Precautions

Patients with renal disease should be watched for hypermagnesemia manifested by tremor and cardiovascular symptoms. Aluminum hydroxide preparations may cause excessive phosphorus depletion.

Drug Interactions

Antacids may inhibit the absorption of tetracyclines, so these antibiotics should be given at least 1 hour before antacid administration. The alkalinization of gastric and renal pH alters the bioavailability of many drugs.

Treatment

Simple withdrawal of the drug is usually all that is necessary.

Chapter 2

ANTIANGINAL AGENTS

Antianginal Agents

Principal Types of Antianginal Agents

Nitrates
Calcium channel blockers
Dipyridamole
Beta blockers (see page 19)

Introduction

All types of drugs in this group produce side effects by inducing hypotension. The calcium channel blockers also have a negative inotropic effect on heart muscle and thus may induce heart failure and various types of heart block. For this reason, the calcium channel blockers deserve a higher toxicity rating.

Nitrates

Nitrates

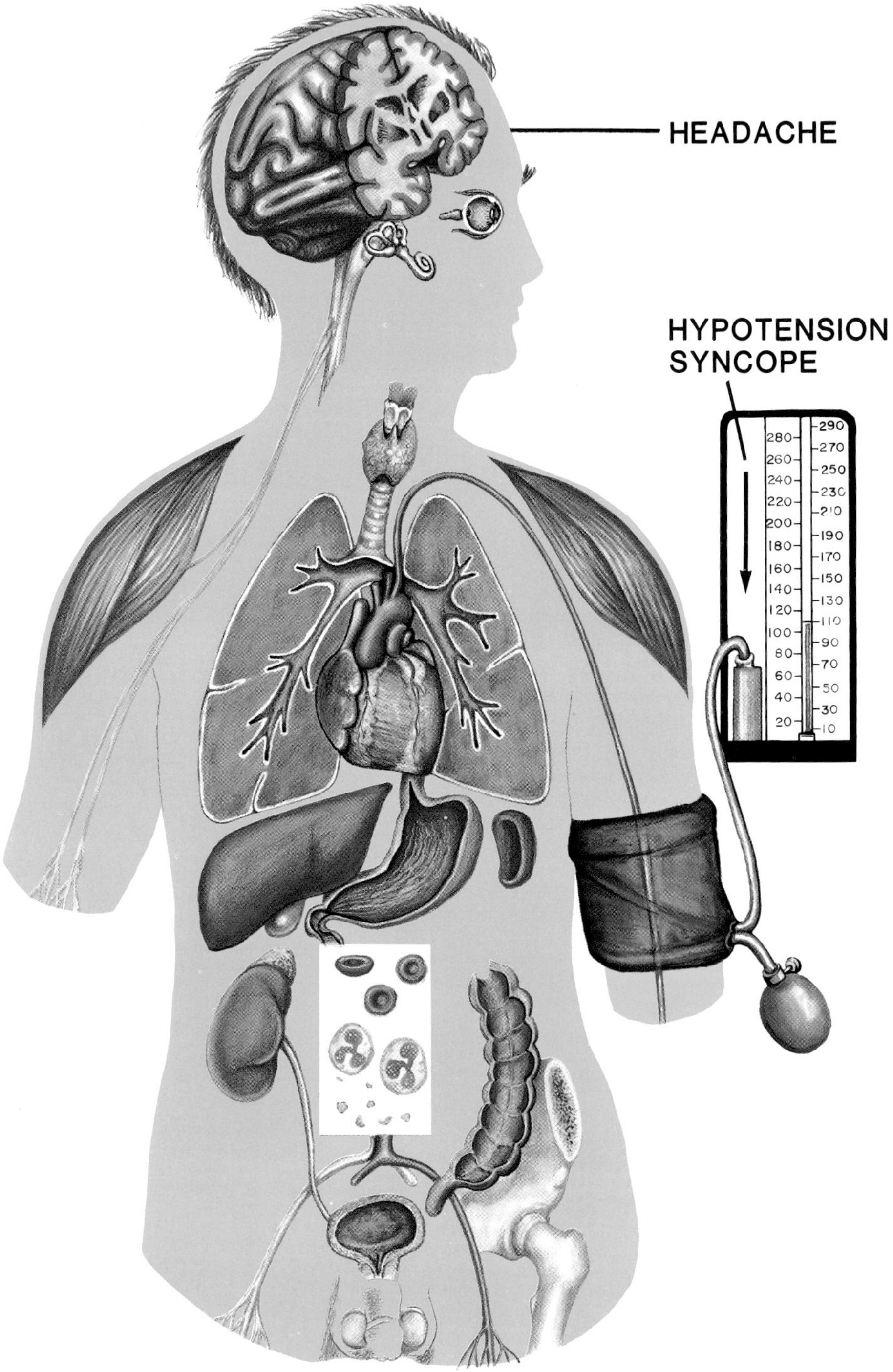

HEADACHE

HYPOTENSION
SYNCOPE

Nitrates

Principal Drugs

Generic Name	Representative Trade Names
Nitroglycerin	Nitrostat
Nitroglycerin ointment	Nitrol Ointment, Nitrodisc, Transderm-Nitro
Isosorbide dinitrate	Isordil, Sorbitrate
Pentaerythritol tetranitrate	Peritrate

Toxicity Rating: Low

Adverse Reactions

Central Nervous System Headache is a common reaction, but is usually transient. There may be transient dizziness, weakness, and even syncope. Syncope is usually due to the associated postural hypotension. Alcohol may potentiate the syncopal attacks.

Skin Transient flushing, sweating, and more persistent rashes such as exfoliative dermatitis have occurred.

Other There may be acute nausea and vomiting, usually associated with the hypotension.

Contraindications

The only real contraindication is known hypersensitivity to the drug.

Treatment

Withdrawal of the drug and administration of oxygen and vasopressors are the major methods of treatment.

Calcium Channel Blockers

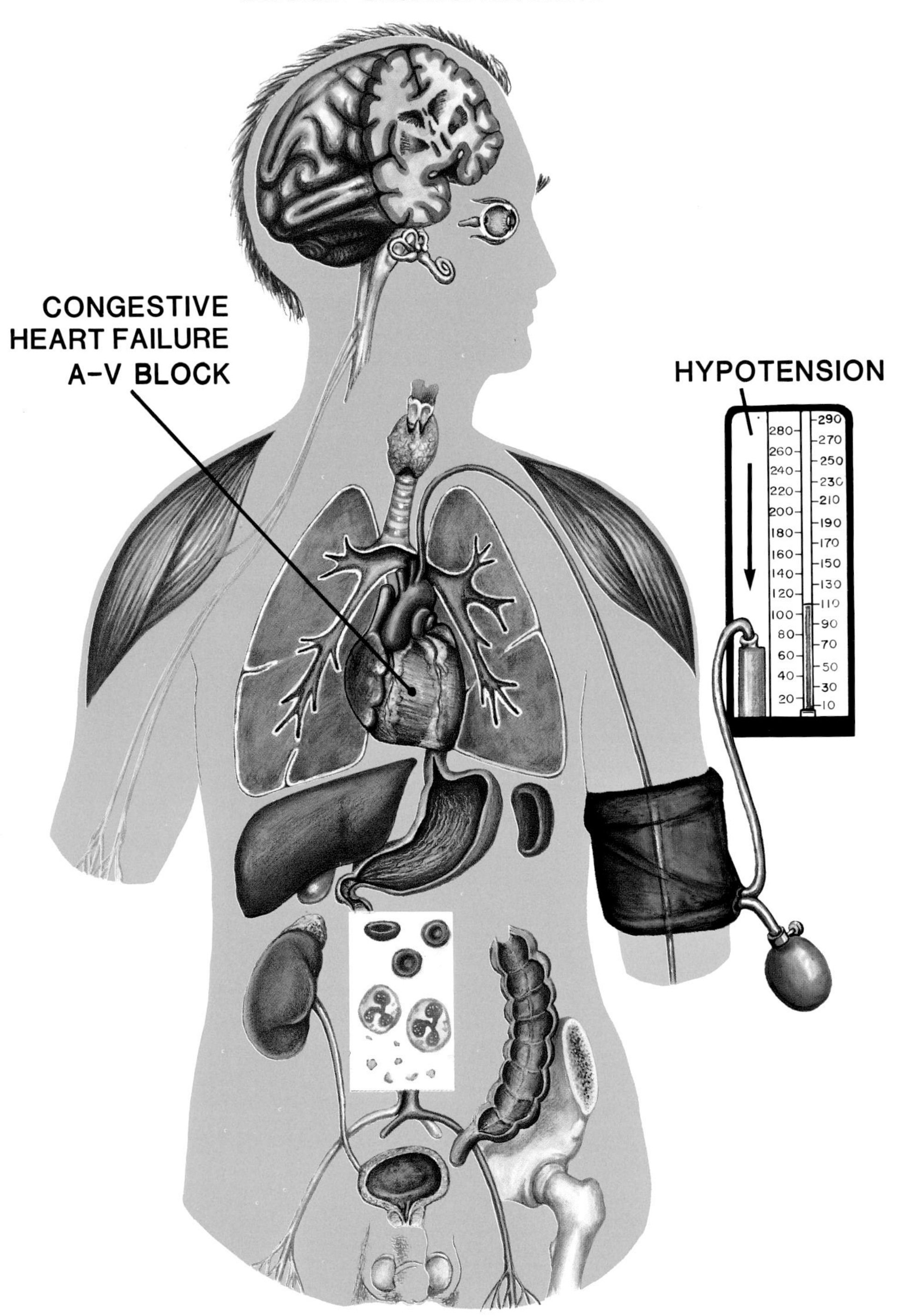

Calcium Channel Blockers

Principal Drugs

Generic Name	Representative Trade Names
Nifedipine	**Procardia**
Verapamil hydrochloride	**Calan, Isoptin**

Toxicity Rating: Medium

Adverse Reactions

Cardiovascular Hypotension is the major side effect of calcium channel blockers, and is responsible for most of the adverse symptoms such as dizziness, weakness, palpitations, and syncope. There may be flushing, peripheral edema, and shortness of breath. Frank *congestive heart failure* may develop, especially in patients with aortic stenosis. Calcium channel blockers occasionally make anginal symptoms worse, especially when verapamil is administered concomitantly with a beta blocker. *Atrioventricular conduction disturbances* including heart block are occasionally encountered, especially with verapamil therapy.

Central Nervous System Many of the CNS side effects are related to the hypotensive effect of calcium channel blockers. However, lightheadedness, mood changes, and muscle cramps have occurred independent of hypotension.

Gastrointestinal Nausea, diarrhea, constipation, cramps, and bloating may occur.

Respiratory Cough, nasal congestion, and shortness of breath have been noted.

Other Allergic skin reactions including urticaria, pruritus, and edema occur. Fever, sweating, and chills have also been seen. No cases of hepatitis have been noted.

Contraindications

Other than known hypersensitivity, there are none.

Precautions

Calcium channel blockers should be given cautiously in patients with known congestive heart failure, hypotension, or heart blocks. Unlike the beta blockers, preexisting asthma is not a contraindication.

Drug Interactions

These drugs, especially verapamil, may potentiate congestive heart failure or heart block and exacerbate angina when used with beta blockers. Patients recently withdrawn from the beta blockers may experience increased anginal attacks and these attacks may be potentiated by administering calcium channel blockers.

Treatment

Withdrawal of the drug is usually all that is necessary. Administration of vasopressors, oxygen, and intravenous fluids is occassionally necessary.

Dipyridamole

Representative Trade Name: Persantine

Toxicity Rating: Low

Adverse Reactions

Cardiovascular Transient hypotension may cause dizziness, weakness, or syncope. Occasionally the hypotension may precipitate anginal attacks—the very condition for which the drug is prescribed.

Other Headache, skin rash, nausea, and flushing have been observed.

Contraindications

Other than known hypersensitivity, there are none.

Treatment

Withdrawal of dipyridamole is usually followed by recovery from the side effects.

Chapter 3

ANTIARRHYTHMIC DRUGS

Table 3-1. Side Effects of Antiarrhythmic Drugs

Drug	Arrhythmias	Heart Block	Congestive Heart Failure	Hypotension	CNS	Gastrointestinal Effects	Hematopoietic Effects	Cinchonism	Respiratory Effects	Allergic Reactions	Other
Digitalis preparations	+	+	−	−	+	+	+	−	−	+	Visual disturbances
Propanolol	−	+	+	+	+	+	+	−	+ (asthma)	+	−
Lidocaine	−	+	−	+	+	−	−	−	−	+	−
Bretylium tosylate	+	−	−	+	+	+	−	−	−	+	−
Disopyramide	−	+	+	+	+	+	−	−	−	+	−
Quinidine	+	+	+	+	+	+	+	+	−	+	−
Procainamide	+	+	+	+	+	−	+ (including "lupus syndrome")	−	−	+	−

Introduction

Principal Types of Antiarrhythmic Drugs

Digitalis preparations
Propranolol
Lidocaine hydrochloride
Bretylium tosylate
Disopyramide phosphate
Quinidine
Procainamide hydrochloride
Calcium channel blockers (see page 11)
Atropine sulfate (see pages 33–34)
Potassium, calcium (see page 314)

Adverse Reactions Common to All Antiarrhythmics

As shown in Table 3-1, many toxic side effects are common in some degree to all the above antiarrhythmic drugs. These shared side effects are discussed here.

Central Nervous System All the above antiarrhythmics may cause central nervous system disturbances including confusion, emotional instability, and psychosis. However, these symptoms are rare with procainamide, and with bretylium they are usually an indirect effect of hypotension.

Gastrointestinal Nausea, vomiting, diarrhea, and constipation may be observed with any of these drugs, but since lidocaine is not given orally, gastrointestinal symptoms are rare. Procainamide causes a low incidence of gastrointestinal effects compared to the other antiarrhythmics under discussion, while quinidine probably causes the highest incidence.

Cardiovascular All the above antiarrhythmics except bretylium may induce varying degrees of heart block and may even lead to asystole. Bretylium and digitalis, on the other hand, may induce ventricular extrasystoles and other arrhythmias. Propranolol and lidocaine are not likely to cause arrhythmias. However, propranolol and disopyramide are more likely to induce congestive heart failure than the other drugs in this group that have negative inotropic effects. Although all the above antiarrhythmics may produce hypotension either directly or indirectly due to their cardiac effects, hypotension is particularly likely to occur with bretylium.

Side Effects of Specific Drugs Some adverse reactions are peculiar to various drugs in this group. *Propranolol* has a bronchoconstrictive effect and can precipitate attacks of bronchial asthma in susceptible individuals. Digitalis preparations are associated with many unusual disturbances including blurred vision, distortion of color vision (particularly yellow vision), halos, and bilateral central scotomata. Quinidine causes cinchonism (dizziness, tinnitus, blurred vision, headache, and tremor). Procainamide may be associated with a reversible "lupus syndrome." Reversible alopecia is not uncommon with propranolol. Bretylium may cause transient hypertension due to catecholamine release.

Other Antiarrhythmics

Not all the antiarrhythmic drugs are discussed in this chapter. The calcium channel blockers (verapamil HCl, etc.) can be found under antianginal drugs (Page 11). Atropine sulfate is discussed with the other anticholinergic drugs (Pages 33–34), and potassium and calcium are discussed under minerals (Page 314).

Digitalis Preparations

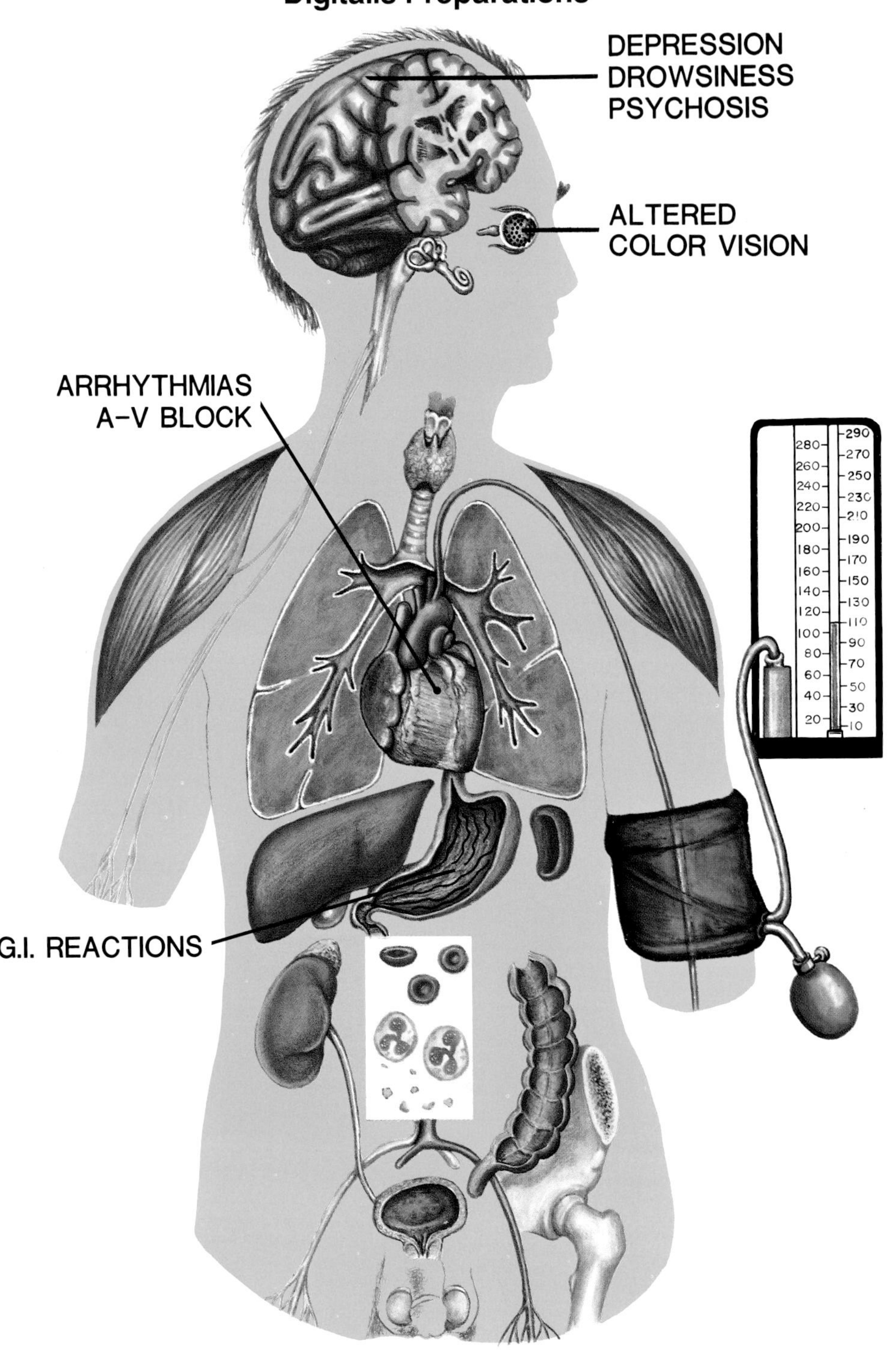

Digitalis Preparations

Principal Drugs

Generic Name	Representative Trade Name
Digitalis leaf	Pil-Digis
Digoxin	Lanoxin
Digitoxin	Crystodigin
Ouabain	Ouabain

Toxicity Rating: Medium because of arrhythmias and heart block.

Adverse Reactions

Cardiovascular Cardiac arrhythmias may occur, including sinus arrest, complete atrioventricular block, atrioventricular dissociation with block, and ventricular fibrillation.

Gastrointestinal Anorexia, nausea, vomiting, diarrhea, and abdominal distention are not uncommon.

Central Nervous System Drowsiness, depression, fatigue, hallucinations, confusion, and frank organic psychosis may occur.

Special Senses Photophobia, altered red-green color perception, and blurred vision occur.

Other Gynecomastia has occasionally been reported.

Contraindications

Contraindications are ventricular fibrillation, known hypersensitivity, and sinus tachycardia not related to congestive heart failure.

Precautions

Use of these drugs to treat obesity may be dangerous. The dose should be lowered and monitored carefully in patients with renal insufficiency or hypokalemia. Hypercalcemia, hypomagnesemia, and hypokalemia may predispose patients to digitalis toxicity. Hypothyroidism may also predispose patients to digitalis toxicity, and hyperthyroid patients require more digitalis. Patients with acute myocardial infarction or emphysema are sensitive to digitalis-induced arrhythmias. Patients undergoing electric cardioversion may need their dose of digitalis reduced: blood levels should be measured before electric cardioversion and the dose adjusted accordingly. Digitalis blood levels should be carefully monitored when this drug is given to patients with any type of heart block or bradycardia. Digitalis may also precipitate ventricular fibrillation in patients with the Wolff-Parkinson-White syndrome. Intramuscular injections of digitalis preparations may be painful.

Drug Interactions

Corticosteroids, IV calcium, and diuretics that cause hypokalemia may precipitate digitalis toxicity. Quinidine may cause an elevation of blood levels of digitalis. Sympathomimetics increase the risk of digitalis-induced arrhythmias. Succinylcholine chloride may induce arrhythmias in digitalized patients. Beta adrenergic blocking agents (e.g. propranolol) may induce heart block or congestive failure in digitalized patients. Amphotericin B, carbenicillin, ticarcillin, and metolazone predispose patients to hypokalemia and digitalis toxicity. Antacids, *p*-aminosalicylic acid salts, cholestyramine, colestipol, kaolin-pectin, and neomycin decrease digitalis absorption.

Treatment

Simple withdrawal of the drug may be all that is necessary, but careful monitoring in the intensive care unit may be wise in patients predisposed to arrhythmias. Ventricular arrhythmias may respond to phenytoin or lidocaine. Hypokalemia should be treated by oral or intravenous potassium (40 mEq/500 mL of 5 percent dextrose in water). Life-threatening digitalis toxicity may be treated by intravenous potassium (40 mEq/500 mL of 5 percent dextrose in water). Edetate disodium (EDTA) infusions have been used to lower the serum calcium and thus combat digitalis toxicity. Frequent measurment of serum electrolytes and digitalis levels must be done.

Propranolol

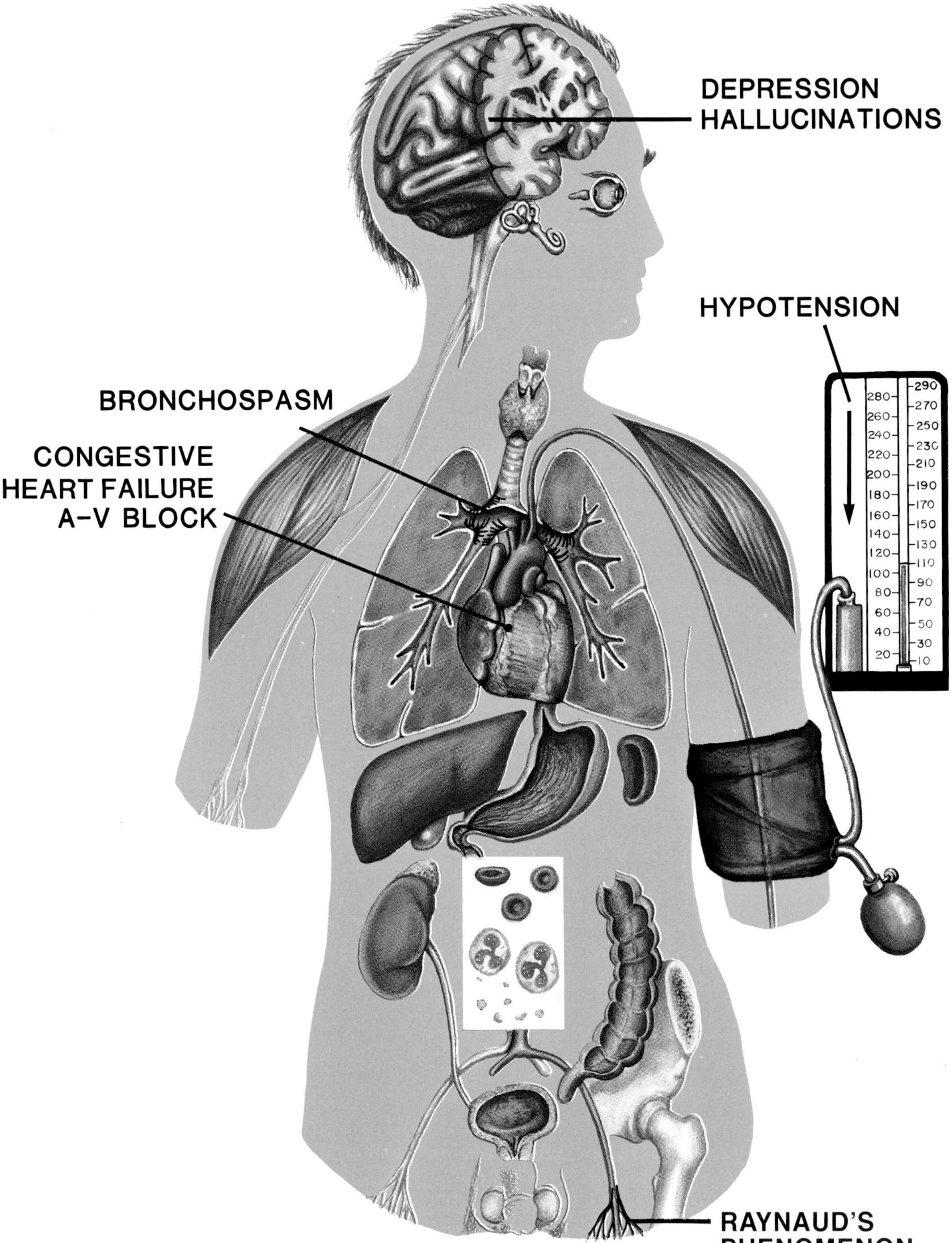

DEPRESSION
HALLUCINATIONS

HYPOTENSION

BRONCHOSPASM

CONGESTIVE
HEART FAILURE
A-V BLOCK

RAYNAUD'S
PHENOMENON

Propranolol

Principal Drugs

Generic Name	Representative Trade Name
Propranolol hydrochloride	Inderal
Related drugs:	
Metoprolol tartrate	Lopressor
Nadolol	Corgard
Timolol maleate	Blocadren

Toxicity Rating: Medium because of hypotension, bronchospasm, atrioventricular block, and congestive heart failure.

Adverse Reactions

Cardiovascular Propranolol depresses the myocardium as well as the conduction system, causing bradycardia, atrioventricular block, and congestive heart failure. It also causes hypotension. It may exert a vasoconstrictive effect on the peripheral vasculature, causing Raynaud's phenomenon.

Central Nervous System Propranolol depresses the nervous system in most cases (mental depression, weakness, catatonia) but may cause hallucinations and emotional lability in some patients.

Gastrointestinal Nausea, vomiting, and diarrhea or constipation — the extremes of hypermotility and hypomotility — are not uncommon. Occasionally ischemic colitis and mesenteric thrombosis (arterial) occurs.

Respiratory Propranolol may intensify bronchospasm in bronchial asthma, and thus should be avoided in asthmatic patients.

Hematologic Agranulocytosis, thrombocytopenia, and vascular purpura have been observed.

Allergic Erythematous rash, fever, aching, and pharyngitis may occur. Acute laryngeal spasm and respiratory distress have also been observed. Conjunctivitis occurs and may be an allergic reaction to propranolol.

Other Reversible alopecia is not uncommon. Blood urea nitrogen may be increased in patients with severe heart disease. Alterations in liver function have occurred.

Contraindications

Propranolol is contraindicated in patients with bronchial asthma, congestive heart failure, bradycardia, bradyarrhythmias, and when adrenergic-augmenting psychotropic drugs are being given.

Precautions

Close monitoring of heart rate and blood pressure is mandatory with intravenous administration and useful upon initiation of oral therapy.

Treatment

Most reactions subside after withdrawal of the drug. Atropine 0.5 – 1 mg IV controls excessive bradycardia in many cases. If atropine is ineffective, intravenous isoproterenol may be necessary to control excessive bradycardia (pulse rate less than 45 beats per minute) or heart block. Hypertensive reactions may be controlled by epinephrine or other sympathomimetics. Heart failure can be treated with digitalis and diuretics. Bronchospasm is reversed in most cases with theophylline or a β_2 antagonist (e.g. terbutaline).

Lidocaine Hydrochloride

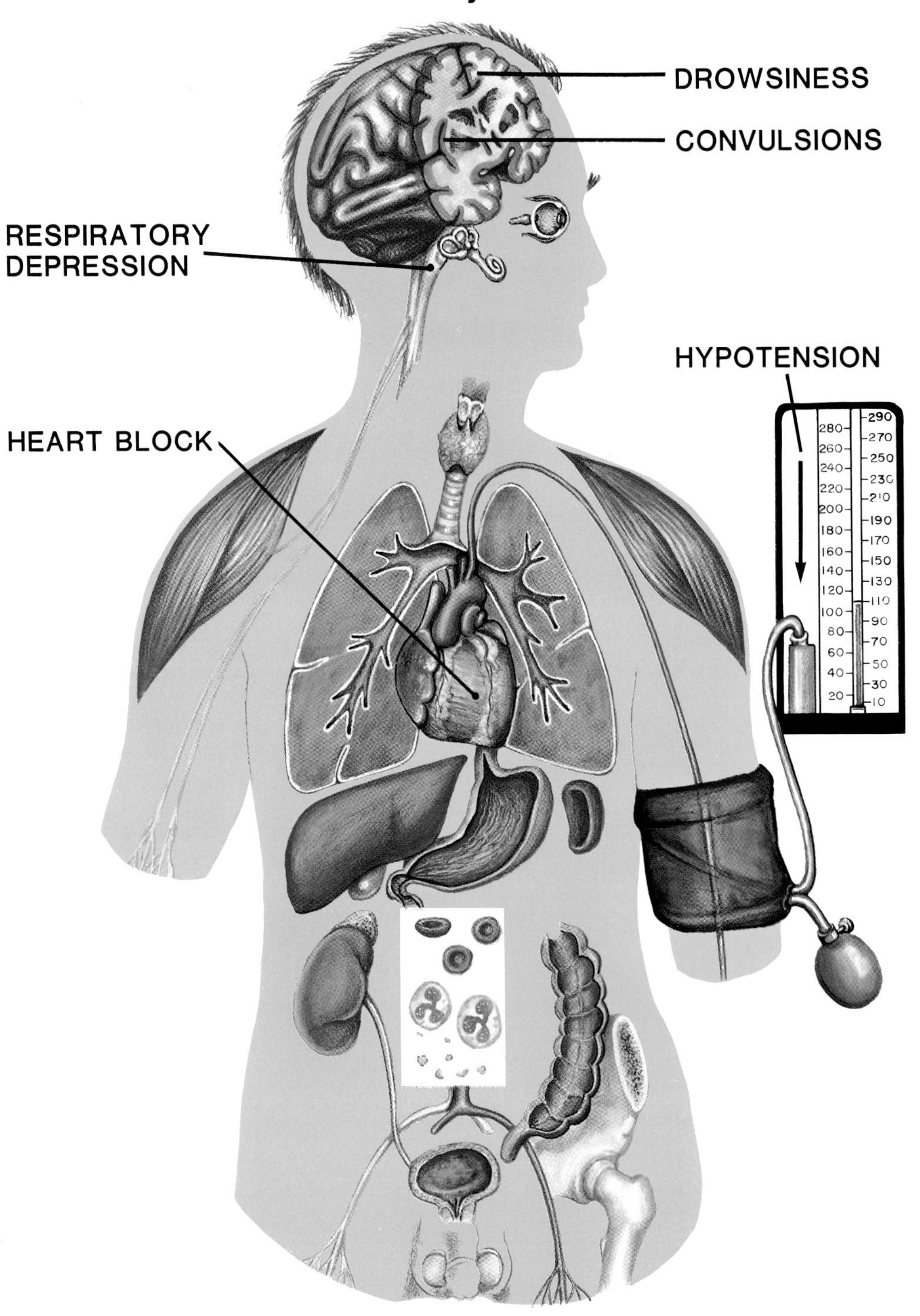

Lidocaine Hydrochloride

Representative Trade Name: Xylocaine

Toxicity Rating: Low

Adverse Reactions

Central Nervous System Depressive effects on the central nervous system include drowsiness, slurred speech, coma, and respiratory depression. Like most drugs that depress the nervous system, an excitatory effect is observed in some patients due to idiosyncracies or a relatively large dose. Thus, twitching, convulsions, tinnitus, and paresthesias may develop.

Cardiovascular Large doses of the drug depress myocardium and atrioventricular conduction, leading to heart block and hypotension.

Allergic Rash, urticaria, and anaphylactoid reactions occur, but are rare.

Contraindications

It is unwise to use lidocaine as a local anesthetic in patients with heart block or in severe shock. This drug should also be avoided in patients with Wolff-Parkinson-White syndrome and in patients with known allergies to lidocaine or related drugs.

Precautions

In pregnant women, the necessity of lidocaine therapy must be weighed against possible adverse effects on the fetus. Caution should be used when giving lidocaine repeatedly to patients in severe shock or with liver or kidney disease, as they may be unable to metabolize the drug rapidly. Lidocaine may induce asystole in patients with bradycardia and incomplete heart block.

Treatment

Routine intravenous administration of lidocaine should be done with cardiac monitoring, and the drug should be stopped immediately upon observing signs of depression on the myocardium or conduction system. Emergency resuscitation equipment must be available in case asystole or fibrillation occurs, as no definite antidote is known.

Bretylium Tosylate

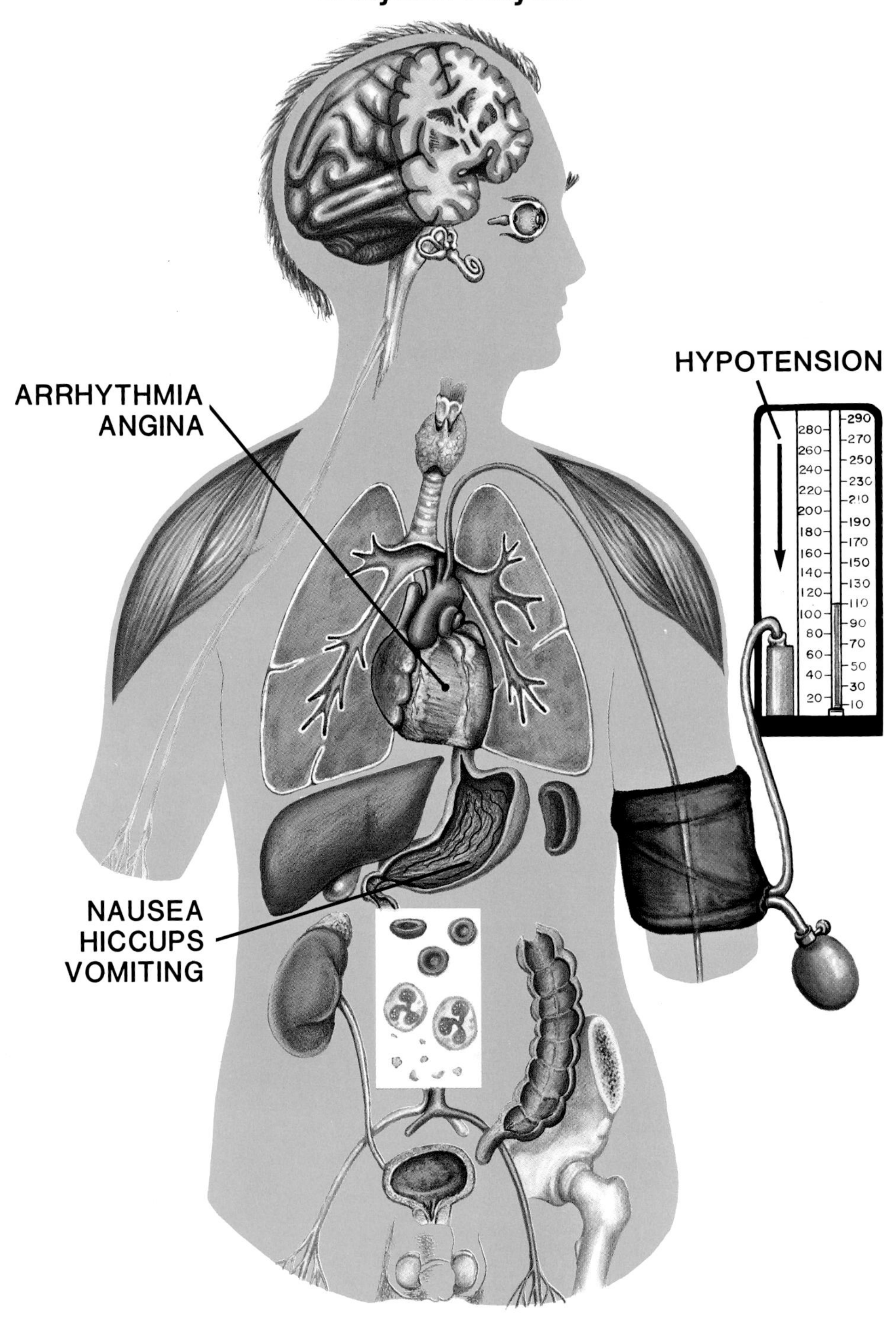

Bretylium Tosylate

Representative Trade Name: Bretylol

Toxicity Rating: Medium because of hypotension, arrhythmias, and angina.

Adverse Reactions

Cardiovascular Hypotension occurs in 50 percent of patients and increases on standing up, so the patient should be kept supine until the degree of hypotension is determined. Transient hypertension and increased premature ventricular contractions or other arrhythmias may be induced by the release of norepinephrine from postganglionic nerve terminals by this drug. This effect may aggravate digitalis toxicity. Angina may be induced by a similar mechanism.

Central Nervous System The hypotension may induce vertigo, lightheadedness, and syncope. Less frequently, confusion, emotional lability, and paranoid psychosis are observed.

Gastrointestinal Nausea, hiccups, and vomiting are precipitated in approximately 3 percent of patients. Diarrhea and abdominal pain also occur.

Allergic An erythematous macular rash is encountered occasionally.

Other Renal dysfunction, diaphoresis, nasal congestion, and conjunctivitis are rare reactions and not clearly related to bretylium tosylate.

Contraindications

When used in life-threatening emergencies, there is no absolute contraindication to this drug.

Precautions

It is wise to avoid using bretylium tosylate in patients with possible digitalis toxicity or fixed cardiac output, for example patients with aortic stenosis or pulmonary hypertension. The dosage should be reduced in patients with renal disease.

Treatment

An intravenous infusion of dopamine or norepinephrine may be given to combat hypotension below 75 mm Hg systolic. Volume expansion may be employed for this purpose also. Withdrawal of the drug is effective in other reactions.

Disopyramide Phosphate

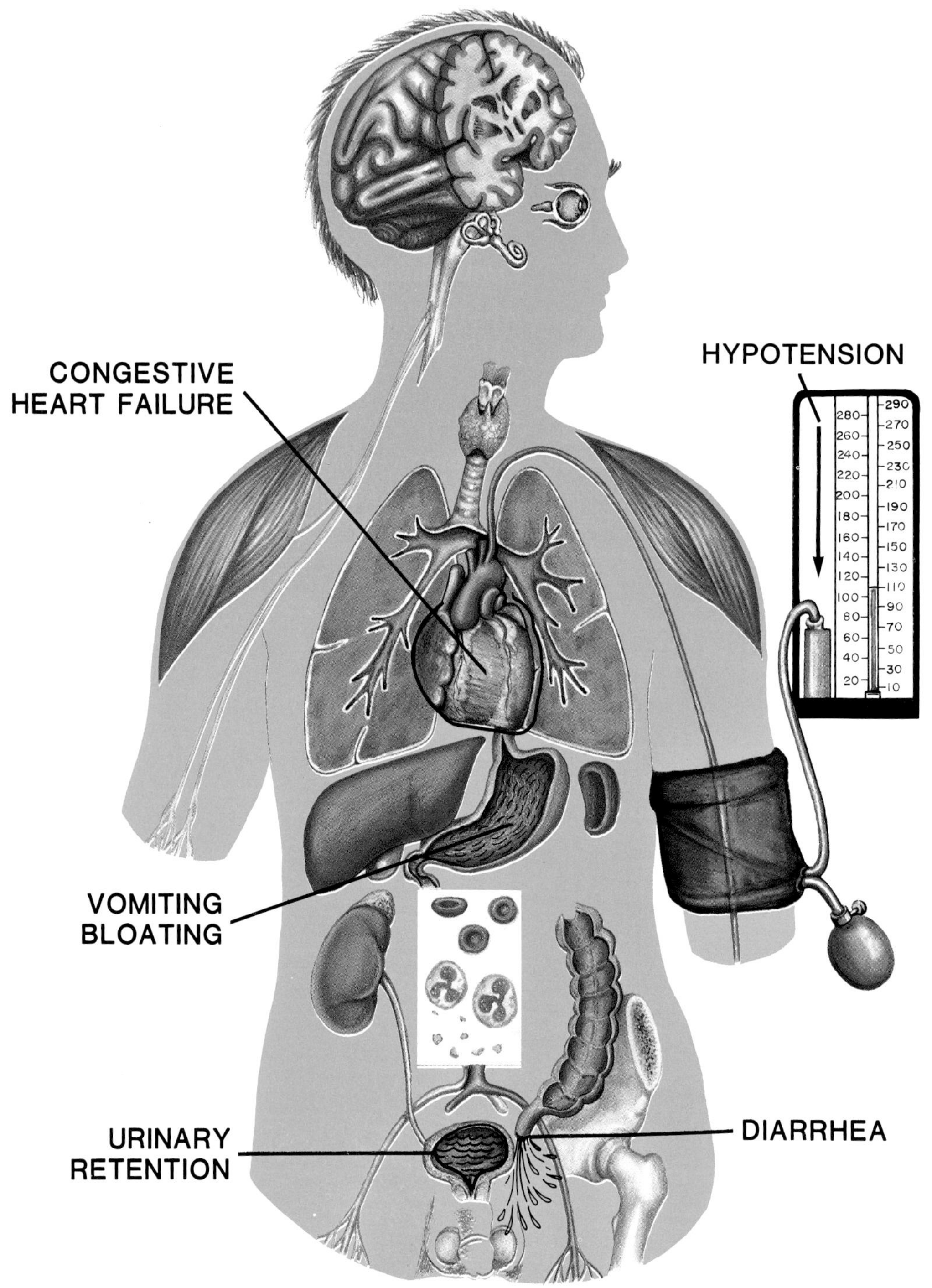

Disopyramide Phosphate

Representative Trade Name: Norpace

Toxicity Rating: Medium because of hypotension, congestive heart failure, and arrhythmias.

Adverse Reactions

Cardiovascular *Hypotension* and congestive heart failure are the major reactions to disopyramide. Cardiac conduction abnormalities (enhancement of ventricular response in artrial fibrillation) may occur.

Gastrointestinal Anticholinergic effects of this drug are manifested by dry mouth and throat, nausea, bloating, gas, vomiting, or diarrhea.

Genitourinary *Urinary retention* is a major anticholinergic effect of this drug.

Other Other infrequently observed adverse effects are blurred vision, dizziness, headaches, fatigue, impotence, nervousness, insomnia, and depression. Hypoglycemia, jaundice, hypokalemia, and increased cholesterol or triglycerides have been reported. Rare instances of thrombocytopenia, agranulocytosis, psychosis, and gynecomastia have also been reported.

Contraindications

Disopyramide is contraindicated in patients with second and third degree heart block, cardiogenic shock, severe congestive heart failure not due to arrhythmias, severe renal insufficiency, or known hypersensitivity to disopyramide. Disopyramide should be discontinued if significant widening of the QRS complex or QT prolongation is observed.

Precautions

Use of disopyramide phosphate should be avoided in patients with atrial arrhythmias without prior digitalization. Caution should be observed when prescribing disopyramide in patients with sick sinus syndrome or other cardiac conduction disturbances including bundle branch block. Patients with cardiomyopathies may develop hypotension on this drug, so a loading dose is usually not given. Patients with hepatic or renal insufficiency should receive lower dosages. Potassium abnormality should be corrected prior to therapy. The anticholinergic effects of the drug may be a hazard to patients with glaucoma and myasthenia gravis.

Drug Interactions

Phenytoin and other hepatic enzyme inducers may lower plasma levels of disopyramide. Simultaneous use of quinidine, procainamide, or propranolol may cause serious negative inotropic effects such as congestive heart failure, and may also prolong atrioventricular conduction time.

Treatment

Simple withdrawal of the drug may be all that is necessary. For severe hypotension, dopamine or isoproterenol infusions may be given. Progressive atrioventricular block may make an endocardial pacemaker necessary. Hemodialysis may be used to reduce serum levels of disopyramide.

Quinidine

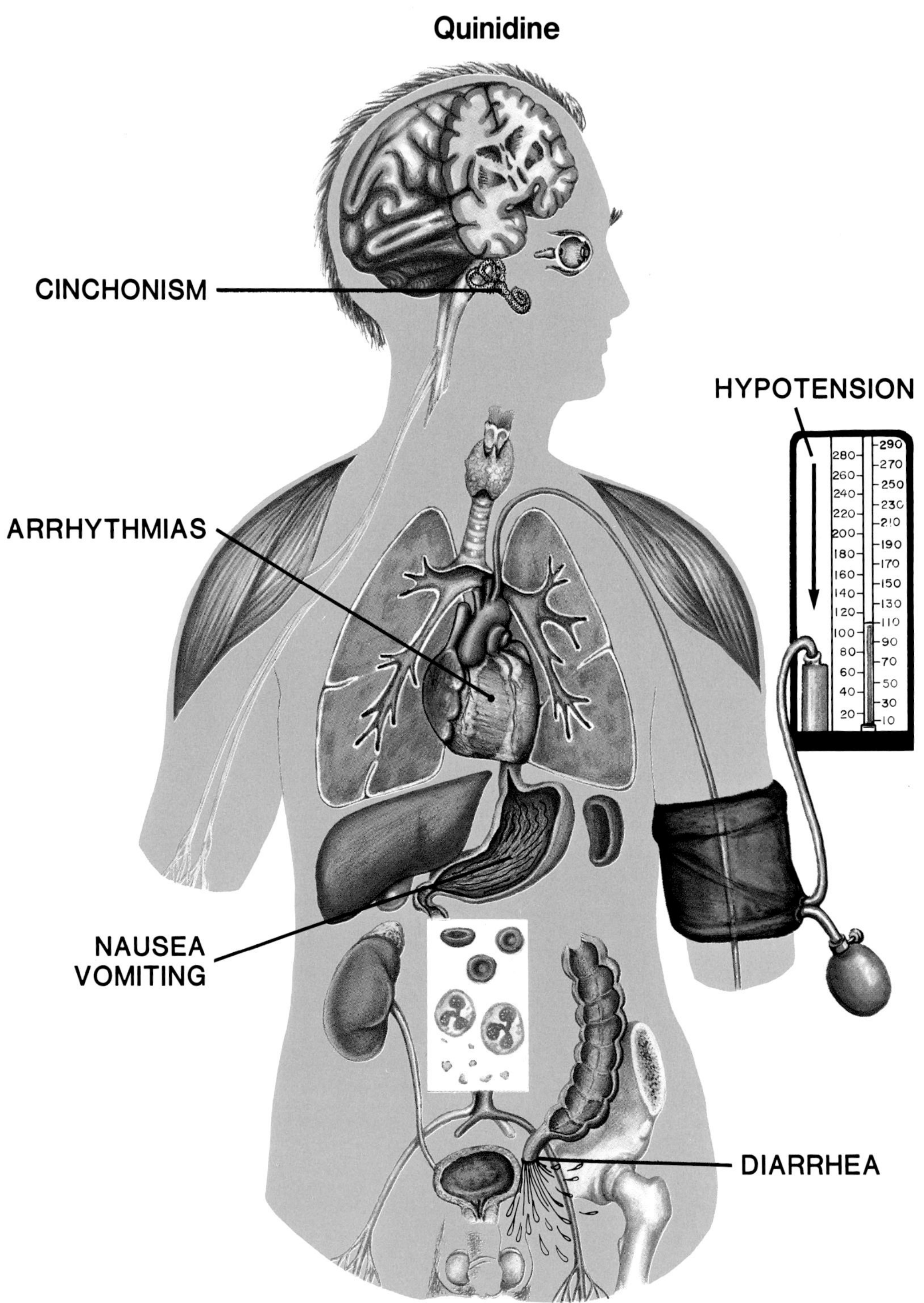
CINCHONISM
HYPOTENSION
ARRHYTHMIAS
NAUSEA
VOMITING
DIARRHEA

Quinidine

Principal Drugs

Generic Name	Representative Trade Names
Quinidine gluconate	Duraquin, Quinaglute
Quinidine sulfate	Quinidex
Quinidine polygalacturonate	Cardioquin

Toxicity Rating: Medium because of hypotension and cardiac arrhythmias.

Adverse Reactions

Cardiovascular As with the other antiarrhythmics discussed in this chapter, the major reactions to quinidine are *cardiac arrhythmias* and *hypotension*. Quinidine may aggravate congestive heart failure, but unlike propranolol does not usually precipitate it. The cardiac arrhythmias caused by quinidine are usually of ventricular origin, and include premature ventricular contractions, idioventricular rhythms, ventricular tachycardia, and fibrillation.

Gastrointestinal The most common side effects of quinidine are gastrointestinal, and include nausea, vomiting, diarrhea, and abdominal pain.

Special Senses Like aspirin, quinidine may induce tinnitus and blurred vision (symptoms of cinchonism).

Central Nervous System Quinidine may cause headache, confusion, syncope, optic neuritis, and cinchonism (tinnitus, headache, blurred vision, dizziness, and tremor).

Hematopoietic Hypoprothrombinemia, thrombocytopenia, agranulocytosis, and hemolytic anemia may occur.

Allergic Angioneurotic edema, pruritus, cutaneous urticaria, acute vascular collapse, and asthma have been observed.

Other Hepatic dysfunction occurs occasionally.

Contraindications

Quinidine is contraindicated in patients with complete heart block, complete bundle branch block, and other intraventricular conduction defects. Patients with a history of hypersensitivity to quinidine or of myasthenia gravis should not receive this drug. Quinidine should not be used to treat arrhythmias that are due to digitalis toxicity.

Precautions

Prior digitalization is advisable when quinidine is used to treat atrial flutter of fibrillation, but digoxin plasma levels may increase to toxic levels when quinidine is given concurrently. Conversion of atrial fibrillation to normal sinus rhythm may dislodge a mural thrombus. Caution should be observed when using quinidine in the presence of any conduction disturbance, of congestive heart failure, or of renal insufficiency. In long-term therapy, periodic hemograms and blood chemistry evaluations should be done. Quinidine should be used with caution in pregnant women and nursing mothers.

Drug Interactions

Concurrent administration of quinidine and coumarin anticoagulants may reduce prothrombin levels. Combining quinidine and anticholinergic drugs (atropine, etc.) may cause additive vagolysis of the myocardium. Concurrent use of quinidine with other cardiac depressant drugs (propranolol, etc.) should be avoided. Phenobarbital and phenytoin cause a 50 percent reduction in the plasma half-life of quinidine. Quinidine may increase the neuromuscular blockade effect of decamethonium, tubocurarine, or succinylcholine.

Treatment

Withdrawal of the drug is the basic treatment. Administration of 1/6 M sodium lactate may reverse cardiotoxicity, and catecholamines and other vasoconstrictors may reverse hypotension.

Procainamide Hydrochloride

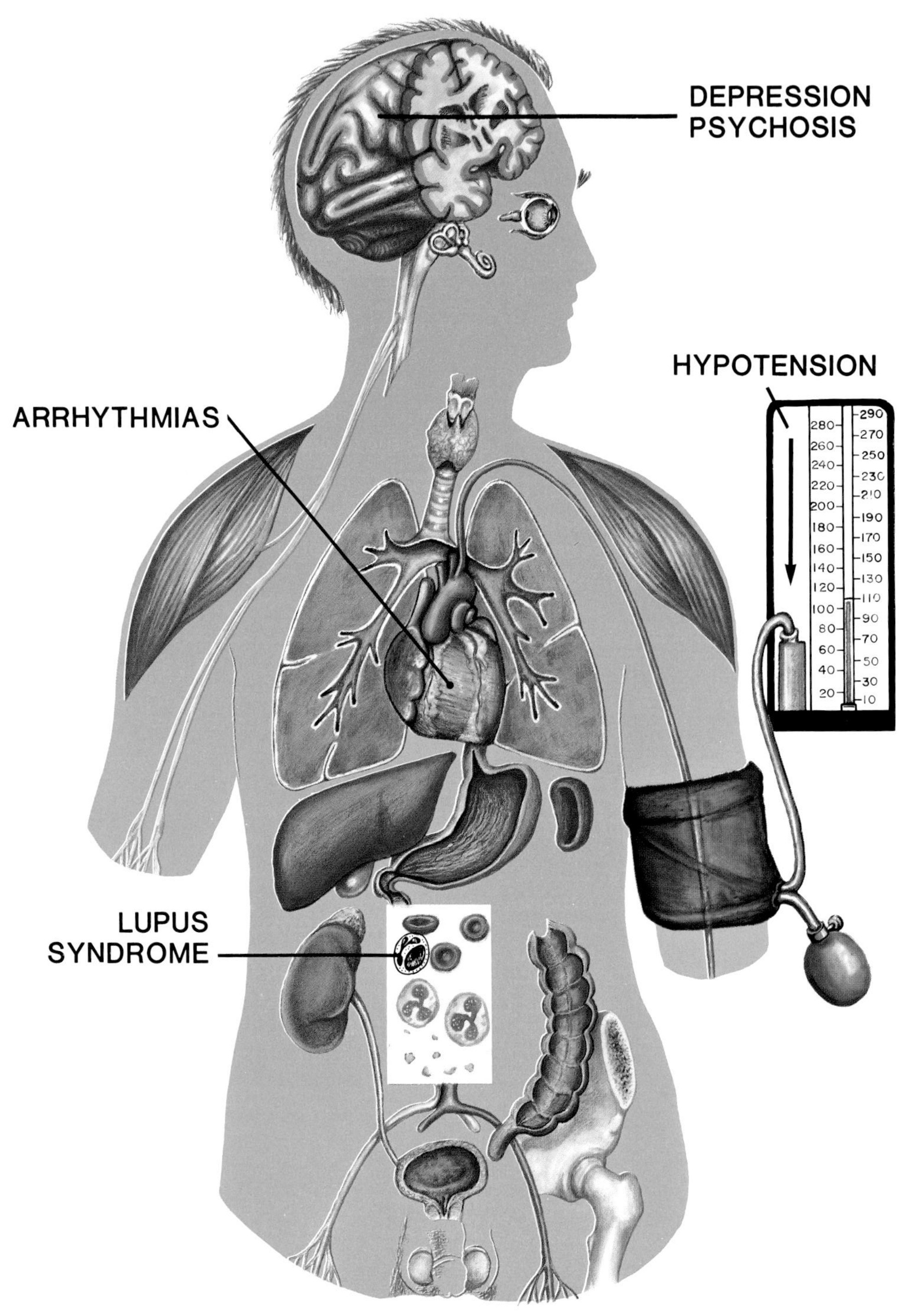

Procainamide Hydrochloride

Representative Trade Name: Pronestyl

Toxicity Rating: Medium because of hypotension and arrhythmias.

Adverse Reactions

Cardiovascular As with quinidine, the major reactions to procainamide are arrhythmias and hypotension, especially if the drug is given intravenously. Hypotension from oral administration is rare.

Hematopoietic The most fascinating reaction of procainamide is a "lupus syndrome," which is usually reversible. Repeated use of procainamide may cause agranulocytosis which is potentially fatal.

Other Unlike quinidine, procainamide is not associated with overt cinchonism, but mental depression, giddiness, and psychosis have been reported. Gastrointestinal reactions are also less frequent than with quinidine and include nausea, vomiting, diarrhea, and abdominal pain.

Allergic Reactions Angioneurotic edema, rash, fever and chills, and hepatomegaly with altered liver function may be seen.

Contraindications

Contraindications for procainamide are similar to those for quinidine and include hypersensitivity to the drug, myasthenia gravis, and complete and significant incomplete heart block.

Precautions

These are also similar to those for quinidine (see page 27). Parenteral administration necessitates electrocardiographic monitoring.

Drug Interactions

Interactions of procainamide are similar to those of quinidine (page 27).

Treatment

The drug should be withdrawn. Catecholamines should be used to counteract its hypotensive effects.

Chapter 4

ANTICHOLINERGIC DRUGS

Anticholinergic Drugs

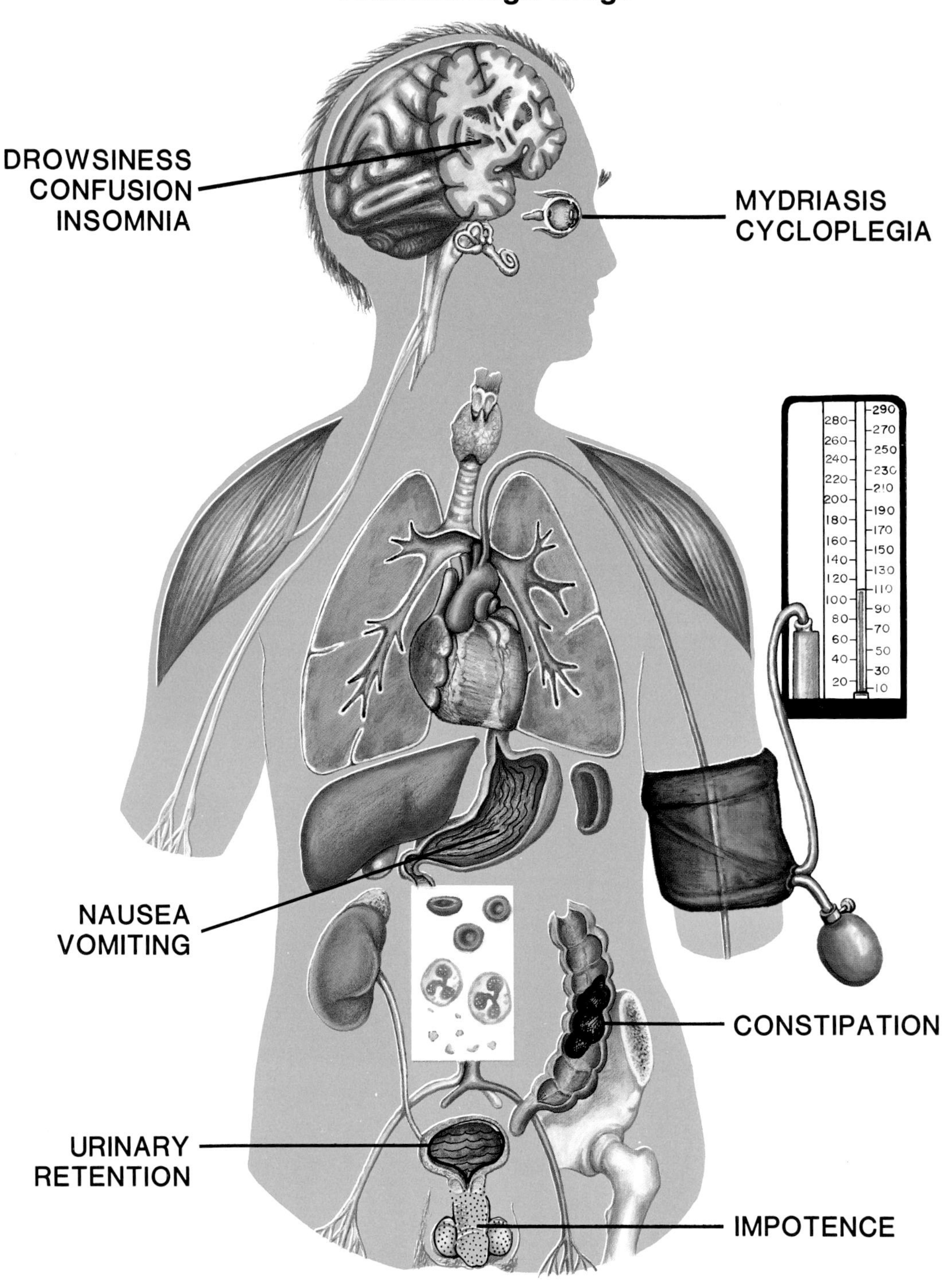

Anticholinergic Drugs

Principal Drugs

Generic Name	Representative Trade Names
Atropine sulfate	Atropine Sulfate
Belladonna alkaloids	Tincture of Belladonna; in Donnatal
Propantheline bromide	Pro-Banthine
Dicyclomine hydrochloride	Bentyl
Isopropamide iodide	Darbid
Tridihexethyl chloride	in Pathibamate
Hyoscyamine sulfate	Levsin
Glycopyrrolate	Robinul
Mepenzolate bromide	Cantil
Anisotropine methylbromide	Valpin
Scopolamine	Transderm Scōp
Scopolamine hydrobromide	in Donnatal

Toxicity Rating: Low as long as preexisting contraindicating conditions (glaucoma, etc.) are recognized.

Adverse Reactions

Ophthalmologic Blurred vision, mydriasis, cycloplegia, and even glaucoma may occur.

Gastrointestinal Constipation, nausea, vomiting, and bloating are common.

Genitourinary Genitourinary effects may occur—urinary retention, impotence, and aggravation of bladder neck obstruction resulting from the same smooth muscle relaxation that is therapeutic in the gastrointestinal tract.

Central Nervous System The nervousness, dizziness, drowsiness, and insomnia that occur are probably due to interference with nerve conduction and synaptic transmission. Mental confusion may occur in the elderly. Headaches have also been reported.

Allergic Severe allergic reactions including anaphylaxis and urticaria may occur.

Other Xerostomia, decreased sweating, and suppression of lactation may occur.

Contraindications

Anticholinergic drugs are contraindicated in the presence of glaucoma, obstructive uropathy, intestinal obstruction, toxic megacolon, myasthenia gravis, and possible heat stroke.

Precautions

These drugs should be used with caution in patients with autonomic neuropathy, ulcerative colitis, nephritis, hepatitis, hyperthyroidism, cardiac disorders, and hiatial hernia with reflux esophagitis. It may not be wise to use these drugs in the presence of biliary tract disease.

Drug Interactions

Antacids may decrease the absorption of anticholinergic drugs. Anticholinergic drugs decrease the therapeutic effect of levodopa; however, they may increase the anticholinergic effects of levodopa and anticholinergic-like CNS depressants.

Treatment

Treatment for adverse effects of anticholinergic drugs is as follows:

1. Discontinue the drug.
2. Administer cholinergic ophthalmic drugs (pilocarpine, etc.) for glaucoma.
3. If necessary, give bethanechol for urinary retention.

Chapter 5

ANTICOAGULANTS

Anticoagulants

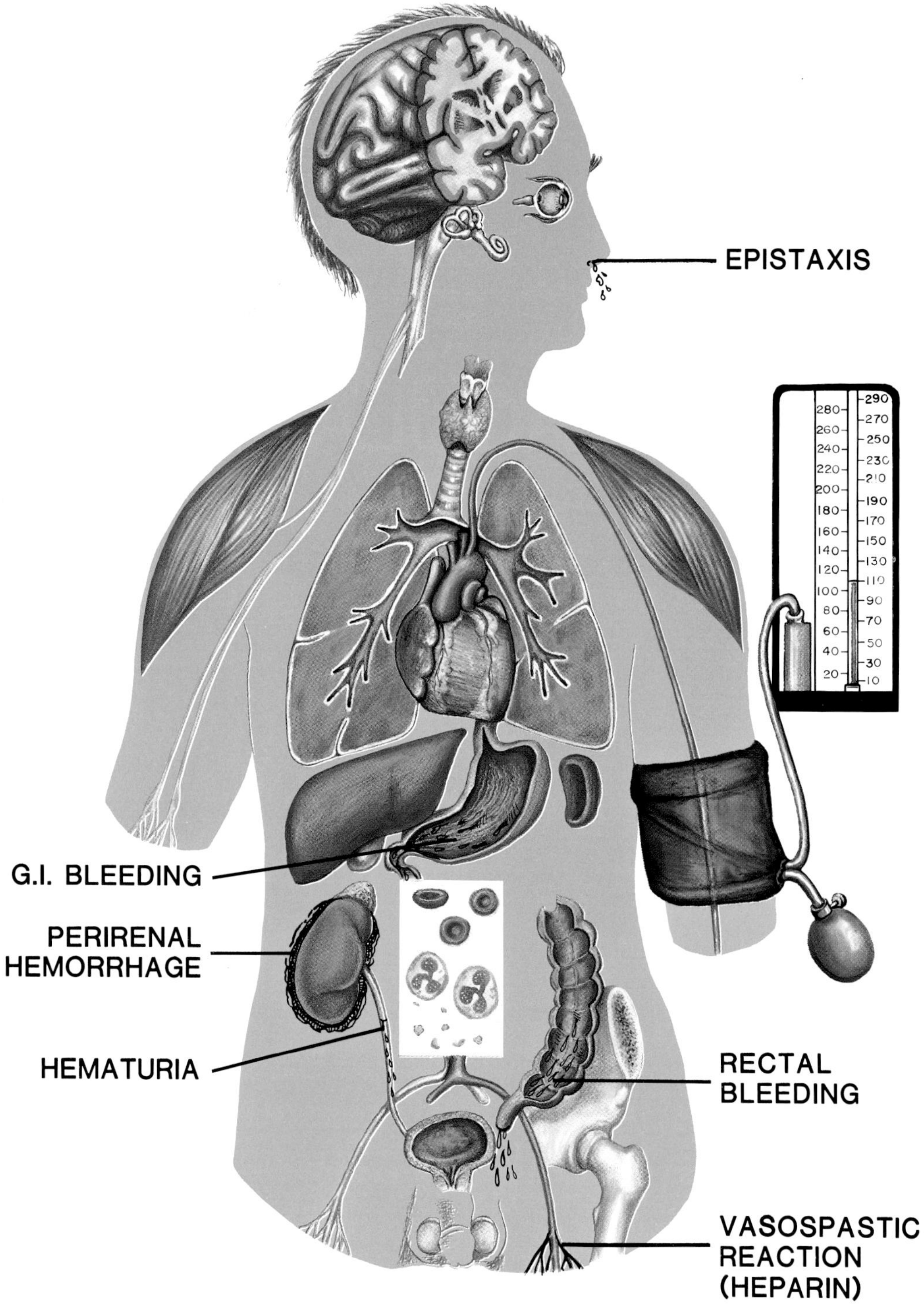

EPISTAXIS

G.I. BLEEDING

PERIRENAL HEMORRHAGE

HEMATURIA

RECTAL BLEEDING

VASOSPASTIC REACTION (HEPARIN)

Anticoagulants

Principal Drugs

Generic Name	Representative Trade Name
Warfarin sodium	Coumadin
Heparin sodium	Heparin Sodium
Low molecular weight dextran	Rheomacrodex
Phenprocoumon	Liquamar

Toxicity Rating: Medium because of hemorrhagic complications.

Adverse Reactions

Gastrointestinal Massive gastrointestinal hemorrhage may occur, especially with patients who have a silent peptic ulcer, esophageal varices, or other undiagnosed lesions of the gastrointestinal tract.

Genitourinary Massive hematuria or perirenal hemorrhage may occur.

Upper Respiratory Epistaxis is not uncommon.

Allergic Drug fever, urticaria, asthma, and anaphylactoid reactions may occur.

Other Adrenal hemorrhage may cause fatal adrenal insufficiency. Local irritation, bruising, and hematomas may occur.

Reactions Peculiar to Heparin:

Vasospastic reactions may affect one limb or progress to a generalized effect with cyanosis, tachypnea, and headache. These reactions may be allergic. Thrombocytopenia, osteoporosis, renal insufficiency, alopecia, priapism, and rebound hyperlipemia have been reported.

Reactions Peculiar to Warfarin Sodium:

Gastrointestinal Nausea, diarrhea, and abdominal cramping occur.

Dermatologic "Purple toe syndrome" and hemorrhages may occur.

Hepatic Hepatitis has occurred.

Contraindications

Anticoagulants are contraindicated in patients with significant hemorrhagic disorders and where the potential danger from hemorrhage is greater than the potential danger from thrombosis. Known hypersensitivity is a relative contraindication. Coumarin drugs are contraindicated in pregnancy.

Precautions

Coagulation profiles should be done frequently during the early stages of therapy and at regular intervals thereafter. Anticoagulants should be used cautiously in patients who have had recent surgical or invasive procedures, in patients with hepatic or renal dysfunction, blood dyscrasias, subacute bacterial endocarditis, or peptic ulcer, and in patients taking drugs that may interfere with coagulation (aspirin, etc.).

Drug Interactions

Digitalis, tetracyclines, antihistamines, and nicotine may interfere with the action of heparin. The anticoagulant effects of coumarin drugs may be potentiated by antibiotics, alcohol, chlorpropamide, aspirin and other nonsteroidal antiinflammatory drugs, phenytoin, chloral hydrate, allopurinol, narcotics, sulfonamides, thyroid drugs, metronidazole, and MAO inhibitors. The anticoagulant effects of coumarin drugs are reduced by corticosteroids, some antihistamines, carbamazepine, barbiturates, chlordiazepoxide, cholestyramine, oral contraceptives, and numerous other drugs.

Treatment

Heparin anticoagulation is reversed by giving a slow infusion of protamine sulfate. Each milligram of protamine sulfate neutralizes approximately 100 units (1 – 1.5 mg) of heparin. Coumarin anticoagulation may be neutralized by intramuscular phytonadione (vitamin K preparation). Coagulation profiles should be done to monitor the response.

Chapter 6

ANTICONVULSANT DRUGS

Table 6-1. Side Effects of Anticonvulsants

Drug	Ataxia, Nystagmus	Drowsiness	Bone Marrow Depression	Megaloblastic Anemia	Pseudolymphoma	Lupus or Other Collagen Disorder	Acne	Other Rashes	Gastrointestinal Symptoms	Myasthenia	Gingival Hypertrophy	Other
Phenytoin sodium	++	+[a]	+	+	+	+	+	+	+	−	+	−
Mephenytoin	+	−	+	+	+	+	−	+	+	−	+ (less than phenytoin sodium)	−
Ethotoin	−	+	+	+	+	+	+	+	+	−	−	−
Phenobarbital	+	++	+	+	−	−	−	+	+	−	−	−
Mephobarbital	+	++	+	+	−	−	−	+	−	−	−	−
Metharbital	+	+	+	+	−	−	−	+	+	−	−	−
Carbamazepine	+	+	++	−	−	+	−	++	+ (jaundice)	−	+	−
Ethosuximide	+	+	+	−	−	+	−	+	+	−	+	−
Phensuximide	−	+	+	−	−	+	−	+	+	−	−	−
Primidone	+	++	−	+	−	−	−	+	+	−	−	−
Valproic acid	+	−	+	−	−	−	−	−	++ (hepatic toxicity)	−	−	−
Trimethadione	−	+	++	−	−	−	−	++	−	−	−	Aplastic anemia
Paramethadione	−	−	−	−	−	−	−	−	−	−	−	−
Clonazepam	+	+	−	−	−	−	−	+	−	−	−	Rarely bone marrow depression
Amobarbital sodium	−	++	−	−	−	−	−	−	+	−	−	Respiratory depression

[a] Other CNS symptoms are rare.

Introduction

Principal Anticonvulsant Drugs

- Phenytoin sodium
  - Related drugs:
    - Mephenytoin
    - Ethotoin
- Phenobarbital
  - Related drugs:
    - Mephobarbital
    - Metharbital
- Carbamazepine
- Ethosuximide
  - Related drug:
    - Phensuximide
- Primidone
- Valproic acid
- Trimethadione
  - Related drug:
    - Paramethadione
- Clonazepam
- Amobarbital sodium (see page 197)
- Diazepam (see page 259)

As might be expected from drugs that are used to decrease CNS excitability and the seizure threshold, anticonvulsants cause drowsiness and depress other areas of the nervous system (particularly the cerebellum) causing nystagmus, ataxia, and slurred speech. Almost all these drugs depress one or more bone marrow elements and may cause a megaloblastic anemia by interfering with folic acid metabolism. As with almost any drug, rashes and other allergic reactions are not uncommon, but acne seems to be more peculiar to phenytoin sodium and its analogs. Since phenytoin, phenobarbital, carbamazepine, primidone, ethosuximide, and valproic acid are the most frequently prescribed drugs in this group, their side effects will be illustrated and described in more detail.

Phenytoin Sodium

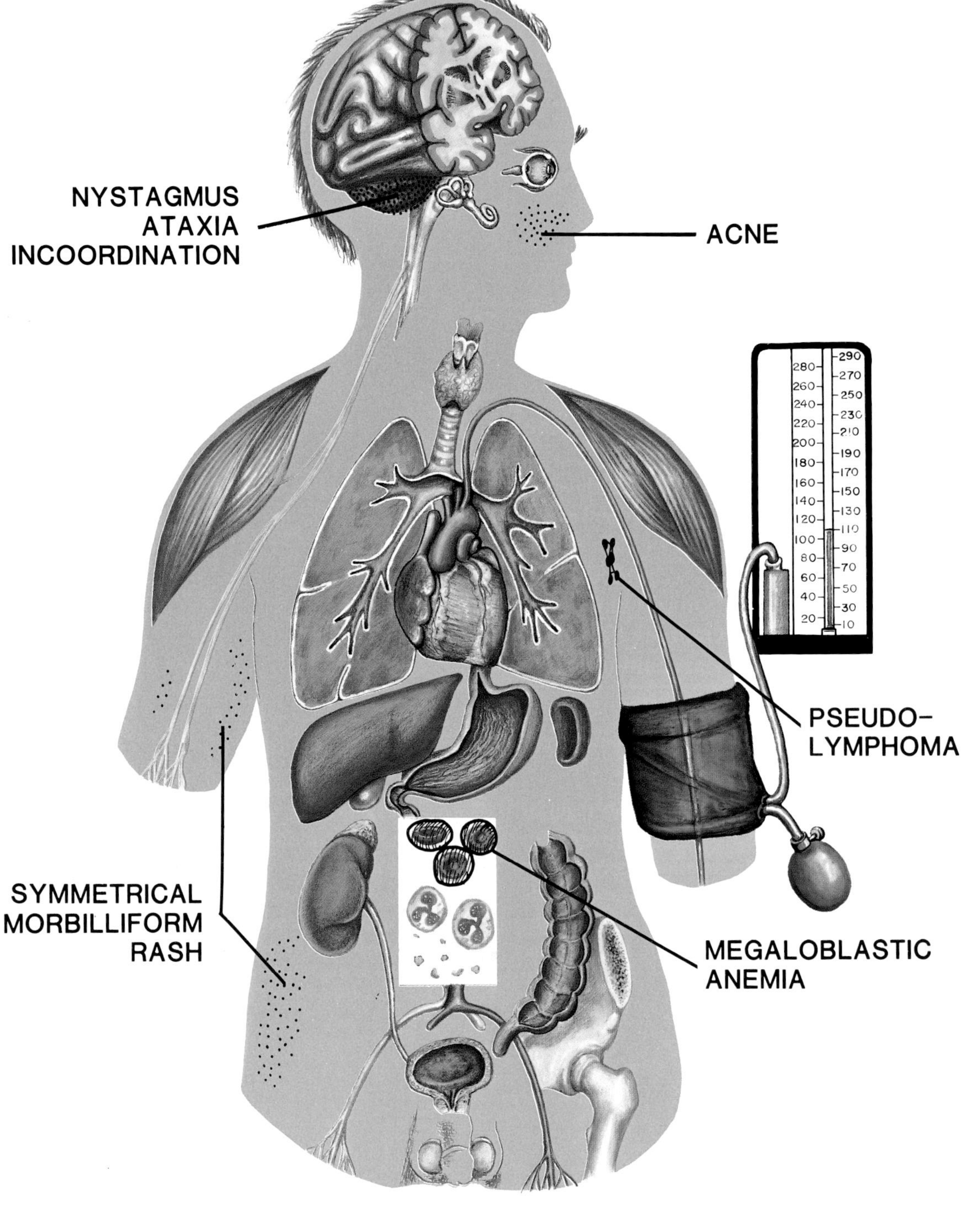

NYSTAGMUS
ATAXIA
INCOORDINATION

ACNE

PSEUDO-
LYMPHOMA

SYMMETRICAL
MORBILLIFORM
RASH

MEGALOBLASTIC
ANEMIA

Phenytoin Sodium

Principal Drugs

Generic Name	Representative Trade Name
Phenytoin sodium	Dilantin
Related drugs:	
Mephenytoin	Mesantoin
Ethotoin	Peganone

Toxicity Rating: Low

Adverse Reactions

Central Nervous System Nystagmus, ataxia, incoordination, and slurred speech are the principle side effects of phenytoin and are dose-related. Other CNS reactions include mental confusion, nervousness, dyskinesias, tremor, and headache.

Skin and Mucous Membrane Acne often develops after prolonged use, but a morbilliform (measles-like) rash is the most common early skin reaction. Gingival hypertrophy frequently occurs after prolonged use.

Hematopoietic Bone marrow depression occasionally causes agranulocytosis, anemia, thrombocytopenia, or pancytopenia, but these effects are reversible. A megaloblastic anemia that responds to folic acid may occur but is more common with mephenytoin. Lymphadenopathy and pseudolymphoma are rarely seen. Lupus erythematosus is occasionally reported.

Metabolic Osteomalacia due to disturbed vitamin D metabolism may occur.

Gastrointestinal Anorexia, nausea, vomiting, and constipation sometimes occur.

Other Hepatitis, hirsutism, and hyperglycemia may occur.

Contraindications

The only absolute contraindication to this drug is known hypersensitivity. The drug must be used with caution in pregnancy as there seems to be a higher incidence of birth defects for pregnant women using this drug. The benefits of keeping the patient seizure-free must be weighed against the unproven danger of fetal malformations. Obviously, seizures have the potential of injuring or destroying the fetus.

Precautions

Patients with decreased liver function, especially the elderly, are more susceptible to toxicity. Phenytoin is not effective in the treatment of petit mal but since a few patients with "absence seizures" actually have temporal lobe seizures, it may be effective. Patients with both true grand mal and petit mal need combined therapy. Phenytoin sodium should not be given for seizures induced by hypoglycemia: rather, the cause of the seizures should be determined.

Drug Interactions

Phenytoin decreases prothrombin time in patients on coumarin anticoagulants. Several drugs may increase or decrease the effectiveness of phenytoin. Phenytoin decreases the effects of corticosteroids, oral contraceptives, and quinidine.

Treatment

Decreasing the dosage is usually adequate treatment for cerebellar signs and other CNS symptoms. Frequent monitoring of phenytoin blood levels will assist in this task; keeping the serum level between 10 and 20 μg/ml will usually prevent CNS symptoms. Some patients will still have toxic reactions at these blood levels, and in these patients the dose must be further reduced. A laboratory test should never replace clinical judgment. With mild rashes (morbilliform, etc.) the drug may be withdrawn and given again after the rash subsides. If the same rash recurs, then the drug must be permanently discontinued. Lupus rashes, Stevens-Johnson syndrome, and exfoliative or purpuric rashes dictate permanent withdrawal of the drug as they are potentially fatal. Pseudolymphoma, bone marrow depression, and hepatitis are obvious reasons to stop the drug, and laboratory results must be carefully followed until recovery is certain. There is no known phenytoin antidote.

Reactions to Related Drugs

Mephenytoin

Since bone marrow depression and folic-acid-related megaloblastic anemia are more common with mephenytoin than with phenytoin, mephenytoin is rarely used in preference to phenytoin. Gingival hyperplasia and ataxia seem to be less frequent with mephenytoin than with phenytoin. Blood counts should be carefully monitored if mephenytoin is given

Ethotoin

This drug seems to have a distinct advantage over phenytoin. Ataxia and gum hypertrophy are rarely reported and have even subsided when ethotoin is substituted for phenytoin. Unlike phenytoin, ethotoin is given in small tablet form. Since blood dyscrasias may be slightly more frequent than with phenytoin therapy, repeated complete blood counts are recommended during the initial stages of therapy. Ethotoin should not be given with phenacemide as paranoid symptoms may develop.

Phenobarbital

Principal Drugs

Generic Name	Representative Trade Name
Phenobarbital	Phenobarbital
Related drugs:	
Mephobarbital	Mebaral
Metharbital	Gemonil

Toxicity Rating: Low

Adverse Reactions

Central Nervous System Drowsiness and frank sedation are the most pronounced CNS side effects of phenobarbital, although they may wear off after 1–2 weeks of therapy. Surprisingly, the opposite effect may occur in children and elderly patients. Ataxia, nystagmus, and slurred speech occur as with phenytoin, but not as frequently. These effects are dose related. Confusion and impaired mentation also occur.

Dermatologic Rashes are rarely a problem but do occur.

Gastrointestinal Anorexia, vomiting, and constipation may occasionally occur.

Hematopoietic While a transient drop in the white count may occur initially, aplastic anemia and persistent leukopenia are rare. Unlike phenytoin, phenobarbital rarely interrupts folate metabolism. Hepatitis is also unusual.

Contraindications

Phenobarbital is contraindicated in patients with porphyria or with known hypersensitivity to the drug.

Precautions

Phenobarbital should be given with caution to pregnant and nursing mothers. The drug should be withdrawn gradually to prevent the development of withdrawal seizures. Drug dependency is uncommon with therapeutic doses.

Drug Interactions

Although phenobarbital may reduce the serum concentration of phenytoin by its effects on absorption and biotransformation, this effect may be neutralized by the inhibition of phenytoin catabolism by phenobarbital. Phenobarbital may increase the effects of other CNS depressants. Serum levels of phenobarbital may be increased by phenytoin and valproic acid: folic acid, on the other hand, may decrease serum phenobarbital levels. Phenobarbital can decrease the action of coumarin drugs, oral contraceptives, quinidine, griseofulvin, and various antibiotics.

Treatment

Simple withdrawal of the drug is usually sufficient, but it should be done gradually unless there is severe CNS depression or coma. In cases of overdosage, rapid perfusion with balanced electrolyte solution may eliminate the drug rapidly. Peritoneal dialysis or hemodialysis may be used in severe cases.

Carbamazepine

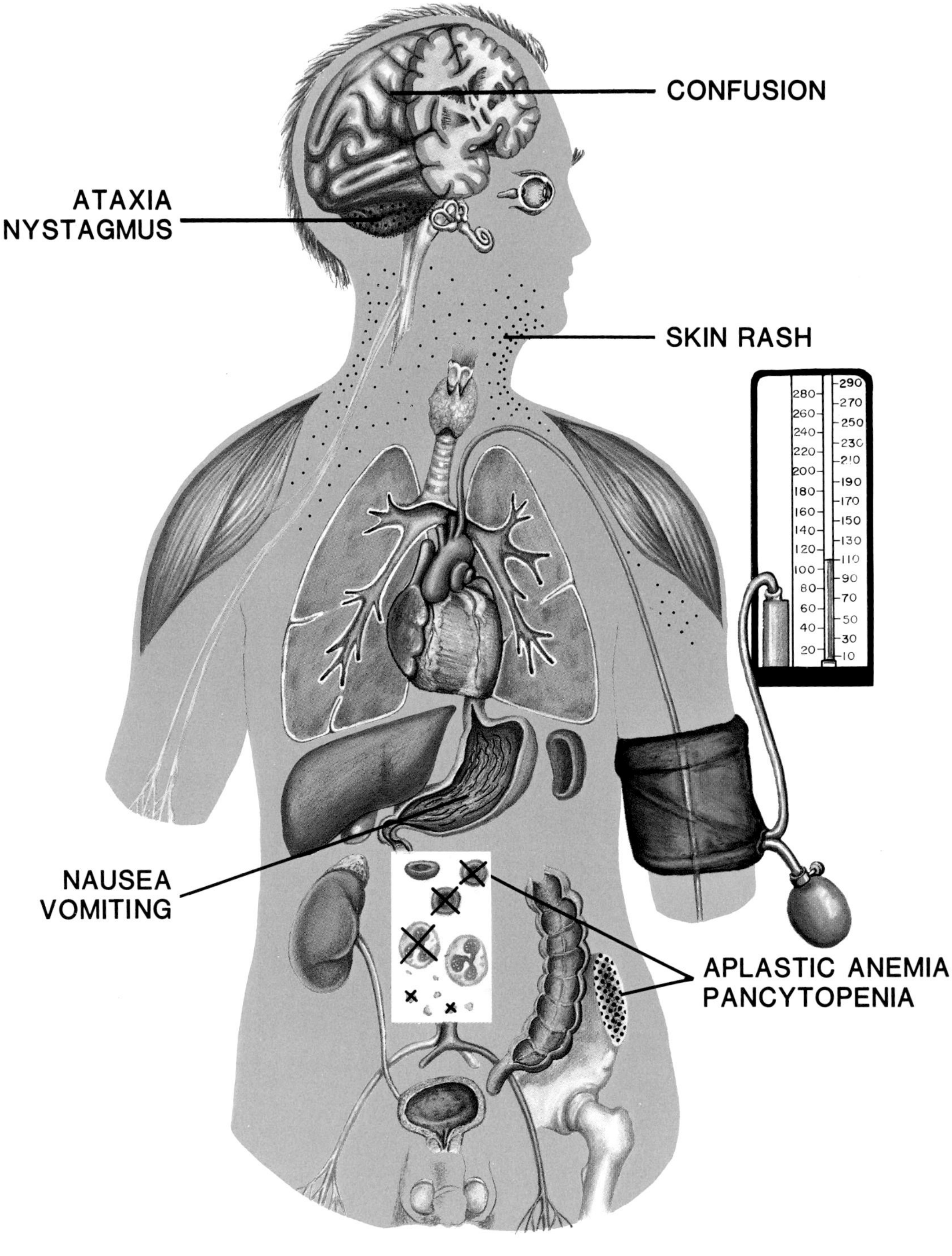

CONFUSION

ATAXIA
NYSTAGMUS

SKIN RASH

NAUSEA
VOMITING

APLASTIC ANEMIA
PANCYTOPENIA

Carbamazepine

Representative Trade Name: Tegretol

Toxicity Rating: Medium to high because fatal aplastic anemia has been reported.

Adverse Reactions

Central Nervous System Dizziness, headache, confusion, ataxia, and occasional nystagmus occur, but are not as common as with phenytoin.

Cardiovascular Almost any type of cardiovascular reaction may occur, including congestive heart failure, hypertension, shock, coronary insufficiency, arrhythmias, and atrioventricular block. Thrombophlebitis has also been reported.

Hematopoietic The most potentially dangerous reactions to carbamazepine involve the hematopoietic system, and include aplastic anemia, agranulocytosis, thrombocytopenia, and eosinophilia. Leukocytosis may occasionally occur.

Gastrointestinal Nausea and vomiting may occur during the initial phase of therapy but often disappear with continued use. Hepatitis has been reported.

Dermatologic Every type of skin reaction may occur, including urticaria, erythema multiforme, exfoliative dermatitis, and skin pigmentation.

Genitourinary Carbamazepine may cause urinary frequency or retention. Severe renal insufficiency with azotemia, albuminuria, and glycosuria may occur.

Respiratory Hypersensitivity pneumonitis with fever and dyspnea may occur.

Other Impotence, testicular atrophy, alopecia, peripheral retinitis, tinnitus, lens opacities, inappropriate ADH secretion, and muscular aches and pains have been reported rarely.

Contraindications

Carbamazepine should not be given to patients with bone marrow depression or with hypersensitivity to this or other tricyclic compounds. It is also inadvisable to give it to patients taking MAO inhibitors or until 14 days after MAO inhibitors have been discontinued.

Precautions

A complete blood count, platelet count, and reticulocyte count should be done before initiating carbamazepine therapy. Some authorities recommend preliminary liver and renal function tests as well. The complete blood count and platelet count should be repeated frequently during the first 3 months of therapy, and monthly thereafter. The patient must be informed of the symptoms of agranulocytosis (glossitis, stomatitis, fever, etc.). Monitoring carbamazepine blood levels is very helpful for determining the optimum dosage. Baseline eye tests and slit-lamp examinations before starting therapy are also recommended.

Drug Interactions

Carbamazepine blood levels may be decreased when phenobarbital, phenytoin, or primidone are given concurrently. Erythromycin may increase carbamazepine blood levels. Carbamazepine decreases the action of coumarin drugs, phenytoin, doxycycline, and oral contraceptives.

Treatment

Withdrawal of the drug, slowly if possible, and careful monitoring of blood counts is indicated if bone marrow depression occurs. Bone marrow aspiration should be done immediately, and severely depressed blood elements replenished by transfusion. Prophylactic antibiotics are often advisable. Physicians not familiar with the treatment of aplastic anemia and other hematologic complications should consult with a hematologist.

Ethosuximide

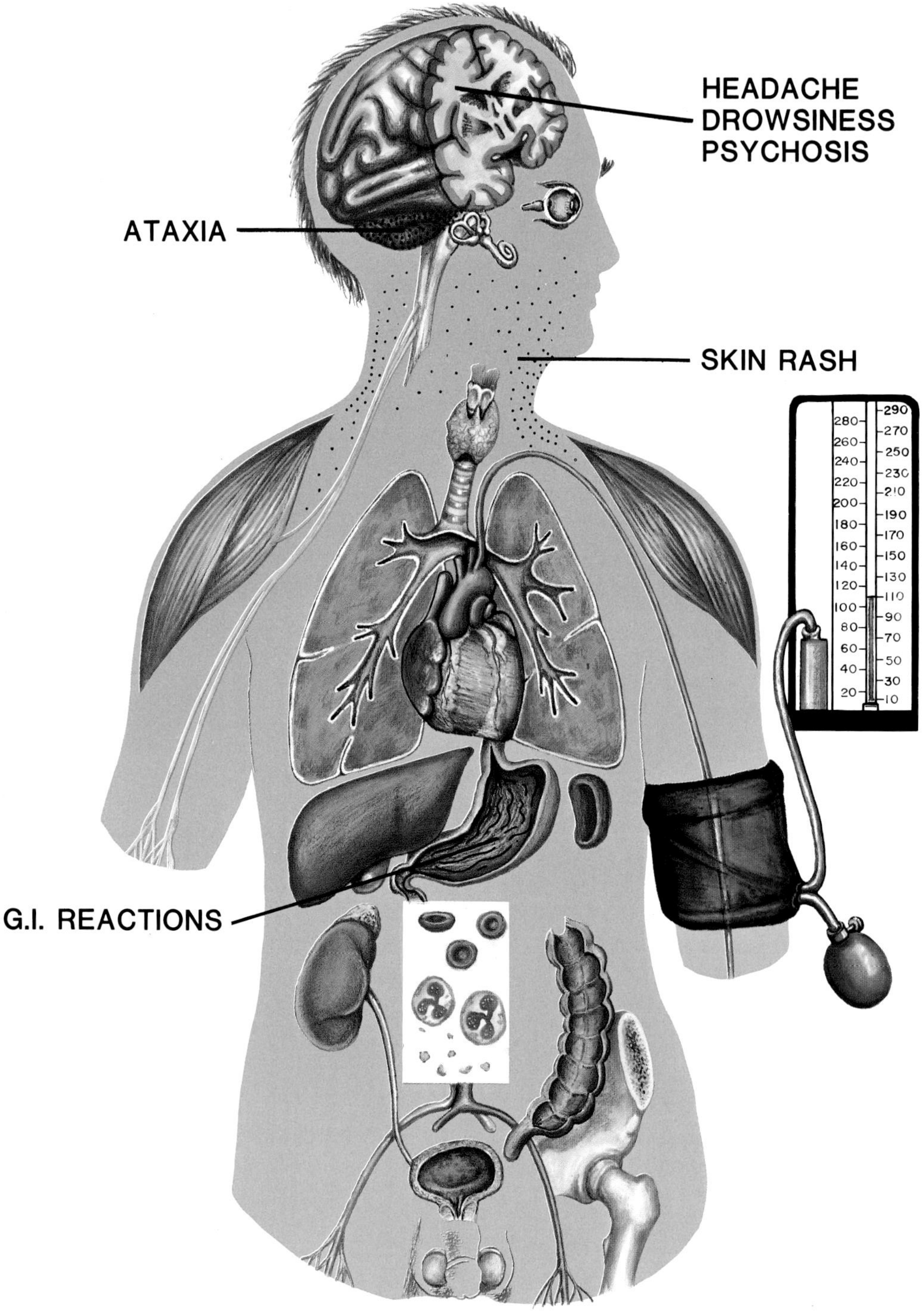

HEADACHE
DROWSINESS
PSYCHOSIS

ATAXIA

SKIN RASH

G.I. REACTIONS

Ethosuximide

Principal Drugs

Generic Name	Representative Trade Name
Ethosuximide	Zarontin
Related drug:	
Phensuximide	Milontin

Toxicity Rating: Low

Adverse Reactions

Central Nervous System Like phenytoin, ethosuximide may cause headache, dizziness, occasional drowsiness, and ataxia. There may also be euphoria, irritability, and behavioral abnormalities including paranoid psychosis. Ethosuximide may increase seizure activity in patients with grand mal or mixed forms of epilepsy.

Gastrointestinal There are frequent reports of nausea, vomiting, abdominal pain, and diarrhea.

Hematologic Bone marrow depression occurs but is much rarer than with carbamazepine.

Dermatologic Like carbamazepine, ethosuximide may cause any type of skin reaction including urticaria and erythema multiforme.

Other Gum hypertrophy, hirsutism, vaginal bleeding, and myopia have occurred.

Contraindications

Grand-mal type epilepsy and known hypersensitivity to ethosuximide are the major contraindications.

Precautions

Since bone marrow depression may occur, periodic blood counts should be done during therapy. Ethosuximide should be used carefully in patients with known hepatic and renal dysfunction. The safety of ethosuximide in pregnancy has not been established. Patients should be warned that working around dangerous machinery or driving may be hazardous while taking this drug.

Drug Interactions

Carbamazepine may decrease the serum level of ethosuximide.

Treatment

Simple withdrawal of the drug is usually all that is necessary. When possible, the drug should be withdrawn slowly to avoid precipitating petit mal.

Primidone

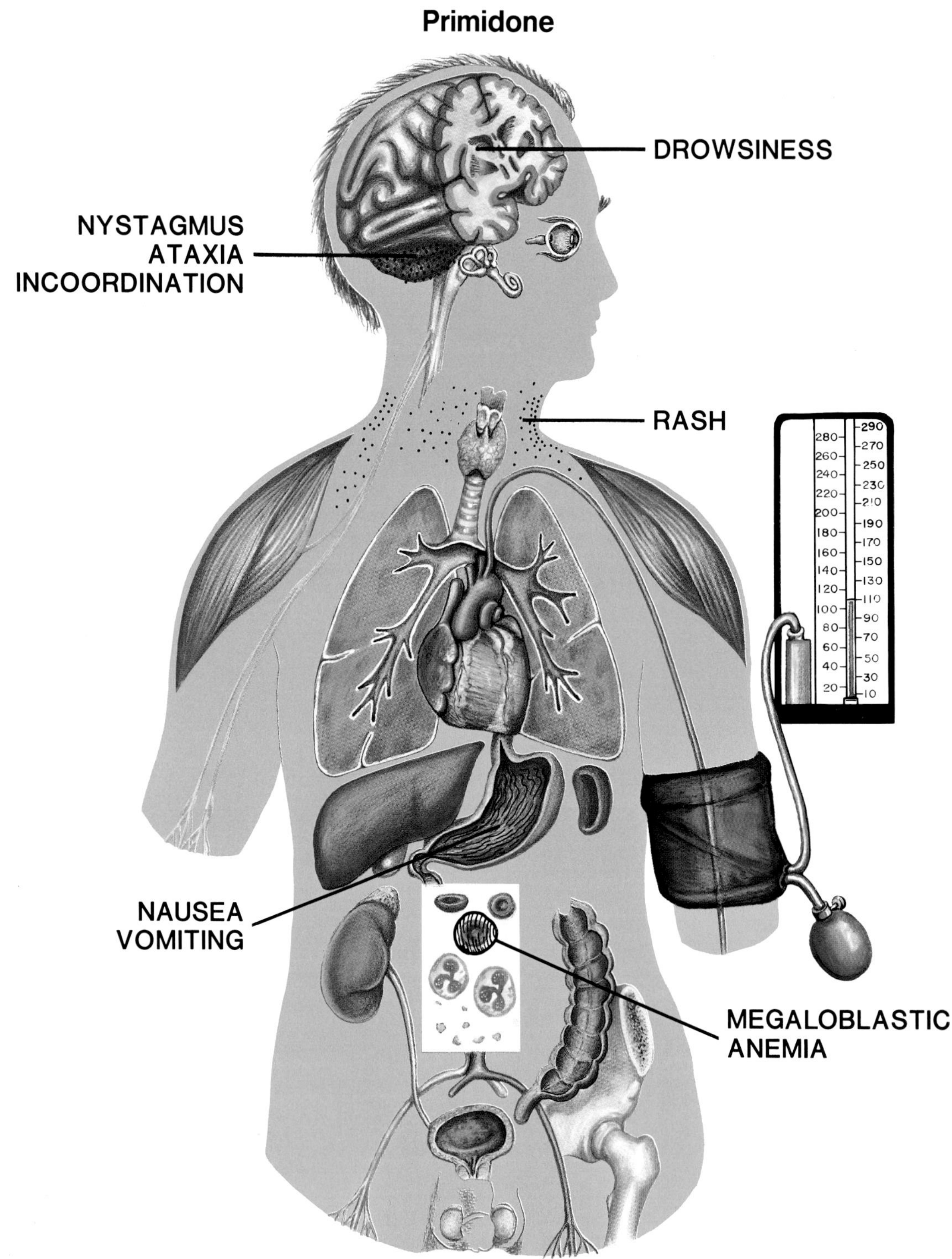

DROWSINESS
NYSTAGMUS
ATAXIA
INCOORDINATION
RASH
NAUSEA
VOMITING
MEGALOBLASTIC
ANEMIA

Primidone

Representative Trade Name: Mysoline

Toxicity Rating: Low

Adverse Reactions

Central Nervous System As with phenytoin, the most frequent reaction is ataxia, occasionally accompanied by nystagmus, irritability, diplopia, and drowsiness. Vertigo is also a frequent reaction.

Gastrointestinal Nausea and vomiting occur.

Hematologic A megaloblastic anemia due to interference with folic acid metabolism occurs rarely.

Other Impotence and skin rashes may occur but are rare.

Contraindications

Primidone is contraindicated in patients with porphyria or known hypersensitivity to phenobarbital.

Precautions

Safety in pregnancy has not been established. Therapy should be initiated with small doses of the drug to prevent severe gastrointestinal or neurological reactions. A comprehensive blood analysis should be done twice a year to detect megaloblastic anemia early. Withdrawal of the drug should be gradual to prevent seizures.

Treatment

Withdrawal of the drug is usually all that is necessary. Folic acid administration will clear up megaloblastic anemia in most cases, but pernicious anemia should be carefully ruled out first.

Valproic Acid

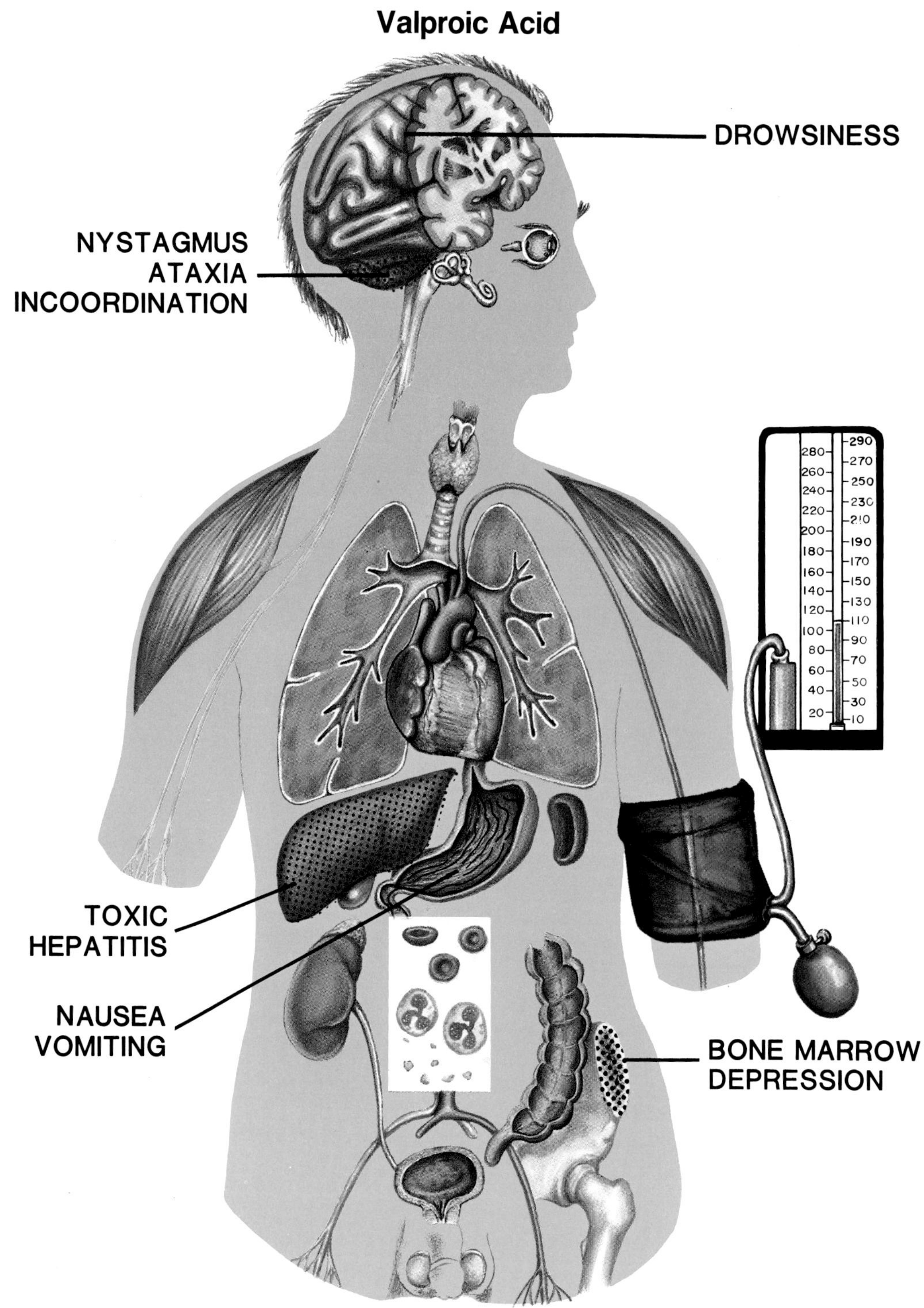

Valproic Acid

Representative Trade Name: Depakene

Toxicity Rating: Medium in view of hepatotoxicity and reports of fatal hepatic failure.

Adverse Reactions

Central Nervous System Like phenytoin, valproic acid may cause nystagmus, ataxia, tremor, dizziness, and headache. Emotional disturbances including depression or psychosis occur.

Hepatic Many patients have alterations in liver function, and a few develop toxic hepatitis and fatal hepatic failure.

Gastrointestinal Nausea, vomiting, diarrhea, abdominal cramps, and constipation have occurred.

Hematologic Like many anticonvulsants, valproic acid can cause bone marrow depression, particularly thrombocytopenia. Valproic acid disturbs platelet aggregation, causing easy bruising. Other coagulation defects may occur.

Other Acute pancreatitis, rare skin rashes, transient hair loss, irregular menses, hyperglycemia, and elevated blood ammonia levels have occurred.

Contraindications

Preexisting hepatic dysfunction and known hypersensitivity to the drug are contraindications for valproic acid therapy.

Precautions

Because of the potential for serious hepatotoxicity, liver function studies should be performed frequently, both before and during valproic acid therapy, especially in the first six months. As with other anticonvulsants, the benefits of valproic acid during pregnancy must be weighed against the possible risk of birth defects. Because of the risk of thrombocytopenia and platelet dysfunction, platelet counts and coagulation studies should be done frequently during therapy.

Drug Interactions

The interactions of valproic acid with other anticonvulsants are especially important. Valproic acid may increase serum levels of phenobarbital or primidone. It may decrease serum phenytoin levels, causing breakthrough seizures: however, it occasionally paradoxically increases serum phenytoin levels. Coadministration of valproic acid and clonazepam may result in breakthrough absence status. Valproic acid has been reported to alter the action of anticoagulants and to affect thyroid function.

Treatment

Simple withdrawal of the drug is sufficient to control most adverse reactions. Naloxone may reverse the CNS effects of valproic acid but should be used with caution. Treatment of hepatic failure should be left to the expert hepatologist or consulting gastroenterologist.

Trimethadione

Principal Drugs

Generic Name	Representative Trade Name
Trimethadione	Tridione
Related drug:	
Paramethadione	Paradione

Toxicity Rating: High because of the potential for fetal malformations and fatal aplastic anemia.

Adverse Reactions

The adverse reactions to trimethadione are very similar to those to ethosuximide (page 49), except there are more reports of fatal bone marrow depression with trimethadione. Furthermore, the ability of trimethadione to produce fetal malformations is well established. Severe forms of erythema multiforme and exfoliative dermatitis are not uncommon. There have been a few reports of hepatitis and nephritis.

Precautions

Frequent blood counts and liver and renal function tests should be done. The drug must be withdrawn at the first sign of skin rash. Scotomata are also an indication to stop the drug. The drug should be withdrawn slowly if possible to prevent petit mal status.

Clonazepam

Representative Trade Name: Clonopin

Toxicity Rating: Low

Adverse Reactions

Central Nervous System Almost half of patients taking clonazepam experience drowsiness, and one third may develop transient ataxia. Like phenytoin, clonazepam may cause nystagmus, tremor, slurred speech, diplopia, and behavior changes. Choreiform movements, dyskinesia, aphonia, hypotonia, and even hemiplegia have been know to occur.

Gastrointestinal Like other anticonvulsants, clonazepam can cause nausea, constipation, and diarrhea.

Respiratory Chest congestion, rhinorrhea, and dyspnea may occur.

Hematologic As with most anticonvulsants, bone marrow depression occurs but is unusual.

Other Palpitations, occasional rash, alopecia, dysuria, enuresis, urinary retention, fever, lymphadenopathy, and weight loss may occur.

Contraindications

Known hypersensitivity to the benzodiazepines, a history of liver disease, and acute narrow-angle glaucoma are contraindications.

Precautions

Driving, use of alcohol, and working around dangerous machinery may be hazardous while on this drug. The benefits of use during pregnancy must be weighed against the possible risk of fetal malformations. Withdrawal symptoms similar to those noted with barbiturates have occurred, so the drug should be withdrawn slowly if possible. Patients with grand mal may experience an increase of their seizures while on this drug.

Drug Interactions

The concurrent use of valproic acid and clonazepam may cause absence status. Almost all other CNS depressants may increase the depressant effects and CNS toxicity of clonazepam, and vice versa.

Treatment

Withdrawal of the drug (gradually if possible) is the principle therapy for reactions.

Chapter 7

ANTIGOUT DRUGS

Colchicine

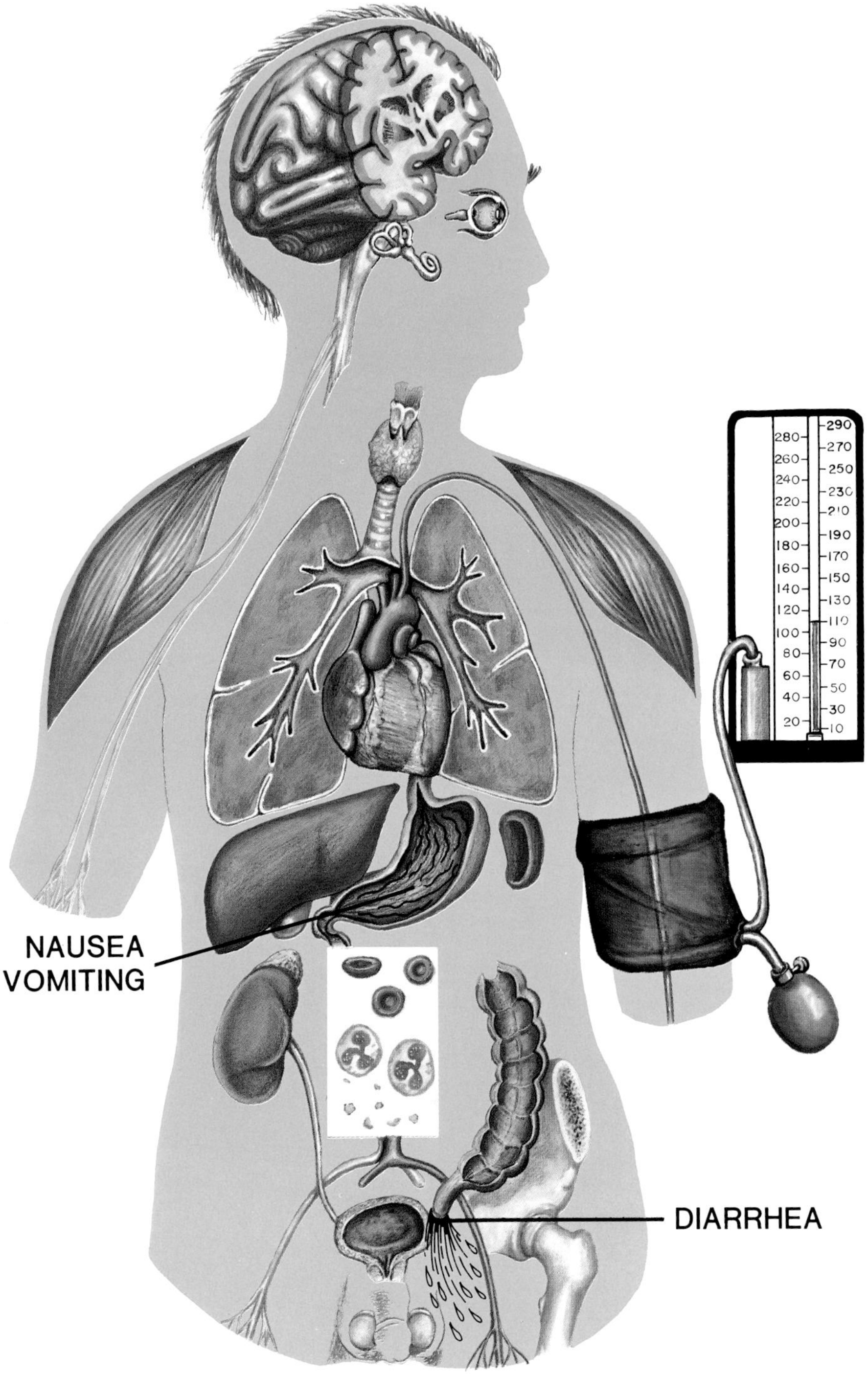

NAUSEA
VOMITING

DIARRHEA

Introduction

Principal Antigout Drugs

Generic Name
Colchicine
Allopurinol
Probenecid
Sulfinpyrazone
Nonsteroidal antiinflammatory drugs (see Chapter 28)
Corticosteroids (see page 181)

Three types of drugs are used in the treatment of gout: the antiinflammatory drugs, drugs that decrease uric acid production, and the uricosuric drugs. The antiinflammatory drugs (colchicine, nonsteroidal antiinflammatory agents, and corticosteroids) have significant gastrointestinal side effects; colchicine causes diarrhea and vomiting, and the steroids and nonsteroidal antiinflammatory drugs cause gastric irritation, peptic ulceration, and GI bleeding. Allopurinol is especially apt to induce hypersensitivity reactions, a characteristic in which it resembles the penicillins. The uricosuric agents can cause growth of uric acid stones as well as hypersensitivity reactions.

Colchicine

Representative Trade Names: Colchicine, ColBENEMID (combination of colchicine and probenecid)

Toxicity Rating: Low

Adverse Reactions

Gastrointestinal The major side effect of colchicine is diarrhea. Nausea, vomiting, and abdominal pain are also frequent and are dose related.

Other Hypersensitivity is rare, but toxic doses of colchicine may cause vascular or renal damage. Skin rashes occur. Agranulocytosis, aplastic anemia, and peripheral neuropathy also occur, but only with prolonged use.

Contraindications

Known hypersensitivity, pregnancy, and preexisting serious gastrointestinal, renal, or cardiac disease are the principal contraindications.

Precautions

This drug should be used with caution in patients with mild to moderate gastrointestinal, renal, or cardiac disorders.

Drug Interactions

Absorption of B_{12} is altered by a direct action on the ileal mucosa. Colchicine may potentiate the action of CNS depressants and sympathomimetic agents.

Treatment

Most reactions from oral colchicine preparations can be handled by simple withdrawal of the drug.

Allopurinol

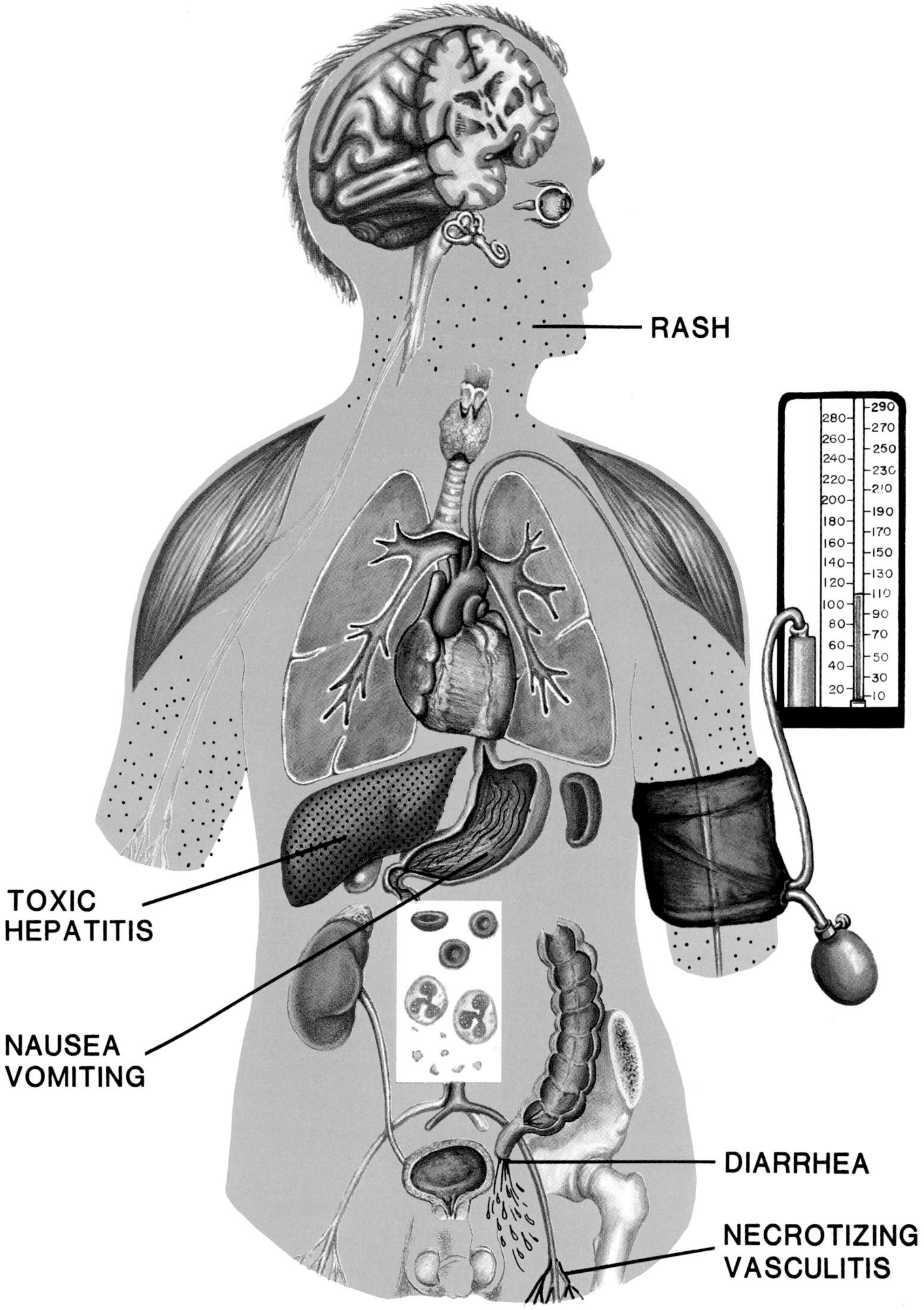

RASH

TOXIC
HEPATITIS

NAUSEA
VOMITING

DIARRHEA

NECROTIZING
VASCULITIS

Allopurinol

Representative Trade Name: Zyloprim

Toxicity Rating: Medium because of occasional severe hypersensitivity reactions.

Adverse Reactions

Dermatologic Allergic skin reactions, particularly a maculopapular rash, are a frequent side effect of allopurinol. Renal disease seems to predispose to these reactions.

Cardiovascular Hypersensitivity to allopurinol may occasionally lead to necrotizing vasculitis.

Gastrointestinal Like colchicine, allopurinol may produce nausea, vomiting, and diarrhea, but these reactions are not as frequently or severe as with colchicine.

Hepatic Hypersensitivity to allopurinol may rarely result in hepatitis and hepatic necrosis.

Other Drug fever and other hypersensitivity reactions occur but are usually preceded by a skin reaction.

Contraindications

Known hypersensitivity is the principle contraindication, but allopurinol is also contraindicated in children unless their elevated uric acid is due to a malignancy.

Precautions

Since a skin rash precedes the more severe hypersensitivity reactions, allopurinol should be withdrawn at the first sign of a skin rash. Patients with preexisting renal or liver disease should bc monitored carefully in the early stages of therapy. Therapy should be initiated with low doses (100 mg/day) because allopurinol has been reported to increase the frequency of gouty attacks during the early stages of therapy. The dose of allopurinol should be reduced in patients with severe renal dysfunction.

Drug Interactions

Allopurinol may enhance the chemotherapeutic action of azathioprine, sometimes to a toxic degree. If a patient receiving azathioprine is to be given allopurinol, the dosage of azathioprine should be reduced by two thirds to three fourths. Concurrent administration of allopurinol with a uricosuric agent may decrease the excretion of oxypurines. Allopurinol can prolong the effect of coumarin drugs.

Treatment

Simple withdrawal of the drug is usually all that is necessary.

Probenecid

Principal Drugs

Generic Name	Representative Trade Name
Probenecid	Benemid
Related drug:	
Sulfinpyrazone	Anturane

Toxicity Rating: Low

Adverse Reactions

Renal Because probenecid increases the excretion of uric acid, uricolithiasis may occur. Nephrotic syndrome has been reported rarely.

Other Skin rashes and other hypersensitivity reactions occur. Occasional nausea, vomiting, and loss of appetite have been observed. Hepatic necrosis and aplastic anemia have been reported.

Contraindications

Probenecid is contraindicated in patients with uric acid stones, known hypersensitivity to probenecid, or blood dyscrasias. It should not be given to children under 2 years old.

Precautions

Probenecid may exacerbate gouty arthritis. If probenecid must be given with methotrexate, the dosage of methotrexate should be decreased. Patients receiving probenecid may need to increase their fluid intake or take sodium bicarbonate to alkalinize their urine to prevent uric acid stone formation. The dosage of probenecid may have to be increased in patients with mild renal dysfunction, and the drug may not be effective at all in moderate to severe renal insufficiency.

Drug Interactions

The interaction of probenecid with methotrexate has been discussed above. Salicylates antagonize the action of probenecid: if analgesia is required in patients on probenecid, acetaminophen is preferred. Probenecid blocks the ability of the kidney to excrete penicillin, cephalosporins, sulfonamides, aminosalicyclic acid, indomethacin, and nitrofurantoin.

Treatment

Withdrawal of the drug is effective treatment for most reactions.

Chapter 8

ANTIHISTAMINES

Antihistamines

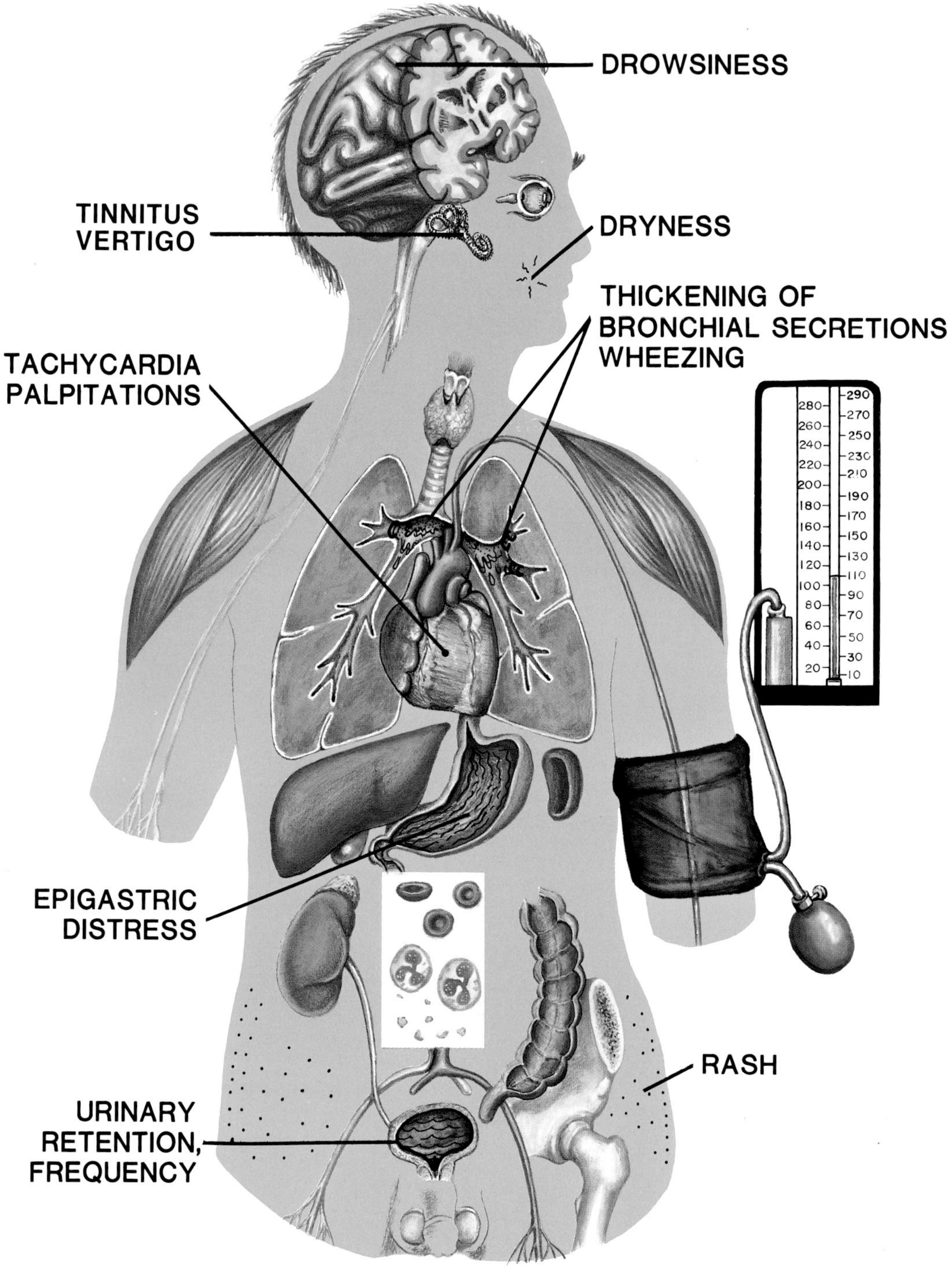

DROWSINESS

TINNITUS
VERTIGO

DRYNESS

THICKENING OF
BRONCHIAL SECRETIONS
WHEEZING

TACHYCARDIA
PALPITATIONS

EPIGASTRIC
DISTRESS

RASH

URINARY
RETENTION,
FREQUENCY

Antihistamines

Principal Drugs

Generic Name	Representative Trade Name
Diphenhydramine hydrochloride	Benadryl
Chlorpheniramine maleate	Chlor-Trimeton
Brompheniramine maleate	Dimetane
Phenindamine tartrate	in Nolamine
Dimenhydrinate	Dramamine
Dexbrompheniramine maleate	in Drixoral
Pheniramine maleate	in Triaminic
Triprolidine hydrochloride	in Actifed-C
Cyclizine lactate	Marezine
Cyproheptadine hydrochloride	Periactin
Meclizine hydrochloride	Antivert

Toxicity rating: Low

Adverse Reactions

Central Nervous System Drowsiness is the most frequent side effect of all antihistamines. Dizziness and disturbed coordination are also frequent, so that it may be hazardous to use these drugs while driving or working around dangerous machinery. In some patients and especially children, instead of drowsiness, there is excitation, nervousness, and restlessness. Other CNS stimulatory effects include euphoria, hallucinations, insomnia, irritability, convulsions, and paresthesias. Frank neuritis has occurred.

Special Senses Antihistamines may affect the inner ear, causing symptoms of tinnitus, vertigo, and even acute labyrinthitis—the very condition for which they may have been prescribed.

Mucous Membranes Dryness of the upper mouth, nose, and throat is not uncommon.

Gastrointestinal Epigastric distress is a common side effect of antihistamines, but almost any gastrointestinal symptom may occur, including nausea, vomiting, diarrhea, and constipation.

Respiratory Tract It may surprise the clinician to learn that these drugs may cause thickening of bronchial secretions, wheezing, nasal stuffiness, and tightness of the chest, even though they are often prescribed in combination with expectorants and sympathomimetics to remedy precisely these symptoms.

Hematologic Hemolytic anemia, thrombocytopenia, agranulocytosis, and hypoplastic anemia are the most severe pathologic reactions to antihistamines, but they are fortunately rare.

Cardiovascular Palpitations, tachycardia, and hypotension may occur.

Genitourinary The effect of antihistamines on the smooth muscle in the gastrointestinal tract is carried over to the urinary tract. Excitation of the smooth muscle produces urinary frequency, while depression of the smooth muscle causes difficulty initiating voiding, poor urinary stream, and frank urinary retention.

Allergic Antihistamines may produce urticaria, rash, anaphylactic shock, and other allergic reactions—often the very conditions they were prescribed for. Early menstruation is also occasionally found.

Table 8-1. Side Effects of Antihistamines

Drug	Drowsiness	Anemia, Thrombocytopenia, Agranulocytosis	Hypotension	Allergic Reactions	Photosensitivity	Dry Mucous Membranes	Special Senses	Urinary Frequency	Other Nervous System Reactions	Respiratory Effects	Cardiovascular	Gastrointestinal
Diphenhydramine hydrochloride	+[a]	+	+	+	+	+	+	+	+	+	+	+
Chlorpheniramine maleate	+[a]	+	+	+	+	+	+	+	+	+	+	+
Brompheniramine maleate	+[a]	+	+	+	+	+	+	+	+	+	+	+
Phenindamine tartrate	+	—[b]	—[b]	+	—[b]	—[b]	—[b]	—[b]	+	—[b]	—[b]	—[b]
Dimenhydrinate	+	—[b]	—[b]	+	—[b]	—[b]	—[b]	—[b]	—[b]	+	—[b]	—[b]
Dexbrompheniramine maleate	+[a]	+	+ (hypertension)	+	+	+	+	+	+	+	+	+
Pheniramine maleate	+[a]	+	+	+	+	+	+	+	+	+	+	+
Triprolidine hydrochloride	+[a]	+	+	+	+	+	+	+	+	+	+	+
Cyclizine lactate	+	+	+	+	+	+	+	+	+	+	+	+ (cholestatic jaundice)
Cyproheptadine hydrochloride	+	−	+	+	+	+	+	−	+	+	−	+
Meclizine hydrochloride	+	−	−	+	−	+	−	−	−	−	−	−

[a] Paradoxical excitation in children
[b] Occur but are rare

Dermatologic In addition to allergic reactions, antihistamines may cause excessive perspiration and photosensitivity.

Contraindications

Antihistamines should not be used in newborn or premature infants, in pregnant women, or in nursing mothers. They must be used with caution in children because of their excitatory effects on the nervous system. They should not be used for diseases of the lower respiratory tract, including asthma. Patients with known hypersensitivity to any of these antihistamines should not be started on a different one.

Precautions

Use antihistamines with caution in patients with glaucoma, prostatic hypertrophy, stenosing peptic ulcer, intestinal obstruction, or epilepsy. These drugs are more likely to cause dizziness, sedation, and hypotension in the elderly. Overdosage may cause hallucination, convulsions, and death in children.

Treatment

Withdrawal of the drug is usually all that needs to be done. Antihistamines should be discontinued if hematologic reactions, neuritis, or labyrinthitis develop. It is not necessary to withdraw the drugs for other symptoms unless they are severe.

Antihistamines that Are Exceptions to the Above

Dimehydrinate

As noted in Table 8-1, only drowsiness, allergic reactions, and respiratory effects are significant reactions to this drug.

Phenindamine Tartrate

As shown in Table 8-1, drowsiness, other central nervous system symptoms and allergic reactions are the only significant side effects of this drug.

Cyclizine Lactate

Cholestatic jaundice has been reported in patients receiving this drug, in addition to the usual antihistamine side effects.

Meclizine Hydrochloride

Reactions other than drowsiness and dry mouth are rare with this drug. It has been used in pregnancy when it was clearly necessary since the potential for fetal harm is slight.

Chapter 9

ANTIHYPERTENSIVES

Table 9-1. Side Effects of Antihypertensive Drugs

Drug	Drowsiness	Other CNS Reactions	Dry Mouth	Gastro-Intestinal Symptoms	Hypotension	Orthostatic Hypotension	Bradycardia	Other Cardiac Reactions	Rash	Male Sexual Dysfunction	Withdrawal Reaction	Edema	Other
Clonidine	+	+	+	+	+	+	+	+	+	+	+	+	–
Guanabenz	+	+	–	+	+	+	–	+	–	+	+	–	–
Hydralazine	–	+	–	+	+	+	–	–	+	–	–	+	Lupus-like syndrome
Prazosin	+	+	+	+	+	++	–	–	+	+	–	+	Syncope
Reserpine	++	++	+	+	+	+	+	+	+	+	–	+	Depression
Methyldopa	+	+	+	+	+	+	–	–	–	+	+	+	Hemolytic anemia
Guanethidine	–	+	+	+	+	++	+	+	+	+	–	+	Syncope
Captopril	–	–	+	–	+	+	–	+	+	–	–	–	Nephrosis, neutropenia
Pargyline	–	+	+	+	+	+	–	–	+	–	–	+	Hypertension
Diazoxide	–	–	–	–	+	+	–	+	+	–	+	+	–
Trimethaphan	–	–	–	–	+	+	–	–	–	–	–	–	–
Sodium nitroprusside	–	+	–	+	+	–	–	–	–	–	–	–	Cyanide toxicity
Propranolol	–	+	–	+	+	–	+	+	+	+	+	+	Bronchospasm

Introduction

Principal Antihypertensive Drugs

Clonidine hydrochloride
- Related drugs:
  - Guanabenz acetate
  - Guanfacine

Methyldopa
Hydralazine hydrochloride
Prazosin hydrochloride
Reserpine
Guanethidine monosulfate
Captopril
Pargyline hydrochloride
Diazoxide
Trimethaphan camsylate
Sodium nitroprusside
Minoxidil
Propranolol (see page 19)

Not all drugs used as antihypertensives are considered in this chapter. Propranolol and the beta blockers are discussed as antiarrhythmics in Chapter 3, and the most commonly used antihypertensives, the diuretics, are considered by themselves in Chapter 18.

Table 9-1 shows the similarities and differences of the side effects of the antihypertensives. None of these drugs is without significant side effects. The most benign antihypertensive (aside from the thiazide diuretics) is probably methyldopa, despite its ability to cause Coomb's positive hemolytic anemia. Most of the antihypertensives discussed in this chapter produce drowsiness, impotence, or other central nervous system reactions. It is necessary to administer a diuretic concomitantly with these drugs to ward off edema due to secondary aldosteronism. Adverse cardiovascular effects are common, ranging from acute syncope induced by prazosin to heart failure caused by propranolol. Hydralazine may cause myocardial ischemia, and many antihypertensives are associated with withdrawal symptoms.

Clonidine Hydrochloride

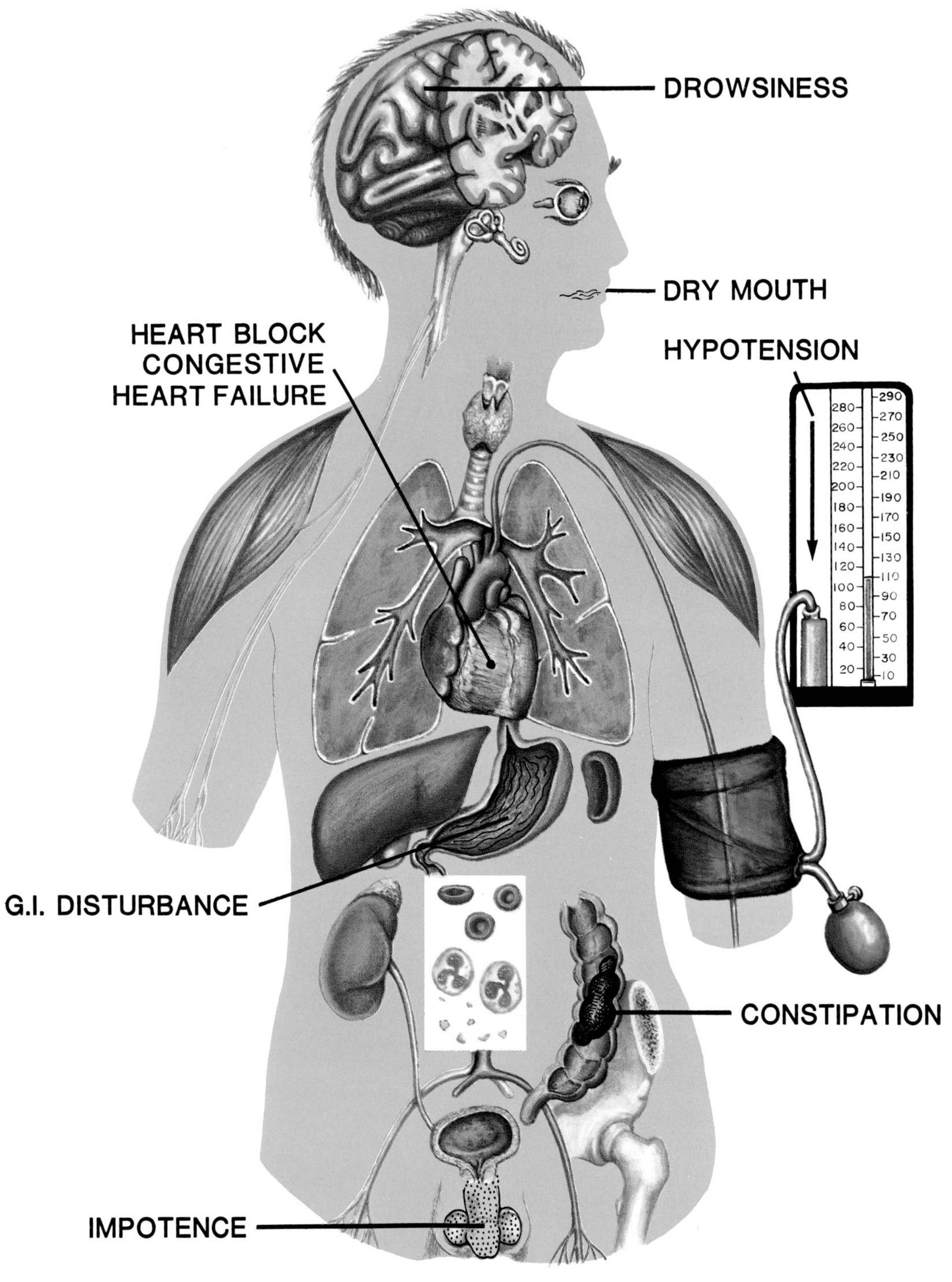

Clonidine Hydrochloride

Principal Drugs

Generic Name	Representative Trade Name
Clonidine hydrochloride	Catapres
Related drugs:	
Guanabenz acetate	Wytensin
Guanfacine	

Toxicity Rating: Medium

Adverse Reactions

Central Nervous System Drowsiness is the most common side effect of clonidine (50 percent of patients). Depression, anxiety, nightmares, and other behavioral changes have been observed.

Gastrointestinal A dry mouth is common. Other gastrointestinal side effects include anorexia, nausea, vomiting, constipation, and adynamic ileus.

Cardiovascular Hypotension, naturally, is an effect of clonidine, and depends on dosage. Postural hypotension may also occur. When the drug is withdrawn abruptly, a hypertensive crisis may be observed. Clonidine affects the cardiac conduction system, causing bradycardia and various degrees of heart block. As with propranolol, congestive heart failure has occurred.

Genitourinary Male impotence and urinary retention have been noted.

Metabolic Unexplained weight gain, transient hyperglycemia, and gynecomastia may be seen.

Allergic Various skin reactions have been observed involving urticaria and angioneurotic edema. Thinning of hair may also occur.

Other Edema may be seen as a result of congestive heart failure or fluid retention due to secondary aldosteronism.

Contraindications

Since experience with clonidine in children and pregnant women is limited, the drug is contraindicated in these patients.

Precautions

Abrupt withdrawal of clonidine may induce a hypertensive crisis, so the drug must be withdrawn slowly. Although no retinal degeneration has been observed in humans, the occurrence of this reaction in laboratory animals makes close ophthamologic observation wise. Patients should be warned regarding the CNS depressive effects and the increased sedation noted when clonidine is combined with alcohol and other sedative drugs. The drug should be used with caution in patients with cardiovascular disease other than hypertension.

Treatment

Gradual withdrawal of the drug is usually all that is necessary. A diuretic is usually administered concomitantly to prevent or resolve edema.

Methyldopa

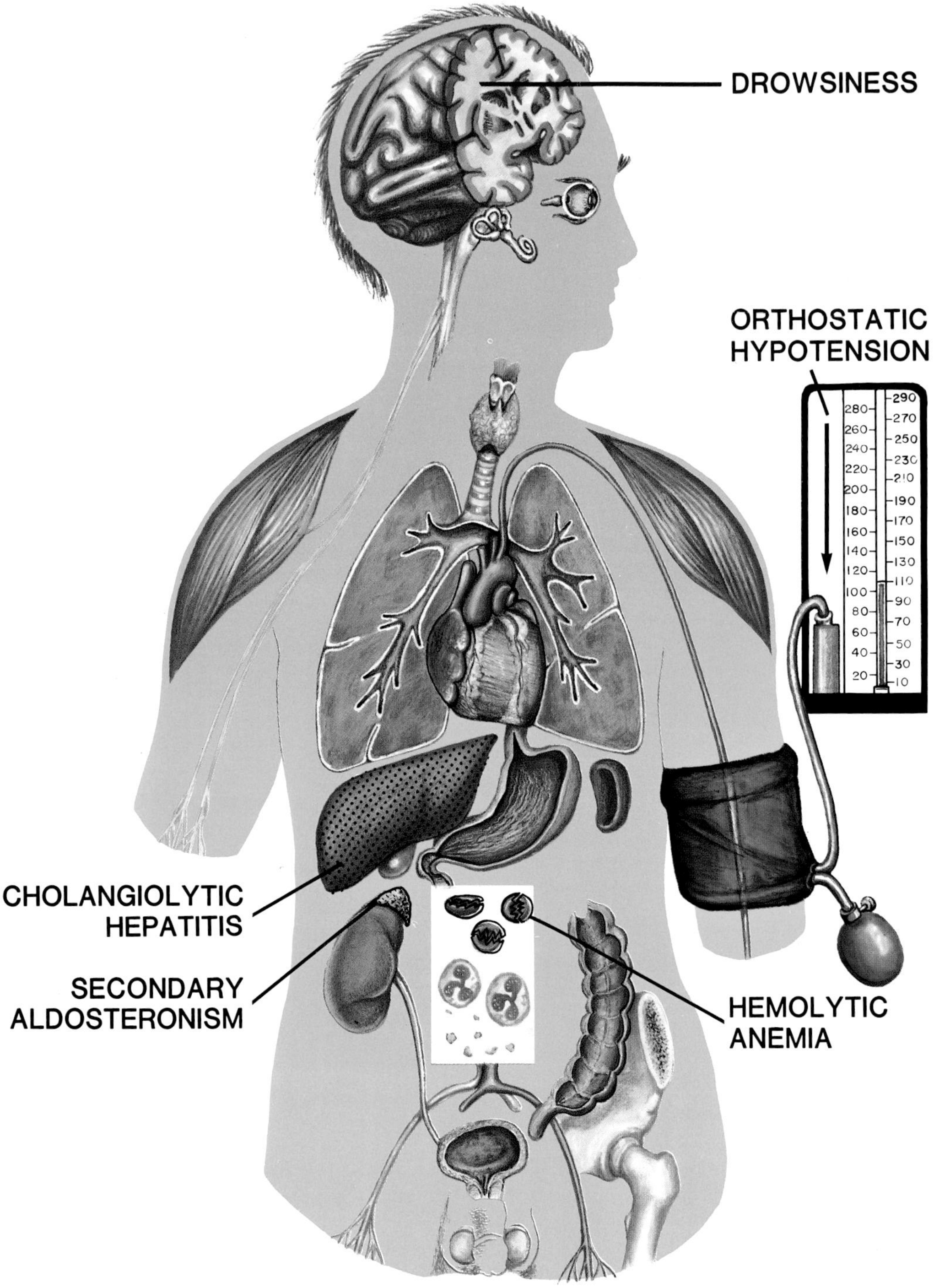

DROWSINESS

ORTHOSTATIC HYPOTENSION

CHOLANGIOLYTIC HEPATITIS

SECONDARY ALDOSTERONISM

HEMOLYTIC ANEMIA

Methyldopa

Representative Trade Name: Aldomet

Toxicity Rating: Low

Adverse Reactions

Hematopoietic A major reaction to methyldopa is hemolytic anemia. The direct Coomb's test is positive in patients with this complication, and tests for antinuclear antigen, L.E. cells, and rheumatoid factor may also be positive. Hemolytic anemia is happily a rare reaction, but 10 to 20 percent of patients on methyldopa develop a positive Coomb's test. Bone marrow depression has also been reported with methyldopa.

Hepatobiliary A second major reaction to methyldopa is hepatitis. This reaction may be due to hypersensitivity cholangitis, as it is with chlorpromazine: it is a serious complication because it can result in potentially fatal hepatic necrosis.

Central Nervous System Transient sedation is common during the first week of therapy, with headache, weakness, and dizziness. If mild, these effects usually subside with time. Bell's palsy, parkinsonism, and other extrapyramidal reactions may occur. Mental and emotional changes, including psychosis and depression, may occur but are very rare.

Cardiovascular Bradycardia and hypotension (especially orthostatic) are the most frequent cardiovascular reactions, but aggravation of angina and edema that is probably due to decreased glomerular filtration and secondary aldosteronism may occur. Fortunately, all of these reactions are infrequent.

Gastrointestinal Any type of gastrointestinal reaction may be seen, including nausea, vomiting, diarrhea, and constipation. A dry mouth and black tongue may be noted.

Allergic Drug fever, rash, hypersensitivity cholangitis, and a lupus-like syndrome are the most frequent allergic side effects. An allergic myocarditis has also been reported.

Other Gynecomastia, hyperprolactinemia, and amenorrhea may occur.

Contraindications

Active hepatic disease and previous hypersensitivity to methyldopa are the most important contraindications. Prior existence of a positive Coomb's test is not a contraindication in itself.

Precautions

Methyldopa should be used carefully in patients with a history of liver disease. Methyldopa may interfere with the measurement of catecholamine, urinary uric acid, serum creatinine, and serum glutamic-oxaloacetic transaminase. The VMA (vanillylmandelic acid) test for pheochromocytoma may be used if it is undesirable to interrupt methyldopa therapy.

Treatment

Withdrawal of the drug is usually all that is necessary. Steroids are occasionally necessary to resolve hemolytic anemia. Fatal hepatitis has occurred even when methyldopa was discontinued when jaundice developed, but this is rare.

Hydralazine Hydrochloride

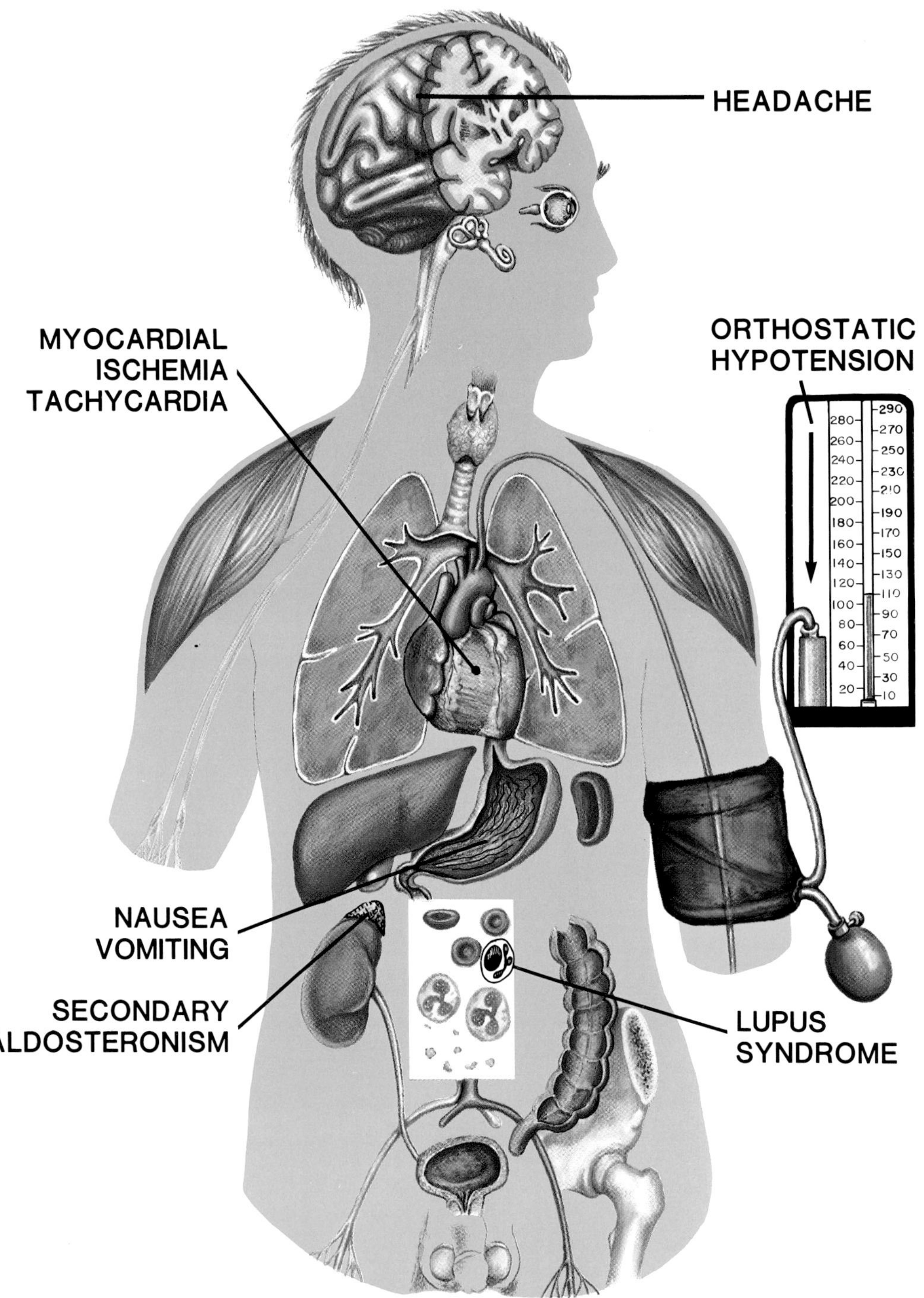

Hydralazine Hydrochloride

Representative Trade Name: Apresoline HCl

Toxicity Rating: This drug deserves a low to medium rating because of its potential to induce myocardial ischemia, peripheral neuritis, and a reversible lupus-like syndrome.

Adverse Reactions

Central Nervous System Headache, tremor, depression, psychosis, and peripheral neuropathy may occur.

Cardiovascular Postural hypotension, myocardial ischemia, tachycardia, and sodium and water retention are the most common reactions.

Hematologic Hydralazine can induce a syndrome that mimics systemic lupus erythematosus, with positive L.E. cell preparations and antinuclear antibody titers. Hydralazine may also cause depression of one or more of the cellular elements of the blood (neutropenia, etc.).

Other Allergic reactions occur but are unusual. There may be a paradoxical pressor response.

Contraindications

Hydralazine is contraindicated where there is known hypersensitivity to it, preexisting coronary artery disease, or mitral valvular disease from rheumatic fever.

Precautions

Hydralazine should be administered with caution to patients with coronary or cerebrovascular insufficiency.

Drug Interactions

The drug is potentially dangerous for patients on MAO inhibitors. Profound hypertension may occur when diazoxide is given with hydralazine.

Treatment

Most of the side effects of hydralazine will subside when the drug is withdrawn. However, occasional patients with the lupus-like syndrome must be maintained on steroids for some time. Myocardial ischemia may be prevented by the concomitant administration of a beta blocker with hydralazine. Peripheral neuropathy can be corrected by administering pyridoxine. A diuretic should be administered with hydralazine to prevent sodium and water retention caused by secondary aldosteronism.

Prazosin Hydrochloride

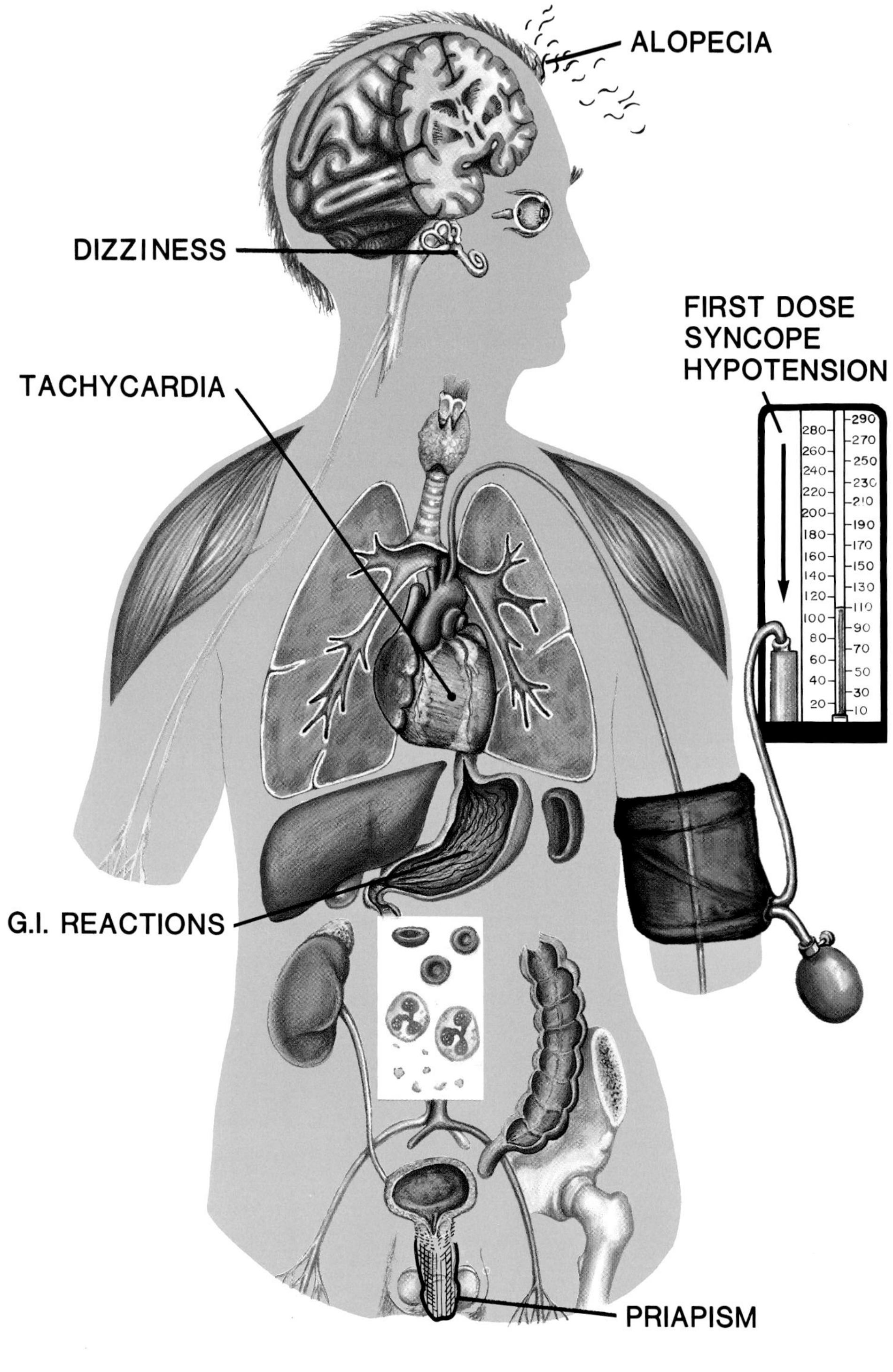

ALOPECIA

DIZZINESS

FIRST DOSE
SYNCOPE
HYPOTENSION

TACHYCARDIA

G.I. REACTIONS

PRIAPISM

Prazosin Hydrochloride

Representative Trade Name: Minipress

Toxicity Rating: Medium because of the marked hypotension and syncope that may occur after the first dose.

Adverse Reactions

Central Nervous System Dizziness, headache, drowsiness, fatigue, depression, and paresthesias have been noted.

Cardiovascular Hypotension (orthostatic or general) and tachycardia are the most common cardiovascular reactions to prazosin. Like other diuretics, prazosin may cause edema due to secondary aldosteronism.

Gastrointestinal Vomiting, diarrhea, constipation, and almost any other gastrointestinal reaction may occur.

Dermatologic Allergic reactions such as pruritus and various rashes occur. More peculiar reactions— alopecia, lichen planus, and diaphoresis—may also occur.

Other Sexual dysfunction, priapism, polyarthritis, and urinary frequency or incontinence occur. Dry mouth, blurred vision, tinnitus, and nasal congestion may also occur.

Contraindications

Other than known hypersensitivity, there are none.

Precautions

Patients must be warned about "first dose" syncope and told to remain recumbent for several hours after the initial dose. The safety of prazosin during pregnancy has not been established.

Treatment Withdrawal of the drug is usually all that is necessary. Permanent pathology is almost nonexistent.

Reserpine

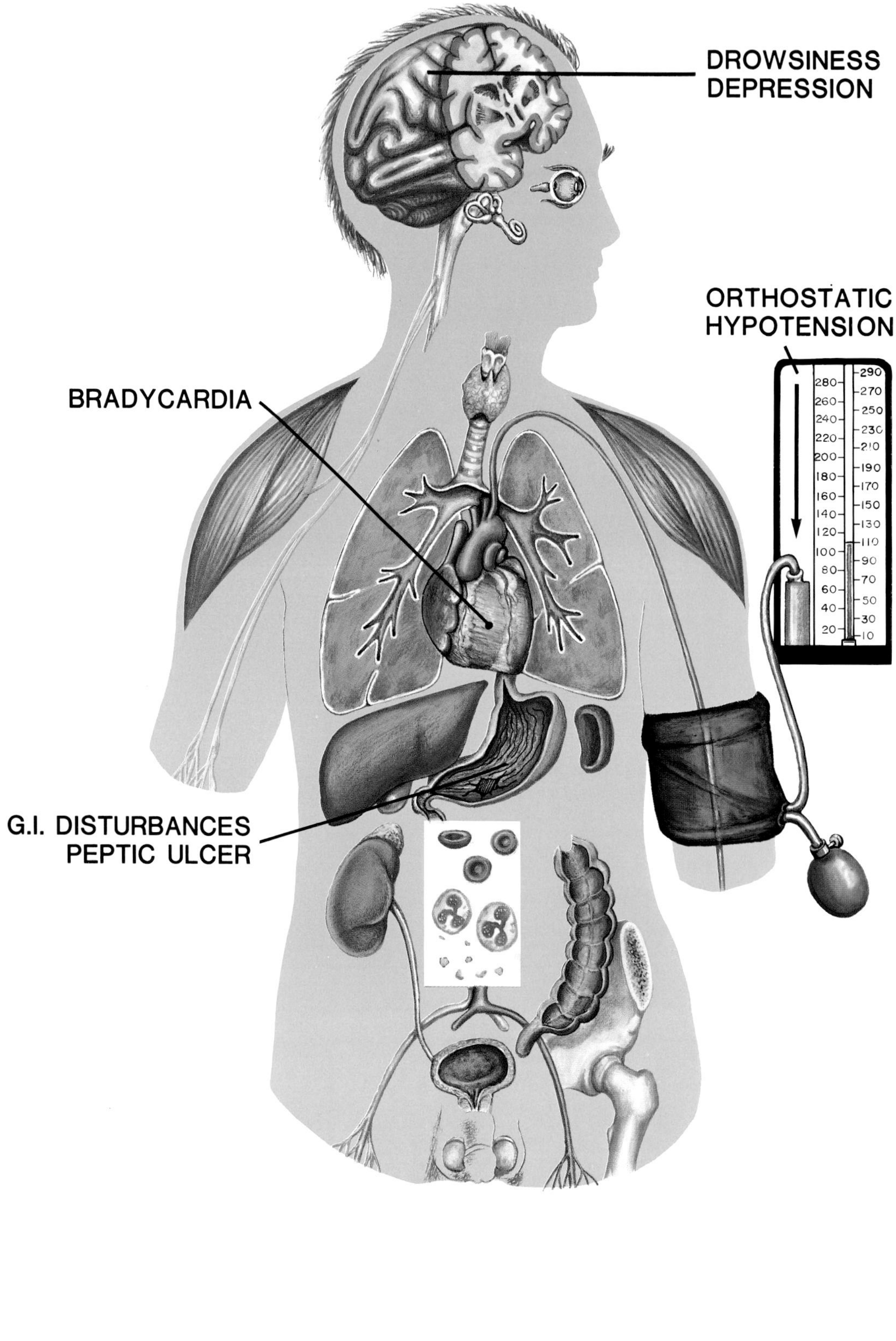

DROWSINESS
DEPRESSION

ORTHOSTATIC
HYPOTENSION

BRADYCARDIA

G.I. DISTURBANCES
PEPTIC ULCER

Reserpine

Representative Trade Name: Serpasil

Toxicity Rating: Low

Adverse Reactions

Central Nervous System Drowsiness and depression, particularly in the elderly, are the worst side effects of reserpine. They may lead to suicide. Other nervous reactions include parkinsonism, nervousness, and nightmares.

Cardiovascular Cardiovascular reactions are not usually serious, but bradycardia, edema, angina, and occasional arrhythmias are encountered.

Gastrointestinal Although not severe, nausea, vomiting, diarrhea, and anorexia are quite common. Peptic ulcer may occur.

Other Pruritus, various rashes, headache, impotence, gynecomastia, blood dyscrasias, glaucoma, deafness, and optic neuritis have occasionally been reported.

Contraindications

Prazosin is contraindicated where there is known hypersensitivity, and also in severely depressed patients and those with active peptic ulcer or ulcerative colitis.

Precautions

Prazosin should be given with caution if at all to depressed patients. Pregnancy is a relative contraindication.

Drug Interactions

MAO inhibitors should probably not be given concomitantly.

Treatment

Cautious withdrawal of the drug is usually effective because almost all the reactions are reversible. Depression, however, may persist for months after the drug is stopped.

Guanethidine Monosulfate

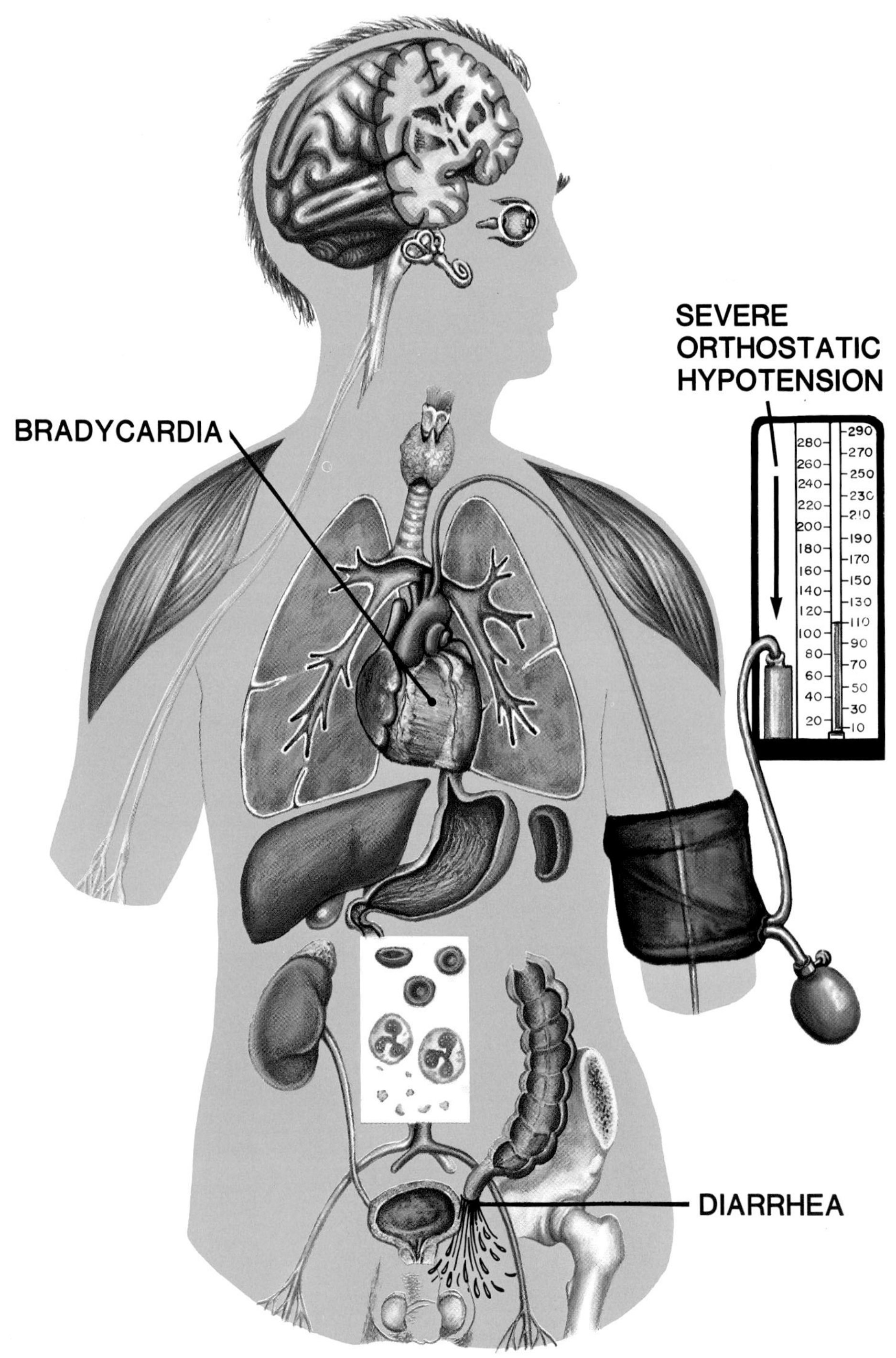

Guanethidine Monosulfate

Representative Trade Name: Ismelin

Toxicity Rating: Medium because of severe hypotension and syncope.

Adverse Reactions

Cardiovascular Severe orthostatic hypotension may occur as in prazosin therapy, but persists beyond the first dose. As a result, dizziness, weakness, syncope, and bradycardia may occur.

Gastrointestinal Diarrhea may be severe.

Other Impotence, edema, alopecia, dry mouth, angina, and ptosis are just a few of many unusual reactions to this drug.

Contraindications

Known hypersensitivity, the presence of a pheochromocytoma, and congestive heart failure are the major contraindications.

Precautions

Patients must be warned of the possibility of severe hypotension. Patients with preexisting renal disease should be watched for rising azotemia. Guanethidine may aggravate coronary or cerebrovascular insufficiency. Peptic ulcer disease and congestive heart failure may also be worsened.

Drug Interactions

It is recommended that guanethidine not be used with MAO inhibitors or rauwolfia derivatives because unusual central nervous system reactions may occur. The hypotensive effect of guanethidine may be reduced by sympathomimetics, tricyclic antidepressants, phenothiazines, and oral contraceptives.

Treatment

Withdrawal of the drug and careful monitoring of blood pressure and vital signs may be necessary. Hospitalization and administration of intravenous fluids, oxygen, and atropine may be necessary. Vasopressors must be given with extreme caution since cardiac arrhythmias may develop.

Captopril

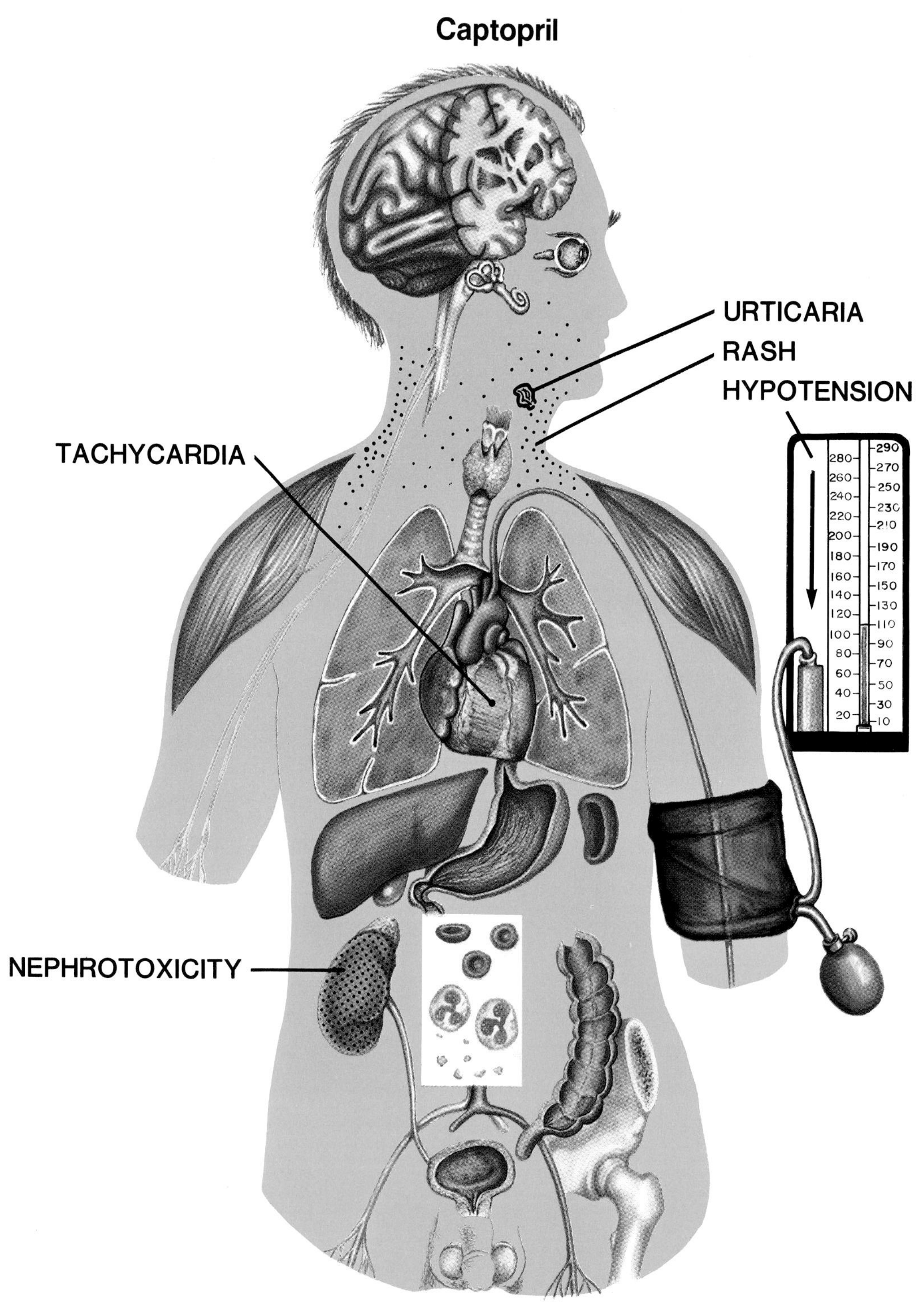
URTICARIA
RASH
HYPOTENSION
TACHYCARDIA
NEPHROTOXICITY

Captopril

Representative Trade Name: Capoten

Toxicity Rating: Medium to high because of renal and hematologic reactions.

Adverse Reactions

Cardiovascular Hypotension is a major reaction to captopril and may aggravate angina, congestive heart failure, and renal failure. Tachycardia and chest pain have occurred.

Renal A number of patients develop proteinuria, but its significance is uncertain. It is certain that the drug must be withdrawn if renal insufficiency develops.

Hematologic Fatal granulocytosis has occurred.

Dermatologic Pruritus, urticaria, and drug fever are among the common allergic reactions that may occur. Positive antinuclear antigen titers are noted, but whether this may lead to a lupus-like syndrome is not known.

Other Loss of taste (dysgeusia) occurs in 7 percent of patients. Potassium and blood urea nitrogen levels may be elevated.

Contraindications and Precautions

Experience with captopril is limited, so it is not clear which factors are positive contraindications for use of the drug and which merely call for caution. Patients with lupus erythematosus, significant renal disease, chronic infections in which neutropenia may pose a hazard, and those who are pregnant should probably not be given this drug.

Drug Interactions

Patients on diuretics may have a dramatic reduction in blood pressure — more than is desired. The effects of captopril may be altered by agents that cause renin release (methyldopa, propranolol, etc.) The concomitant use of captopril with guanethidine and beta blockers should be avoided, as here again the antihypertensive effects may be horrendous. Since captopril decreases aldosterone production, it may cause potassium depletion: consequently, the clinician may not want to administer spironolactone concomitantly.

Treatment

Withdrawal of the drug and careful monitoring of blood pressure, electrolytes, and blood urea nitrogen may be necessary.

Pargyline Hydrochloride

Representative Trade Name: Eutonyl

Toxicity Rating: Medium to high because the drug is an MAO inhibitor.

Adverse Reactions

Cardiovascular Hypotension and orthostatic hypotension are responsible for the most frequent side effects (dizziness, weakness, and fainting). Severe headache may occur if pressor amines are ingested.

Other Dry mouth, nausea and vomiting, arthralgia, headache, and insomnia are just a few of the rare side effects that may be encountered with pargyline.

Contraindications and Precautions

The many situations in which pargyline is contraindicated or dangerous are the main reason the drug deserves a moderate to high toxicity rating. Pargyline cannot be used in patients with a pheochromocytoma, paranoid schizophrenia, hyperthyroidism, malignant hypertension, or renal failure. Patients must be warned against using the drug with sympathomimetics and substances containing tyramine. Numerous foods must be eliminated from the diet because they contain pressor amines. Pargyline may induce hypoglycemia. The drug should not be given to patients with severe renal insufficiency.

Drug Interactions

As an MAO inhibitor, pargyline potentiates sympathomimetic drugs. See page 267 for more interactions applicable to pargyline.

Treatment

Withdrawal of the drug and administration of fluids and electrolytes and pressors or antihypertensive drugs to maintain a normal blood pressure is the goal of therapy. The drug should be withdrawn two weeks before an operation when possible.

Diazoxide

Representative Trade Name: Hyperstat

Toxicity Rating: Medium, primarily because the drug is administered intravenously.

Adverse Reactions

Cardiovascular Hypotension, edema, myocardial ischemia, cerebral ischemia, and arrhythmias may occur. Convulsions, cerebral infarctions, and other neurologic symptoms may occur as a result of hypotension.

Other Acute pancreatitis, papilledema, flushing, headache, and many other reactions are occasionally reported.

Contraindications

Known hypersensitivity to this or other thiazides or sulfonamides is the major contraindication.

Precautions

Careful monitoring of blood pressure and blood sugar is essential. The blood pressure must be lowered carefully in patients with known myocardial ischemia or cerebrovascular insufficiency.

Drug Interactions

Diazoxide raises blood levels of coumarin. Diazoxide may also reduce phenytoin seizure control. Simultaneous use of diazoxide and other diuretics may cause severe hypotension, hyperglycemia, and hyperuricemia. The drug must also be given with caution when the patient has already received antihypertensives.

Treatment

If severe hypotension develops, norepinephrine or other pressor amines may be given with careful blood pressure monitoring. Oral antihypertensives, such as methyldopa, should be begun gradually. Excessive hyperglycemia in diabetics may necessitate insulin administration.

Trimethaphan Camsylate

Representative Trade Name: Arfonad

Toxicity Rating: Medium to high, primarily because of the dramatic hypotensive effects when the drug is given intravenously.

Adverse Reactions

Cardiovascular Hypotension may be precipitous and lead to myocardial ischemia, cerebrovascular insufficiency, and even infarction. Renal insufficiency may also develop.

Other Allergic reactions are not uncommon, and pupillary dilation sometimes occurs.

Contraindications

Known hypersensitivity to the drug is the only contraindication.

Precautions

Any patient with possible cerebrovascular, coronary, or renal insufficiency may be compromised by the hypotension induced by trimethaphan. The drug may liberate histamine in allergic individuals. Since anesthetics may also induce hypotension, the effects of anesthetics and trimethaphan may be additive. Vigilant monitoring of blood pressure is mandatory.

Treatment

Withdrawal of the drug will allow the blood pressure to return to normal (or to pretreatment levels) within ten minutes in most cases. If not, phenylephrine HCl or mephentermine sulfate may be given.

Sodium Nitroprusside

Representative Trade Name: Nipride

Toxicity Rating: Medium to high because severe, life-threatening hypotension may occur unless blood pressure is carefully monitored (preferably by an intraarterial line).

Adverse Reactions

Central Nervous System Dizziness, restlessness, headache, muscle twitching, and apprehension may be observed.

Gastrointestinal Nausea, vomiting, and abdominal pain are frequent.

Cardiovascular Severe hypotension, angina, and palpitations may occur.

Contraindications

This drug should not be used in patients with hypertension due to coarctation of the aorta or arteriovenous shunts. Known hypersensitivity and inadequate facilities for blood pressure monitoring are other contraindications.

Precautions

Cyanide toxicity can occur. It is essential to monitor acid-base balance during prolonged infusion, especially if there is known renal dysfunction. Sodium nitroprusside should be given with caution to patients with hepatic insufficiency. Hypothyroidism may develop. Vital signs and blood pressure must be frequently monitored, and an infusion pump should be used if possible to carefully control the rate of infusion. The solution of nitroprusside should be kept from exposure to light.

Treatment

Overdosage should be treated by discontinuing the drug and by amyl nitrite inhalation followed as soon as possible by 3 percent sodium nitrite IV infusion with careful monitoring of blood pressure. If necessary, an injection of 12.5 g of sodium thiosulfate in 50 ml of 5 percent dextrose can then be given over a 10 minute period. If the blood pressure drops during the administration of nitrites, vasopressor agents may be given.

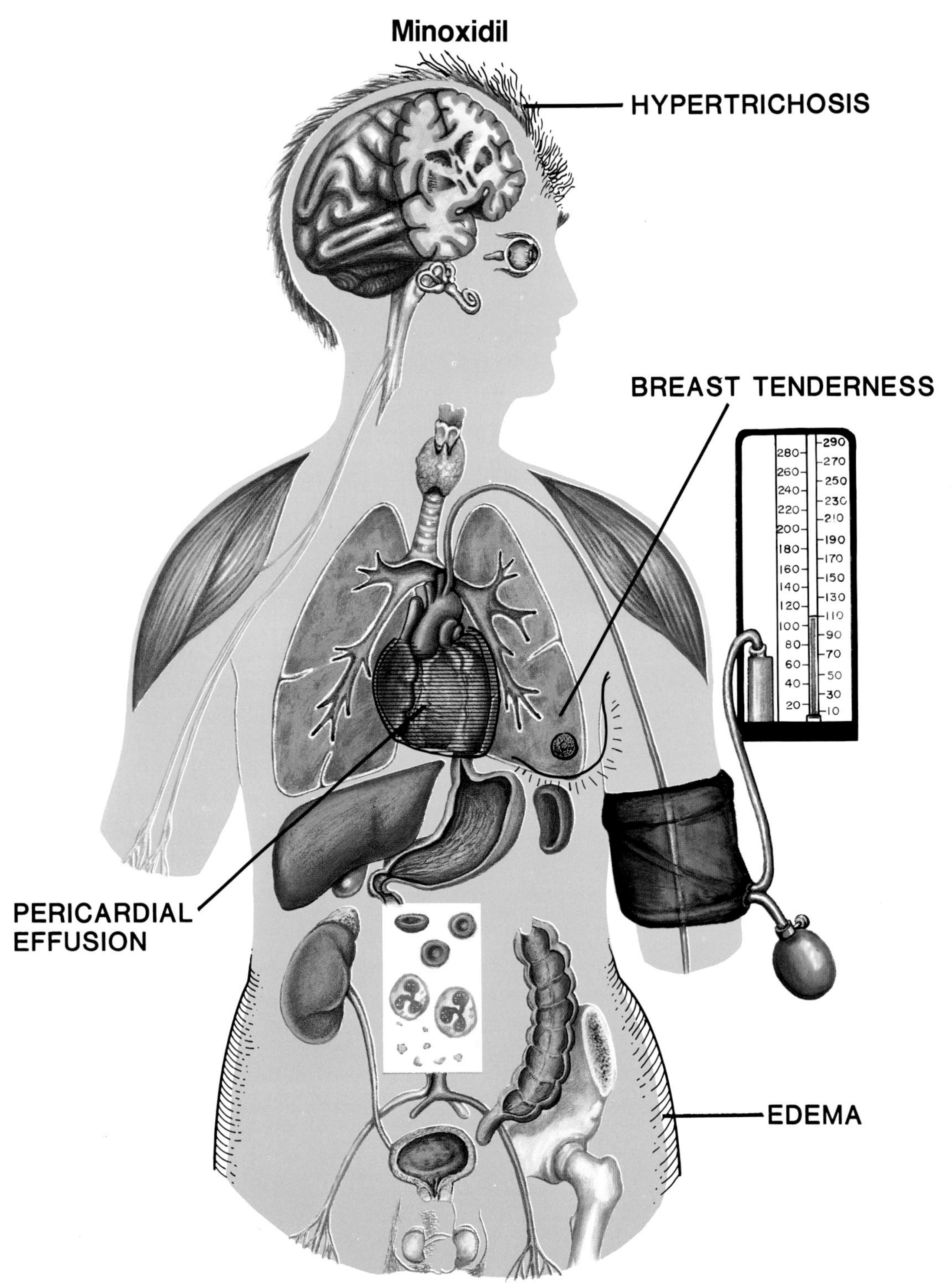
Minoxidil
HYPERTRICHOSIS
BREAST TENDERNESS
PERICARDIAL
EFFUSION
EDEMA

Minoxidil

Representative Trade Name: Loniten

Toxicity Rating: Medium to high because of pericardial effusion which occasionally progresses to tamponade.

Adverse Reactions

Cardiovascular Edema, pericardial effusion, and occasional tamponade have occurred. EKG changes are frequently noted. Tachycardia may also occur.

Endocrinologic Hypertrichosis, secondary aldosteronism, and breast tenderness have been reported.

Contraindications

Known hypersensitivity and pheochromocytomas are the principle contraindications.

Precautions

A diuretic should be given with minoxidil to prevent edema, especially in the presence of congestive heart failure. This drug should be used with caution in patients with angina pectoris or cerebrovascular insufficiency.

Drug Interactions

Minoxidil administration with guanethidine sulfate can result in severe orthostatic hypotension.

Treatment

Withdrawal of the drug is usually sufficient to treat most complications. When severe hypotension develops, intravenous saline and volume expansion is usually adequate treatment; sympathomimetic drugs such as norepinephrine and epinephrine should be avoided. Dopamine may be used if perfusion of a vital organ becomes necessary.

Chapter 10

ANTIMICROBIAL AGENTS

Table 10-1. Common Toxic Reactions of Some Antimicrobial Agents

Drug	Frequent allergic reactions	Bone Marrow Depression	Ototoxicity	Nephrotoxicity	Hepato-toxicity	Pseudo-membranous colitis	Neurotoxicity
Penicillins	+	−	−	−	−	−	−
Cephalosporins	+	−	−	+	−	+	−
Tetracyclines	−	−	+ (minocycline)	−	−	−	−
Sulfonamides	+	+	−	+	−	−	−
Erythromycins	−	−	−	-	+ (primarily with erythromycin estolate)	−	−
Aminoglycosides	−	−	+	+	−	+	−
Chloramphenicol	−	+	−	−	−	−	−
Nitrofurans	−	+	−	−	−	−	+
Clindamycin	−	−	−	−	−	+	−
Isoniazid	−	−	−	−	+	−	+
Rifampin	−	−	−	−	+	−	−

Introduction

Principal Antimicrobial Agents

ANTIBACTERIAL AGENTS

- Penicillins
- Cephalosporins
- Tetracyclines
- Sulfonamides
- Erythromycins
- Aminoglycosides
- Chloramphenicol
- Nitrofurans
- Clindamycin and lincomycin
- Polymixins
- *Miscellaneous antibacterial agents*
  - Bacitracin
  - Nalidixic acid
  - Trimethoprim
  - Spectinomycin hydrochloride
  - Methenamine preparations
  - Vancomycin hydrochloride
- *Antimycobacterial agents*
  - Isoniazid
  - Ethambutol hydrochloride
  - Rifampin
  - *Miscellaneous antimycobacterial agents*
  - Aminosalicylic acid
  - Cycloserine
  - Capreomycin sulfate
  - Ethionamide

SYSTEMIC ANTIFUNGAL AGENTS

- Amphotericin B
- Flucytosine
- Griseofulvin
- Ketoconazole
- Miconazole

Certain toxic reactions are common to all the antimicrobial agents. All of them may cause allergic reactions, and anaphylaxis is a particular danger when antimicrobials are administered parenterally. Allergic reactions are the major side effect of the penicillins; consequently, these drugs should be given orally whenever possible. All antibiotics may produce superinfections and overgrowth by nonsusceptible organisms.

Erythromycin is the least toxic of all the antibiotics; even allergic reactions are rare with this drug. At the other end of the spectrum are the aminoglycosides. Their ototoxicity and nephrotoxicity make it mandatory that they be used only when clearly indicated. Chloramphenicol deserves the same restrictions because of its ability to cause fatal aplastic anemia.

In between these extremes are a number of drugs that deserve "honorable mention" because of their toxicity. The estolate derivative of erythromycin may produce cholestatic hepatitis. One wonders why this drug should be used at all when there are so many excellent alternatives. Minocycline hydrochloride causes reversible ototoxicity in a large percentage of patients, which opens its continued use to question. Finally, clindamycin produces pseudomembranous colitis frequently enough that its indiscriminate use is unwarranted. Table 10-1 shows additional similarities and differences in the toxicities of the most commonly used antimicrobial agents.

Penicillins

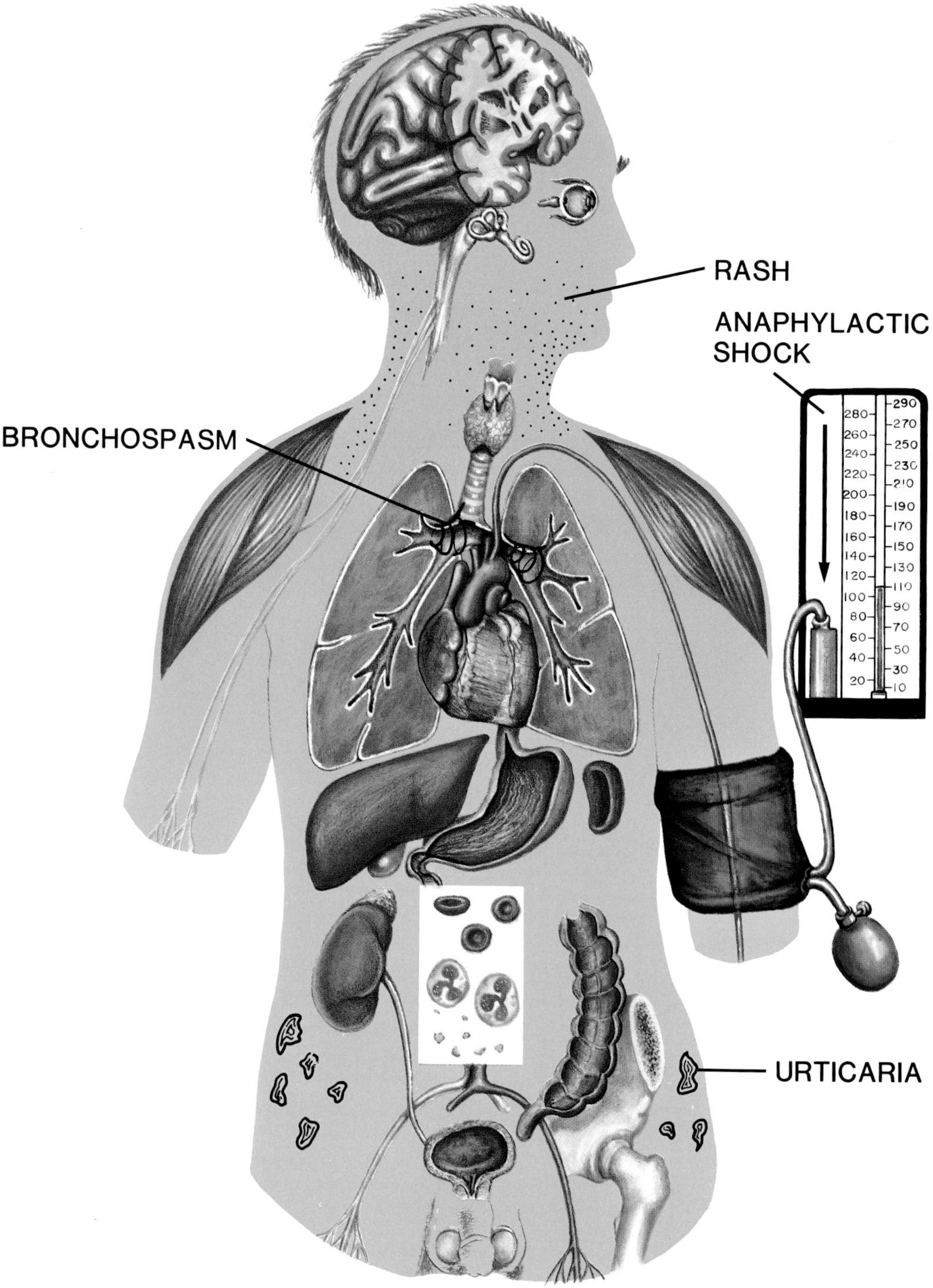

RASH

ANAPHYLACTIC SHOCK

BRONCHOSPASM

URTICARIA

ANTIBACTERIAL AGENTS

Penicillins

Principal Drugs

Generic Name	Representative Trade Name
Penicillin V potassium	Pen-Vee K
Penicillin G procaine	Crysticillin A.S.
Penicillin G benzathine	Bicillin L-A
Ampicillin sodium	Polycillin-N
Amoxicillin trihydrate	Amoxil
Cloxacillin sodium	Tegopen
Dicloxacillin sodium	Dynapen
Methicillin sodium	Staphcillin
Nafcillin sodium	Unipen
Carbenicillin disodium	Geopen
Mezlocillin sodium	Mezlin
Oxacillin sodium	Prostaphlin
Ticarcillin disodium	Ticar

Toxicity Rating: Medium because of rare anaphylactic shock and death, especially from parenteral use.

Adverse Reactions

Allergic Anaphylaxis—sometimes fatal—is the major adverse reaction to all penicillins. Angioneurotic edema and bronchospasm may lead to death by respiratory failure. Urticara, maculopapular eruptions, and other types of allergic dermatitis also occur. A transient mild eruption may occur with oral ampicillin, which may disappear with continued use.

Central Nervous System Convulsions and neuropathy may occur with large doses, especially if they are given intravenously.

Gastrointestinal Nausea, vomiting, and diarrhea are rare but do occur, especially with ampicillin.

Genitourinary Interstitial nephritis occasionally occurs, especially with methicillin.

Hematologic Thrombocytopenia, neutropenia, anemia, and eosinophilia may occur but almost always subside when the drug is discontinued.

Local Pain at the site of injection and thrombophlebitis (with intravenous administration) occur.

Other Glossitis, vaginitis, hypokalemia, and hepatitis may occur.

Contraindications

Known hypersensitivity to penicillins is the major contraindication.

Precautions

Dosage of intravenous preparations may need to be lowered in patients with significant renal insufficiency. These patients should be observed for signs of bleeding. Periodic hematologic, renal, and liver profiles may need to be done with prolonged (especially intravenous) use.

Drug Interactions

Erythromycin, chloramphenicol, and the tetracyclines may inhibit the action of penicillins, and neomycin decreases absorption of penicillins. Probenecid is well known to increase penicillin blood levels.

Treatment

Anaphylactic shock and bronchospasm are treated with 5–10 ml of intravenous or intracardiac epinephrine 1/10,000. Sublingual application may be useful when an intravenous line cannot be established. An adequate airway must be established and maintained even if a tracheotomy is required. An intravenous line must also be established and maintained. Epinephrine administration is followed by 500 mg of hydrocortisone intravenously. If bronchospasm continues, intravenous aminophylline (500 mg in 500 ml of 5 percent dextrose in water) should be given. Cardiopulmonary resuscitation may be necessary in severe cases. It is the author's recommendation that penicillins not be given parenterally (including intramuscularly) unless all necessary equipment for cardiopulmonary resuscitation is available (including a crash cart, Ambu bag, and defibrillator).

Other reactions can usually be managed by simple withdrawal of the drug. Patients who require a penicillin drug but have a history of possible penicillin allergy should be skin tested with penicilloyl-polylysine and minor determinant mixture. Careful desensitization may be necessary if penicillin administration is potentially life-saving.

Cephalosporins

Cephalosporins

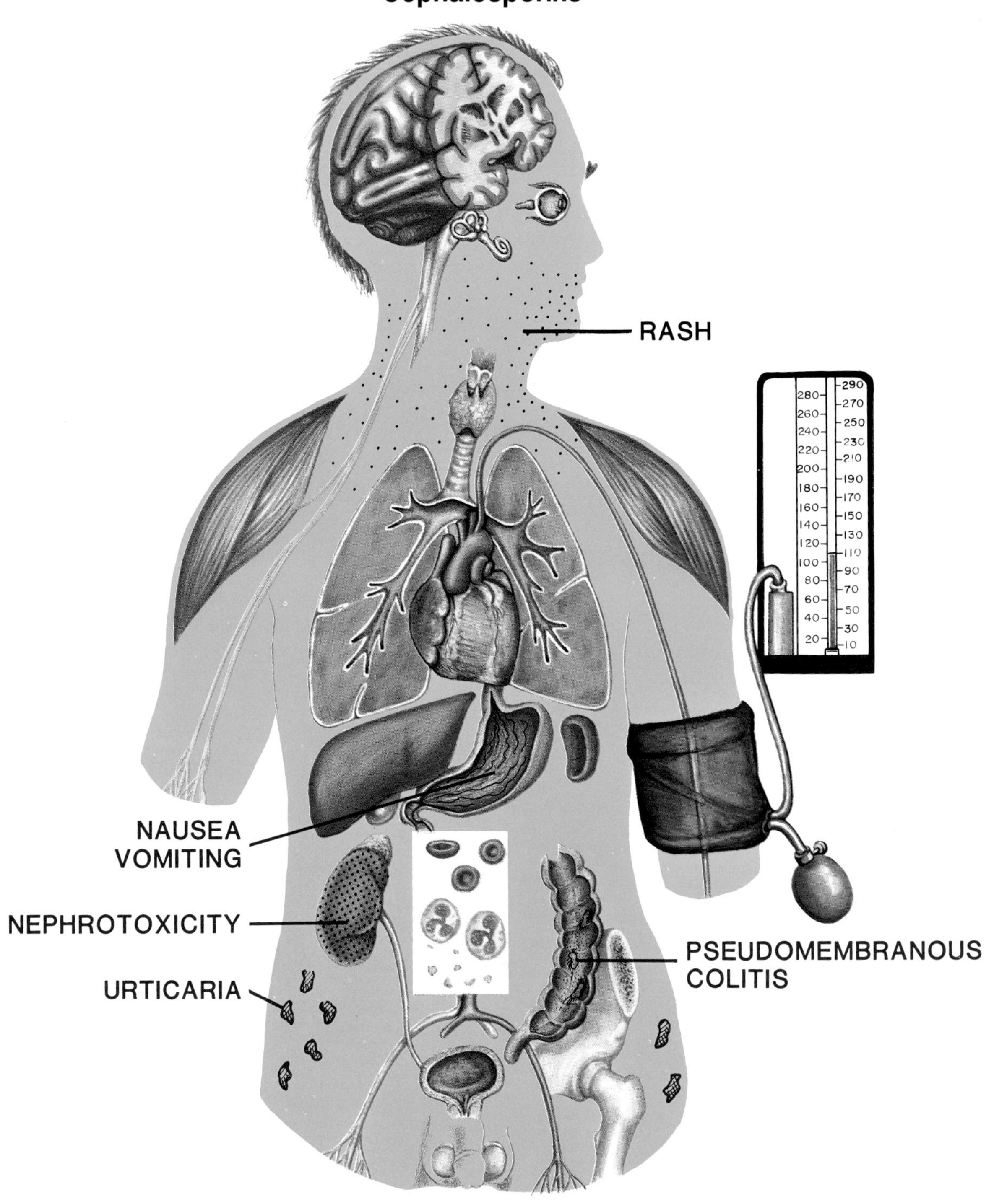

Cephalosporins

Principal Drugs

Generic Name	Representative Trade Name
Cephalexin	Keflex
Cephradine	Anspor, Velosef
Cephapirin sodium	Cefadyl
Cephalothin sodium	Keflin
Cefadroxil	Duricef
Cefamandole nafate	Mandol
Cefaclor	Ceclor
Cefotaxime sodium	Claforan
Moxalactam disodium	Moxam

Toxicity Rating: Low

Adverse Reactions

Allergic As with the penicillins, hypersensitivity reactions are the most common side effects of cephalosporins, and include urticara, drug fever, and anaphylaxis.

Gastrointestinal Nausea, vomiting, and diarrhea occur frequently. Pseudomembranous colitis may result from the overgrowth of *Clostridium difficile.*

Hematologic Any one of the formed elements of the blood may be reduced, but these reactions are infrequent. Hemolytic anemia may occur but is usually reversible. Hypoprothrombinemia caused by reduction of the gastrointestinal flora that produce vitamin K is reported.

Renal Nephrotoxicity occurs but is usually reversible.

Other Like other antibiotics, the cephalosporins may precipitate superinfections or overgrowth by nonsusceptible organisms. Transient alterations of liver function may occur.

Contraindications

The major contraindication is known hypersensitivity to any of the cephalosporins. Patients who have experienced severe or immediate hypersensitivity reactions to a penicillin should not be given a cephalosporin because there is cross-reactivity in 4–5 percent of persons. Cross-reactivity is rare with cefotaxime.

Precautions

Patients should be observed for hypersensitivity. Patients with marked renal impairment need to be given this drug cautiously and often at reduced dosages. The safety in pregnancy has not been established. Patients with known penicillin allergy should be given these drugs with care.

Drug Interactions

Combined use of a cephalosporin with an aminoglycoside enhances the renal toxicity of each. Patients with a history of penicillin allergy may be allergic to cephalosporins as mentioned above.

Treatment

Simple withdrawal of the drug is usually all that is necessary. Hypersensitivity reactions may require antihistamines, epinephrine, or corticosteroids. Pseudomembranous colitis may require IV fluids and oral vancomycin.

Tetracyclines

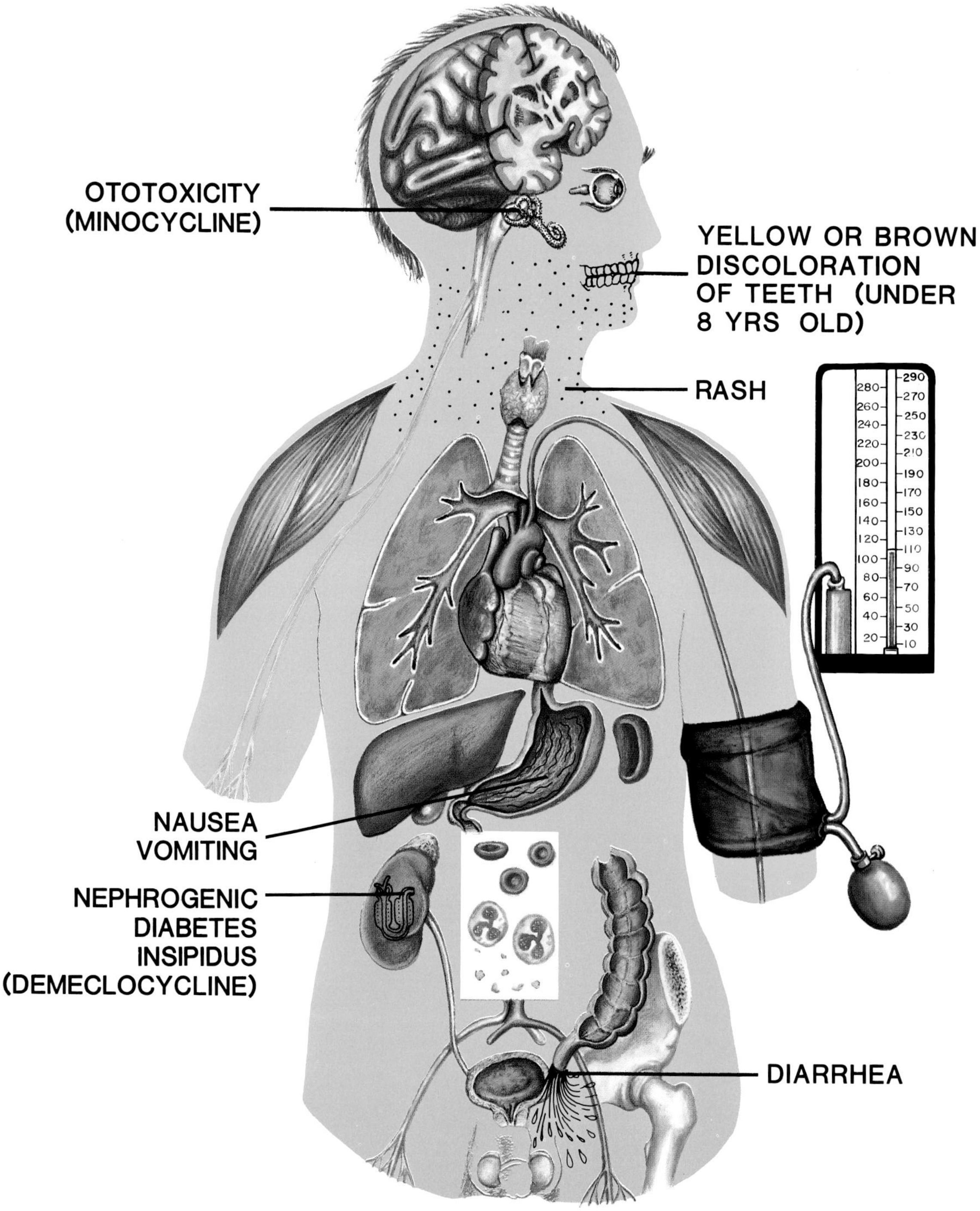

OTOTOXICITY (MINOCYCLINE)

YELLOW OR BROWN DISCOLORATION OF TEETH (UNDER 8 YRS OLD)

RASH

NAUSEA VOMITING

NEPHROGENIC DIABETES INSIPIDUS (DEMECLOCYCLINE)

DIARRHEA

Tetracyclines

Principal Drugs

Generic Name	Representative Trade Name
Tetracycline	Achromycin V
Tetracycline hydrochloride	Robitet, Sumycin; in Mysteclin-F
Minocycline hydrochloride	Minocin
Tetracycline phosphate	Tetrex
Demeclocycline hydrochloride	Declomycin
Doxycycline	Vibramycin

Toxicity Rating: Low except for minocycline, which causes ototoxicity, and consequently deserves a medium rating.

Adverse Reactions

Gastrointestinal As with most oral antibiotics, nausea, vomiting, and diarrhea are frequent. Overgrowth of nonsusceptible organisms and fungi may occur throughout the gastrointestinal tract causing glossitis, enterocolitis, and proctitis.

Allergic Skin rashes, angioneurotic edema, drug fever, and anaphylactic reactions occur but are infrequent. The drug may cause bulging fontanelles in infants but this is reversible. Pseudotumor cerebri may rarely occur.

Other Hemolytic anemia and pancytopenia can occur but are rare. Nephrotoxicity and hepatotoxicity have been reported, but usually in patients with preexisting renal or hepatic dysfunction. A yellow or brown discoloration of the teeth may occur in children under 8 years of age. Photosensitivity may be induced by tetracyclines. Ototoxicity is a reaction peculiar to minocycline but may occur in up to 90 percent of patients taking this drug. Demeclocycline may cause nephrogenic diabetes insipidus, but this is usually reversible.

Contraindications

The major contraindication is known hypersensitivity to tetracyclines.

Precautions

Tetracyclines should not be used in children less than 8 years old or during the last half of pregnancy because of the potential for permanent yellow or brown discoloration of the teeth. The dose should be reduced in patients with renal insufficiency. Patients with known hepatic insufficiency should be followed carefully using liver function tests. Patients should be warned to avoid undue exposure to sunlight while taking the drug because of the phototoxicity.

Drug Interactions

Tetracycline neutralizes the bactericidal action of penicillin. Tetracyclines also lower plasma prothrombin, potentiating the action of anticoagulants. Barbiturates, phenytoin, and carbamazepine may considerably reduce the plasma half-life of doxycycline by increasing its catabolism in the liver. Antacids may impair the absorption of tetracyclines. Methoxyflurane significantly potentiates the renal toxicity of the tetracyclines, and deaths have occurred.

Treatment

The best treatment is withdrawal of the drug. Hepatic and renal failure may necessitate additional supportive measures.

Sulfonamides

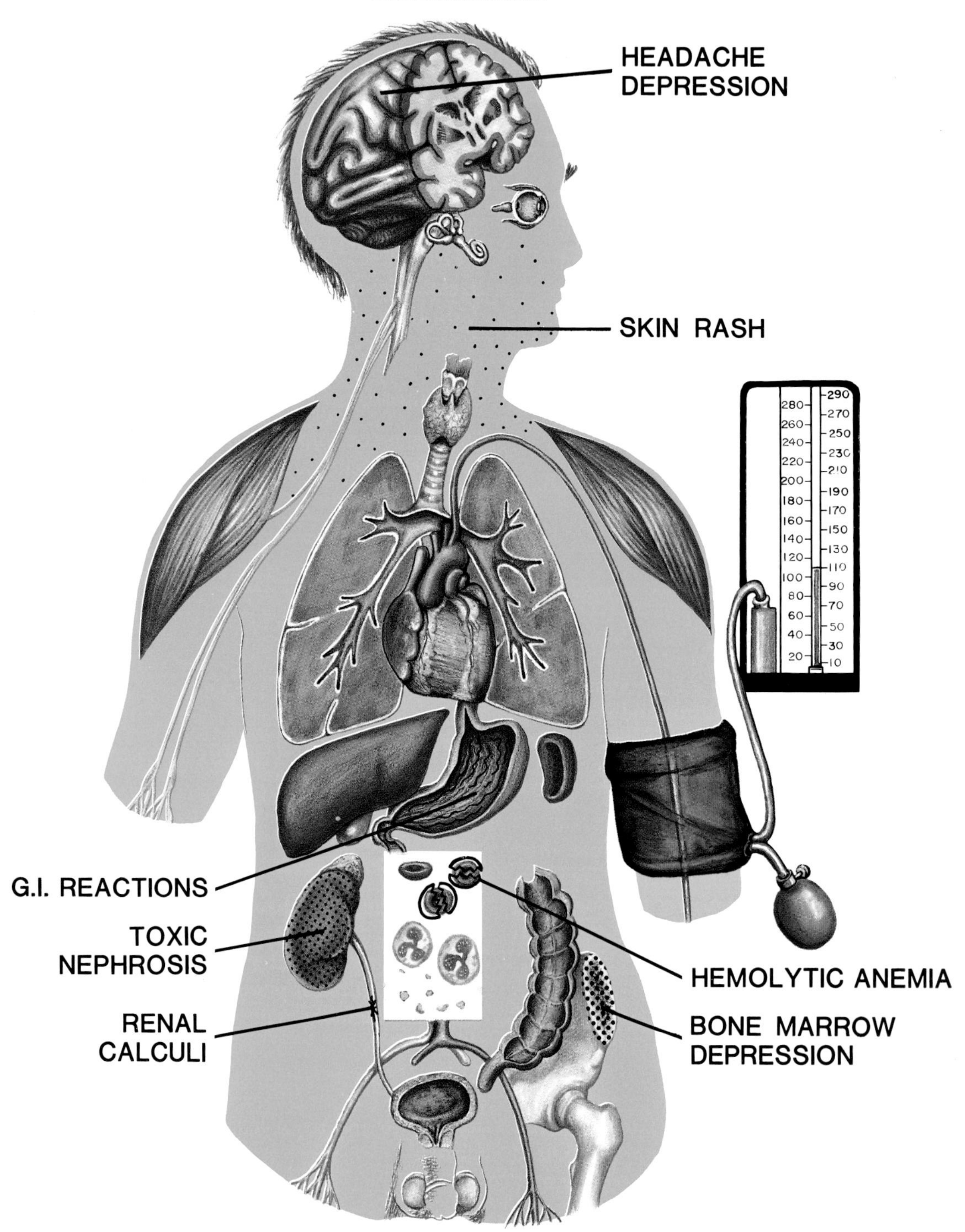

Sulfonamides

Principal Drugs

Generic Name	Representative Trade Name
Sulfamethoxazole	Gantanol, Septra DS
Sulfasalazine	Azulfidine
Sulfanilamide	AVC Cream
Sulfacetamide sodium	Sodium Sulamyd Ophthalmic
Sulfadiazine	Microsulfon
Sulfapyridine	Dagenan

Toxicity Rating: Low

Adverse Reactions

Hematologic Significant bone marrow depression, hemolytic anemia, and megaloblastic anemia may occur.

Genitourinary Fortunately, toxic nephrosis, renal calculi, and hematuria are infrequent with the most commonly used sulfonamide preparations.

Dermatologic Skin rashes of every description may occur, including urticaria, erythema multiforme, and exfoliative dermatitis.

Gastrointestinal Nausea, vomiting, diarrhea, and abdominal pain occur.

Central Nervous System Headache, depression, convulsions, and hallucinations have been reported.

Other Jaundice, serum sickness, and anaphylaxis have occurred. Peripheral neuropathy and a sterile meningitis have been reported.

Contraindications

Pregnancy and known hypersensitivity are the major contraindications. Severe renal insufficiency is another contraindication. Children under two months of age should not receive this drug, nor should nursing mothers.

Precautions

These drugs are inadequate to eradicate Group A beta-hemolytic streptoccal infections. Patients on sulfonamides should be observed for bone marrow and renal toxicity, especially with long-term therapy. Patients with known renal insufficiency, glucose-6-phosphate dehydrogenase deficiency, or blood dyscrasias should be watched carefully.

Drug Interactions

Drugs that acidify the urine (ammonium chloride, ascorbic acid, paraldehyde, etc.) may cause crystalluria. PABA-containing local anesthetics and other PABA drugs may inhibit the action of sulfonamides.

Treatment

Simple withdrawal of the drug is usually all that is necessary. Toxic nephrosis and severe hematologic reactions may require consultation with a nephrologist or hematologist for appropriate management.

Erythromycins

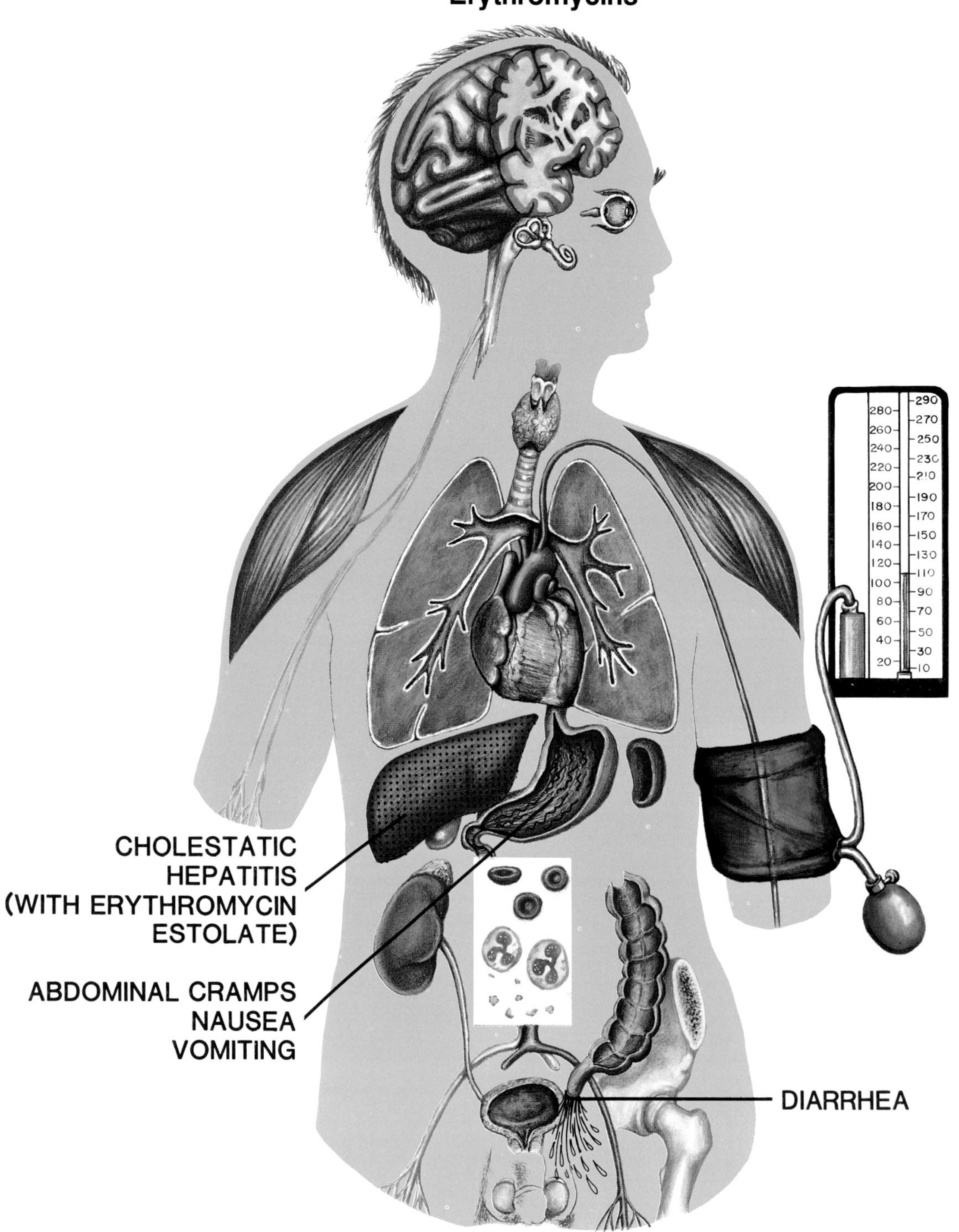

Erythromycins

Principal Drugs

Generic Name	Representative Trade Names
Erythromycin	Erythromycin Base Filmtabs, Ilotycin
Erythromycin estolate	Ilosone
Erythromycin gluceptate	Ilotycin Gluceptate
Erythromycin lactobionate	Erythrocin Lactobionate-I.V.
Erythromycin stearate	Bristamycin, Erythrocin Stearate Filmtabs
Erythromycin ethylsuccinate	E.E.S., Pediamycin

Toxicity Rating: Low

Adverse Reactions

Gastrointestinal The most frequent side effects of erythromycins are gastrointestinal: these include abdominal cramps and less frequently nausea, vomiting, and diarrhea.

Hepatic Cholestatic hepatitis may occur with erythromycin estolate but is almost always reversible.

Allergic Allergic reactions including urticaria and even anaphylaxis may occur but are rare.

Other Rare cases of ototoxicity have been reported. Superinfection with nonsusceptible organisms and fungi (e.g., moniliasis) may occur as with other antibiotics.

Contraindications

The only contraindication is known hypersensitivity to any of the erythromycins.

Precautions

Other than severe liver disease there are none.

Drug Interactions

Erythromycin may increase serum theophylline levels by interfering with its excretion. The drug may also neutralize the action of lincomycin and clindamycin.

Treatment

Simple withdrawal of the drug is usually all that is necessary.

Aminoglycosides

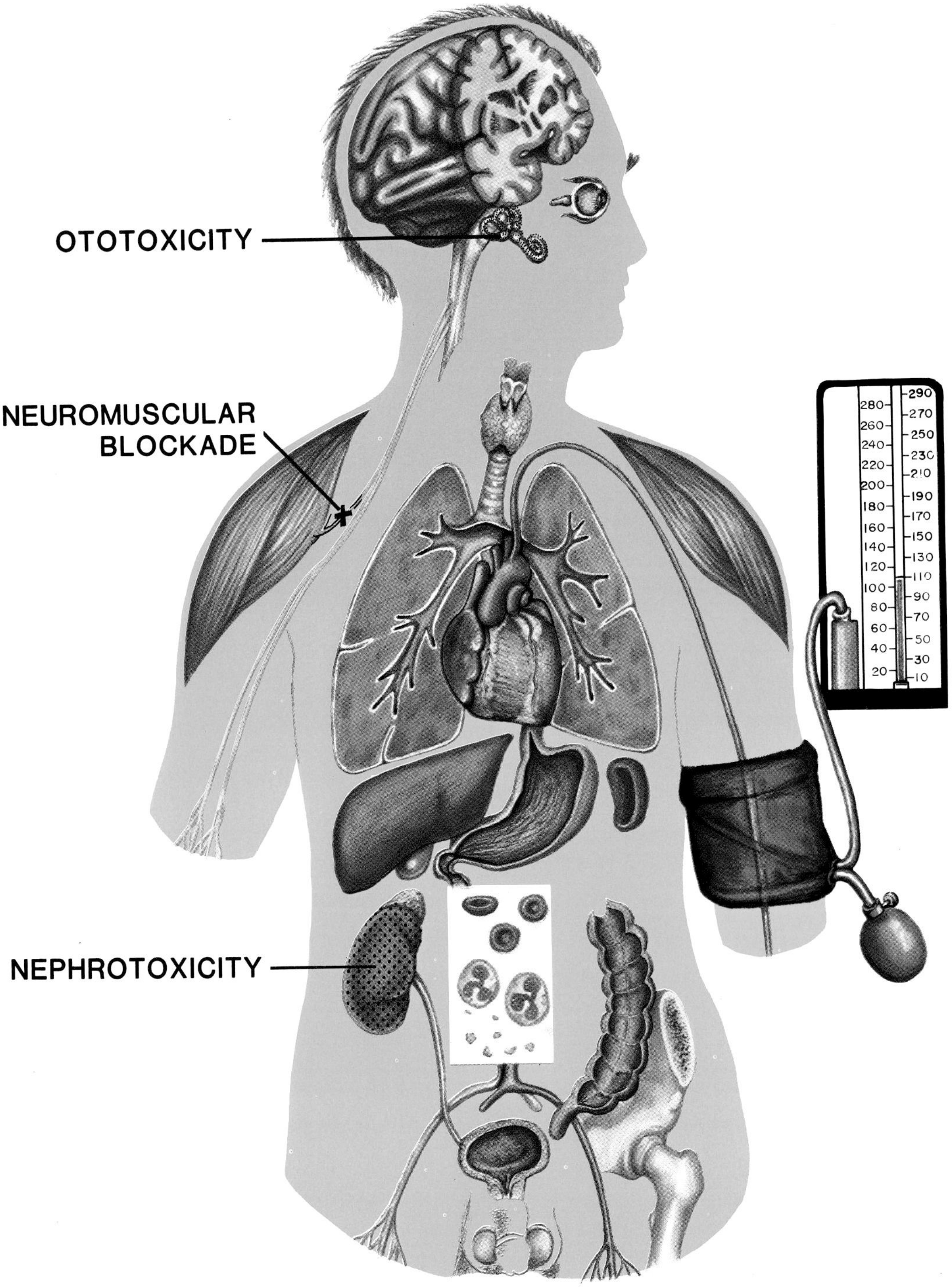

OTOTOXICITY

NEUROMUSCULAR BLOCKADE

NEPHROTOXICITY

Aminoglycosides

Principle Drugs

Generic Name	Representative Trade Name
Gentamicin sulfate	Garamycin
Tobramycin sulfate	Nebcin
Amikacin sulfate	Amikin
Kanamycin sulfate	Kantrex
Neomycin sulfate	Mycifradin
Streptomycin sulfate	

Toxicity Rating: Medium to high due to the ototoxicity and nephrotoxicity of these drugs.

Adverse Reactions

Special Senses Ototoxicity may be manifested by tinnitus, deafness, or vertigo. Some aminoglycosides (e.g., kanamycin) preferentially affect the cochlea while others (e.g., gentamicin) preferentially affect the semicircular canals.

Renal Nephrotoxicity is the most severe side effect of aminoglycosides. It is manifested by azotemia; elevated creatinine; and casts, red cells, and protein in the urine. It is usually reversible.

Gastrointestinal Mild nausea, vomiting, and diarrhea occur. Proctitis and enterocolitis occur but are uncommon.

Allergic Reactions Allergic reactions including urticaria, fever, and anaphylaxis occur but are usually not serious unless the patient has had a previous allergic reaction to these drugs.

Other Neuromuscular blockade may occur leading to progressive flaccid paralysis and respiratory arrest. Blood dyscrasias and bone marrow depression are relatively rare.

Contraindications

Known hypersensitivity is the only real contraindication, but severe renal insufficiency and pregnancy are relative contraindications.

Precautions

These drugs should be given with caution in patients with myasthenia gravis, as acute neuromuscular blockade may occur. Patients receiving succinylcholine or other neuromuscular blockers should be given aminoglycosides with caution. Patients with preexisting renal disease must be given these drugs cautiously and usually at lower dosages. The dosage should be regulated according to the serum creatinine level.

Drug Interactions

Ethacrynic acid and furosemide may potentiate the ototoxicity of aminoglyosides. Aminoglycosides enhance the neuromuscular blockade effect of succinylcholine, tubocurarine, and many other neuromuscular blockers. Carbenicillin may reduce the serum half-life of aminoglycosides; thus, if carbenicillin and aminoglycosides are to be given to a patient with severe renal impairment, they should not be administered in the same solution. Cephalosporins and methoxyflurane may potentiate aminoglycoside nephrotoxicity.

Treatment

Most reactions clear up when the drug is discontinued. Nephrotoxicity may necessitate peritoneal dialysis to remove the drug. Neuromuscular blockade will respond to calcium salts or neostigmine.

Chloramphenicol

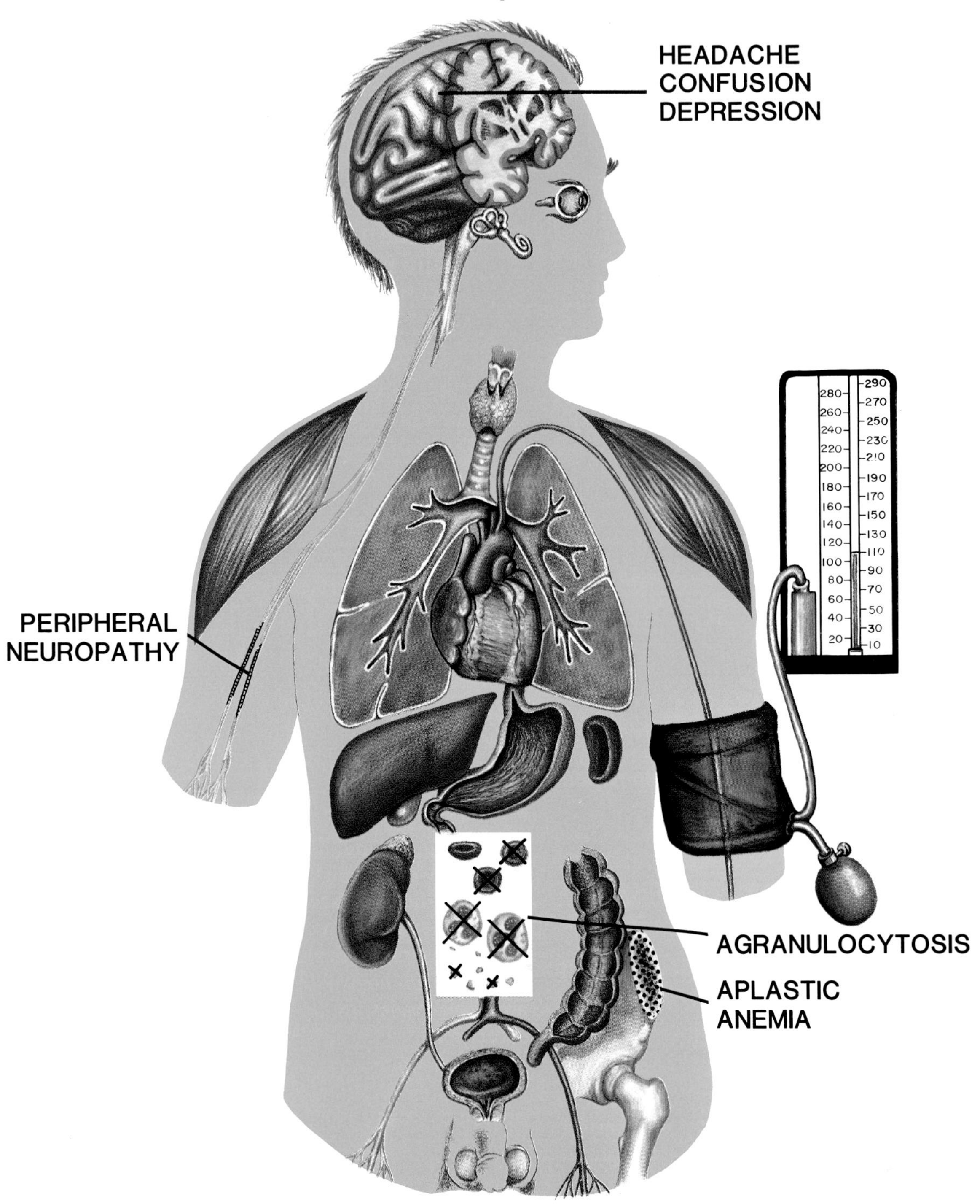

Chloramphenicol

Representative Trade Name: Chloromycetin

Toxicity Rating: High because it may cause fatal aplastic anemia.

Adverse Reactions

Hematologic Aplastic anemia, agranulocytosis, and thrombocytopenia are the most dangerous reactions to this drug because they are occasionally irreversible.

Gastrointestinal Nausea, vomiting, diarrhea, and abdominal pain may occur, as with almost all the antibiotics.

Central Nervous System Headache, depression, confusion, and optic or peripheral neuropathy may occur.

Other Glossitis, allergic skin reactions, and anaphylaxis are rare. A potentially fatal "gray syndrome" has occurred in premature infants and neonates.

Contraindications

This drug is contraindicated in patients with known hypersensitivity, in pregnancy, and when there is no threat to life or "limb."

Precautions

Frequent hematologic profiles are essential during therapy to detect bone marrow depression early. Other drugs that may cause bone marrow depression should not be given if possible.

Drug Interactions

Penicillin antagonizes the action of chloramphenicol, so the two should not be given simultaneously unless necessary. Acetaminophen elevates blood levels of chloramphenicol.

Treatment

In many cases of bone marrow depression, the blood counts will return to normal after withdrawal of the drug. When they do not, fresh whole blood or blood fractions must be given to maintain adequate counts of erythrocytes, leukocytes, and platelets. Prophylactic antibiotics may be necessary. Other symptoms usually subside once the drug is withdrawn.

Nitrofurans

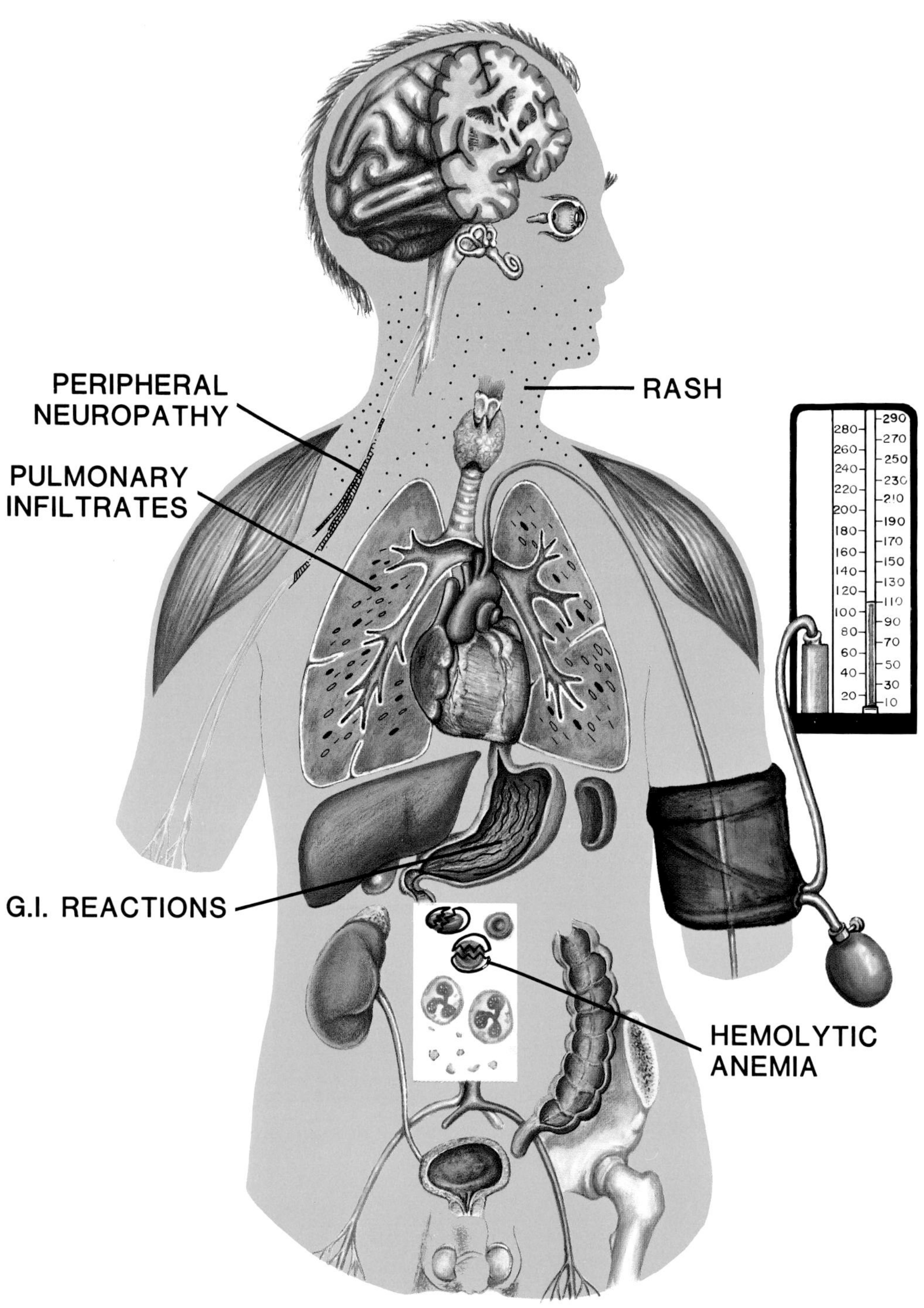

Nitrofurans

Principal Drugs

Generic Name	Representative Trade Name
Nitrofurantoin	Furadantin
Nirofurantoin macrocrystals	Macrodantin
Furazolidone	Furoxone
Nitrofurazone	Furacin

Toxicity Rating: Medium because of peripheral neuropathy and pulmonary fibrosis.

Adverse Reactions

Dermatologic Maculopapular or urticarial eruptions are the second most common side effects. These are seen in as many as 1 percent of patients.

Gastrointestinal Anorexia, nausea, and vomiting are very frequent in patients receiving nitrofurans. These effects are less common with macrocrystalline nitrofurantoin.

Hematologic Nitrofurans may precipitate a hemolytic anemia in patients with glucose-6-phosphate dehydrogenase deficiency or with enolase or glutathione peroxidase deficiency. Depression of one or more of the cytologic elements of the blood, including aplastic anemia, has also been reported.

Neurologic One of the most serious reactions to the nitrofurans is peripheral neuropathy. It is seen most often with associated azotemia. Paresthesias and dysesthesia should be a signal to discontinue the drug.

Hepatic Toxic hepatitis and even liver failure may occur but are fortunately rare. This may be an allergic reaction because it is not dose-related and is associated with antinuclear antibodies and chronic active hepatitis.

Pulmonary An acute onset of fever, chills, muscular pain, shortness of breath, rales, and pulmonary infiltrates has been noted. This may be an allergic reaction as eosinophilia frequently develops. Subacute and chronic forms of these reactions may also occur. These may progress to interstitial fibrosis.

Other Almost any type of hypersensitivity reaction may occur, including anaphylaxis.

Contraindications

Nitrofurans should not be used in patients with impaired renal function (creatinine clearance less than 40 ml per minute), nor in pregnant patients at term. Infants under one month old may develop hemolytic anemia. Nitrofurans should not be used for acute pyelonephritis, chronic bacterial prostatitis, or when there is known hypersensitivity.

Precautions

Anemia, diabetes, and malnutrition predispose to neuropathy.

Treatment

Almost all the above reactions resolve when the drug is withdrawn. Recovery from peripheral neuropathy may take weeks to months, and occasionally there is little or no recovery at all. The hepatotoxicity also usually resolves, but occasional chronic active hepatitis ensues requiring steroid therapy. Steroids have been helpful in persistent pulmonary disease, but the acute pulmonary reactions almost always resolve when the drug is discontinued.

Clindamycin and Lincomycin

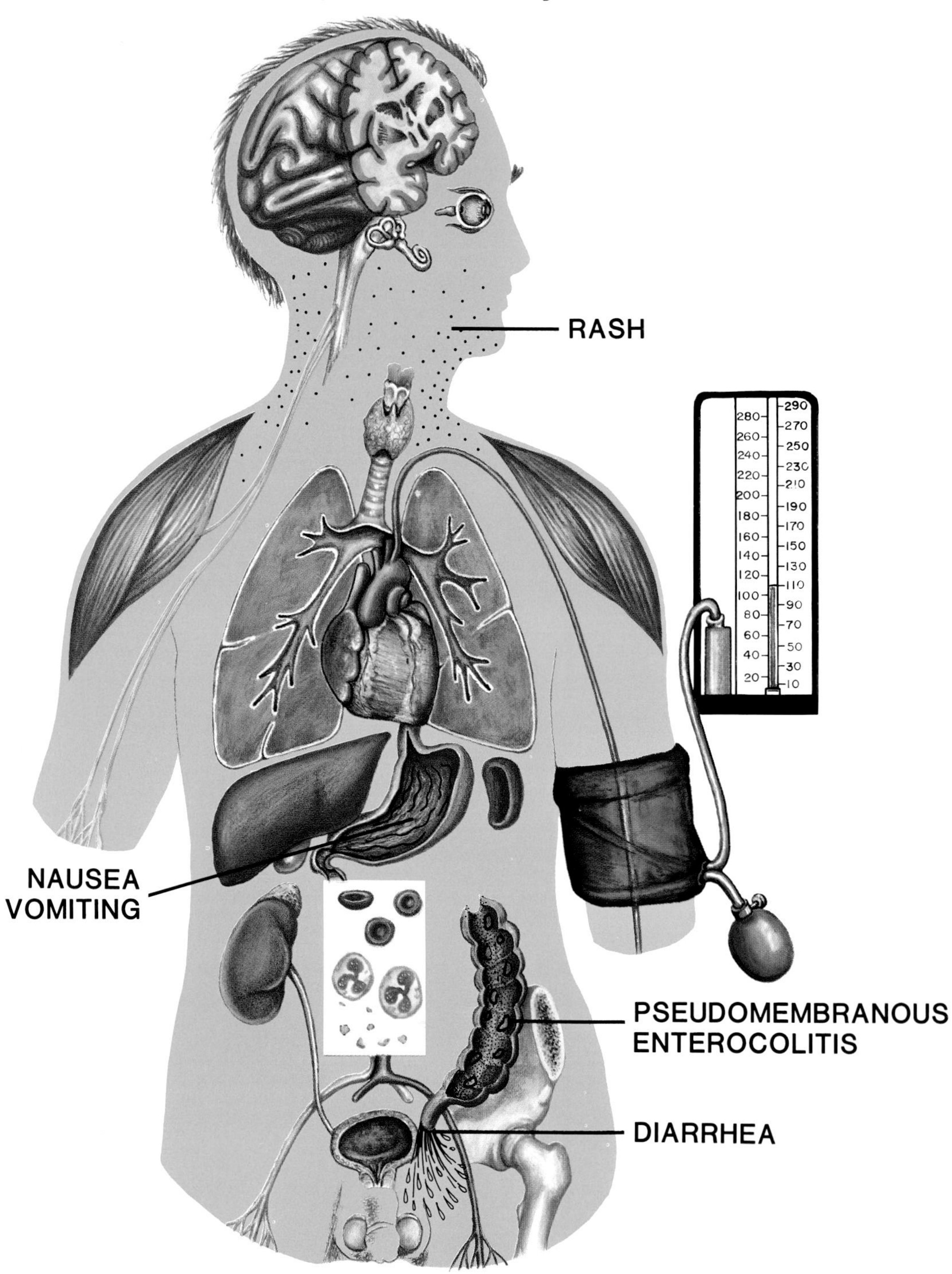

Clindamycin and Lincomycin

Representative Trade Names: Cleocin (clindamycin), Lincocin (lincomycin)

Toxicity Rating: Medium because of the risk of pseudomembranous enterocolitis.

Adverse Reactions

Gastrointestinal Diarrhea develops in as many as 20 percent of patients, and a good percentage of these develop *Clostridium difficile* pseudomembranous enterocolitis. Abdominal pain, nausea, and vomiting may also occur.

Allergic Reactions Maculopapular rash and urticaria are not uncommon (3–5 percent of patients) but the more severe allergic reactions (i.e., fever, anaphylaxis) are rarer than with penicillin.

Hepatic Transient alterations in liver function and jaundice occur.

Other Leukopenia, thrombocytopenia, and eosinophilia have been reported. Rapid intravenous administration of clindamycin or lincomycin may precipitate hypotension and EKG changes. A medicinal taste occasionally occurs with large doses. Polyarthritis has been reported.

Contraindications

As with most antibiotics, known hypersensitivity is the major contraindication. The safety in pregnancy has not been established.

Precautions

Old or debilitated patients are more prone to develop pseudomembranous enterocolitis. The drugs should be given with caution also to patients with liver or renal disease. Frequent hematologic, renal, and liver profiles should be obtained during long-term therapy.

Drug Interactions

Clindamycin and lincomycin may potentiate the neuromuscular effects of succinylcholine and other neuromuscular blockers. Simultaneous administration of clindamycin or lincomycin with ampicillin, phenytoin, and other drugs is prohibited.

Treatment

The drug should be withdrawn. Pseudomembranous colitis can be treated with a course of oral vancomycin, 0.5–2 g daily for 7–10 days. Metronidazole (Flagyl) may also be used. Cholestyramine and steroids may be of value. Other reactions usually subside when the drug is withdrawn.

Polymyxins

Principal Drugs

Generic Name	Representative Trade Name
Polymyxin B sulfate	Aerosporin
Colistin sulfate	Coly-Mycin S
Colistimethate sodium	Coly-Mycin M

Toxicity Rating: Low if given topically. High if given systemically due to nephrotoxicity and neuromuscular blockade.

Adverse Reactions

Renal Anuria and tubular necrosis are the most serious reactions to polymixins and occur frequently when these drugs are given parenterally to patients with preexisting renal disease.

Central Nervous System Vertigo, ataxia, confusion, slurred speech, and paresthesias occur but are usually reversible. Polymixins can cause neuromuscular blockade.

Allergic Allergic reactions are rare.

Other Administration of large doses intravenously may cause apnea.

Contraindications

The major contraindications are known hypersensitivity and (if the drugs are to be given parenterally) severe renal insufficiency.

Precautions

Polymixins must be given carefully in patients with known renal disease. Frequent testing of renal function is advised.

Drug Interactions

Polymixins potentiate the neuromuscular blockade produced by succinylcholine and tubocurarine. They also enhance the neuromuscular effects of aminoglycosides.

Treatment

Neuromuscular blockade and apnea may respond to intravenous calcium gluconate but not to neostigmine. Withdrawal of the drug is usually all that is needed to treat most reactions. Renal or peritoneal dialysis may be necessary if anuria and azotemia are prolonged.

Miscellaneous Antibacterial Agents

Bacitracin

Representative Trade Name: Poly-Mycin

Toxicity Rating: Since this drug is almost invariably used locally, its toxicity is very low.

Adverse Reactions

A full discussion of the adverse reactions to topical antibiotics can be found in Chapter 40.

Nalidixic Acid

Representative Trade Name: NegGram

Toxicity Rating: Low

Adverse Reactions

The most common side effects are nausea, vomiting, rash, and urticaria. Diarrhea, fever, and photophobia are less frequent. Reversible neurologic and visual disturbances occur occasionally.

Contraindications

Nalidixic acid should not be given to patients with known hypersensitivity, nor to children less than 3 years old because it can cause pseudotumor cerebri in infants.

Precautions

Nalidixic acid must be used cautiously in patients with renal or hepatic insufficiency because it may accumulate in the system.

Drug Interactions

Nitrofurantoin may interfere with the action of nalidixic acid. Nalidixic acid enhances the action of coumarin derivatives, thus prolonging the prothrombin time.

Treatment

Simple withdrawal of the drug is usually all that is necessary.

Trimethoprim

Representative Trade Names: Proloprim; in Bactrim and Septra

Toxicity Rating: Low

Adverse Reactions

Allergic reactions (rash, pruritus, etc.) are the most frequent side effects. Next in frequency are gastrointestinal reactions (nausea, vomiting, etc.) which are reversible. Pancytopenia and megaloblastic anemia from folate deficiency can occur with long-term therapy.

Contraindications

Known hypersensitivity, pregnancy, and preexisting folate deficiency are the most significant contraindications.

Precautions

This drug must be given with caution to patients with known renal or hepatic insufficiency, to children under 2 months of age, and to nursing mothers.

Treatment

Simple withdrawal of the drug is usually all that is necessary.

Spectinomycin Hydrochloride

Representative Trade Name: Trobicin

Toxicity Rating: Low

Adverse Reactions

Adverse reactions to this drug are infrequent and include nausea, vomiting, abdominal pain, pruritus, and urticaria. The results of laboratory tests including hematologic profiles and liver and renal function tests may be altered, but these effects are almost invariably reversible. There is no evidence of renal or otologic toxicity. Anaphylaxis has not been reported.

Contraindications

Known hypersensitivity is the major contraindication.

Precautions

Use of spectinomycin may mask the onset of syphilis. A follow-up serology should be done. Spectinomycin is of no value in the treatment of other bacterial infections because they may quickly develop resistance. This drug should be used with caution in pregnant women, infants, and children.

Treatment

Simple withdrawal of the drug is usually effective.

Methenamine Preparations

Representative Trade Names: Mandelamine (methenamine mandelate): Hiprex, Urex (methenamine hippurate)

Toxicity Rating: Low

Adverse Reactions

As with trimethaprim, gastrointestinal and allergic reactions are the most frequent side effects of methenamine preparations, but they are usually mild. Large doses can cause dysuria and acute urinary tract inflammation.

Contraindications

Severe renal insufficiency and known hypersensitivity are the most significant contraindications.

Precautions

Patients must be adequately hydrated to prevent crystalluria. It is unwise to give methenamine preparations to patients with gout because urate stones may develop in an acid urine.

Drug Interactions

Administering methenamine preparations with sulfonamides may precipitate crystalluria.

Treatment

Hydration and withdrawal of the drug are usually sufficient therapy.

Vancomycin Hydrochloride

Representative Trade Name: Vancocin HCl

Toxicity Rating: Medium because fatal uremia and permanent deafness have developed from prolonged use or excessive doses parenterally.

Adverse Reactions

Ototoxicity and nephrotoxicity are the major serious side effects of this drug. Marked hypotension and anaphylactic shock are rarely reported. The most common reactions are paresthesias, rash, and eosinophilia. High fever and chills are uncommon with the new preparations.

Contraindications

Known hypersensitivity is the major contraindication.

Precautions

Vancomycin should be avoided in patients with a history of deafness or renal damage. Renal function tests and audiograms should be performed in all patients before vancomycin therapy to establish function baselines: and the tests should be repeated at intervals during therapy, especially in the elderly. Vancomycin can only be given intravenously when used for systemic infections, and as a result careful observation for phlebitis is necessary.

Drug Interactions

Vancomycin can cause the crystal forms of chloramphenicol, corticosteroids, and methicillin to precipitate if mixed with them in solution.

Treatment

Withdrawal of the drug is usually all that is required to treat adverse reactions.

Isoniazid

Isoniazid

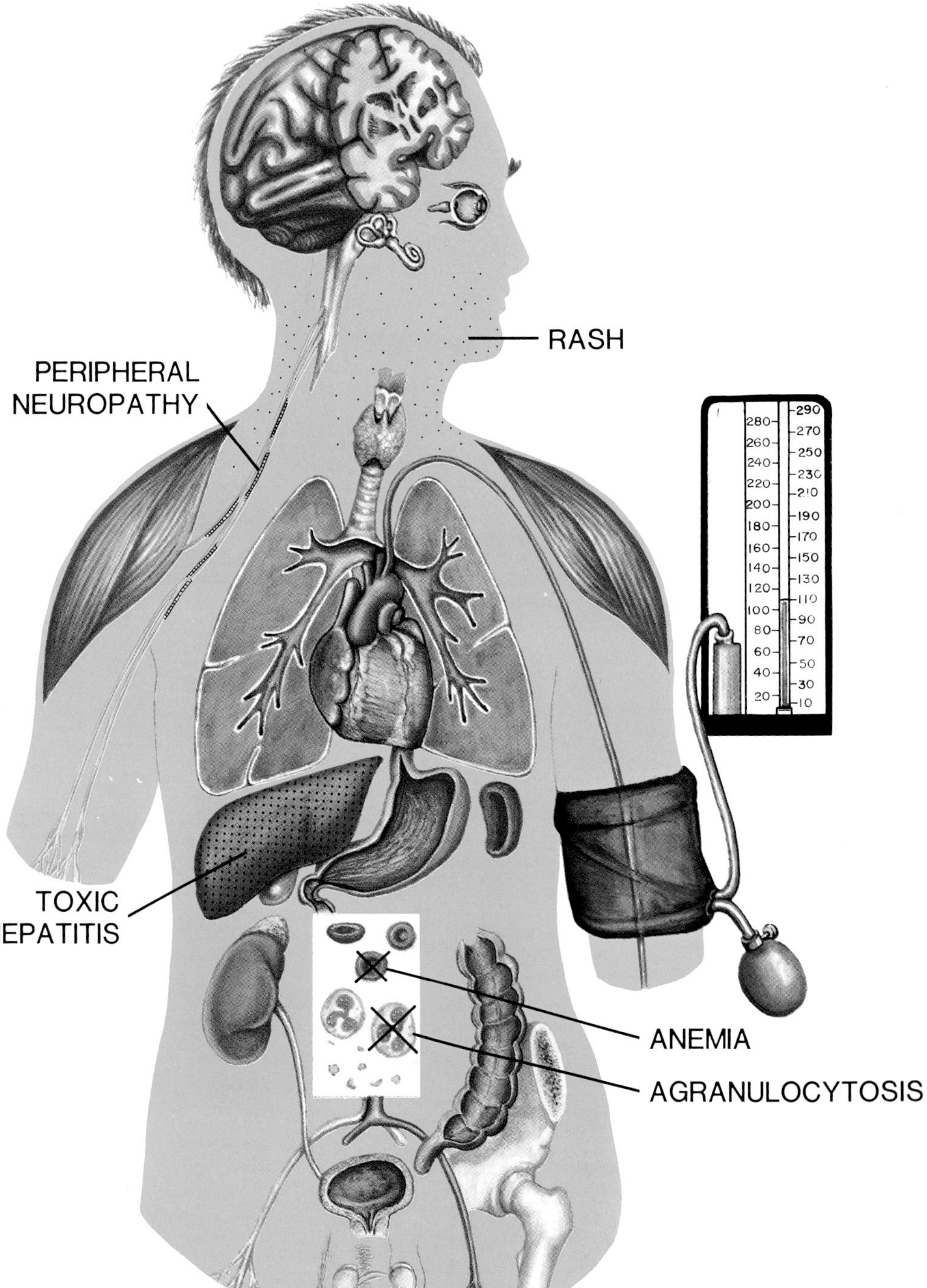

RASH

PERIPHERAL NEUROPATHY

TOXIC HEPATITIS

ANEMIA

AGRANULOCYTOSIS

Isoniazid

Representative Trade Name: INH

Toxicity Rating: Medium

Adverse Reactions

Allergic Fever, rash, eosinophilia, and arthralgias are common. Lymphadenopathy and vasculitis have occurred.

Hepatic Transient alterations in liver enzymes occur in 10–20 percent of patients, and in a small percentage of these (up to 2–3 percent of patients over 50 years old) progressive hepatocellular damage with occasional liver atrophy and death occur. The risk of hepatitis increases with age.

Neurologic Peripheral neuropathy is the most common side effect of isoniazid, and is more likely to occur in alcoholics and patients with severe malnutrition. Occasional convulsions, depression, and manic depressive psychosis are also seen.

Optic Optic neuritis may occur.

Hematologic Isoniazid may cause hemolytic anemia, pyridoxine-responsive anemia, agranulocytosis, red-cell aplasia, and lupus syndrome.

Other A rheumatoid syndrome may occur. Occasional nausea, vomiting, and epigastric distress are seen. Gynecomastia, metabolic acidosis, and hyperglycemia may also be seen.

Contraindications

Hypersensitivity to the drug and severe liver disease are the major contraindications.

Precautions

Isoniazid must be used carefully in patients with preexisting liver or renal diseases or with other severe disorders, and in alcoholics and the elderly. Hepatic function tests should be performed early in the course of therapy. Patients should avoid cheese as it may precipitate a hypertensive crisis.

Drug Interactions

Antacids and laxatives that contain aluminum may decrease isoniazid absorption. Disulfiram should not be given with isoniazid as it may cause ataxia and behavioral changes.

Treatment

If tests show any alteration in liver function, the drug should be withdrawn and an alternative drug started. If isoniazid must be used it may be reintroduced in gradually increasing doses after all liver function test results have returned to normal, but liver enzymes must be carefully monitored and the drug withdrawn if any indications of recurrence of liver involvement appears. Pyridoxine may be given to prevent neuropathy or at the first sign of paresthesias.

Ethambutol Hydrochloride

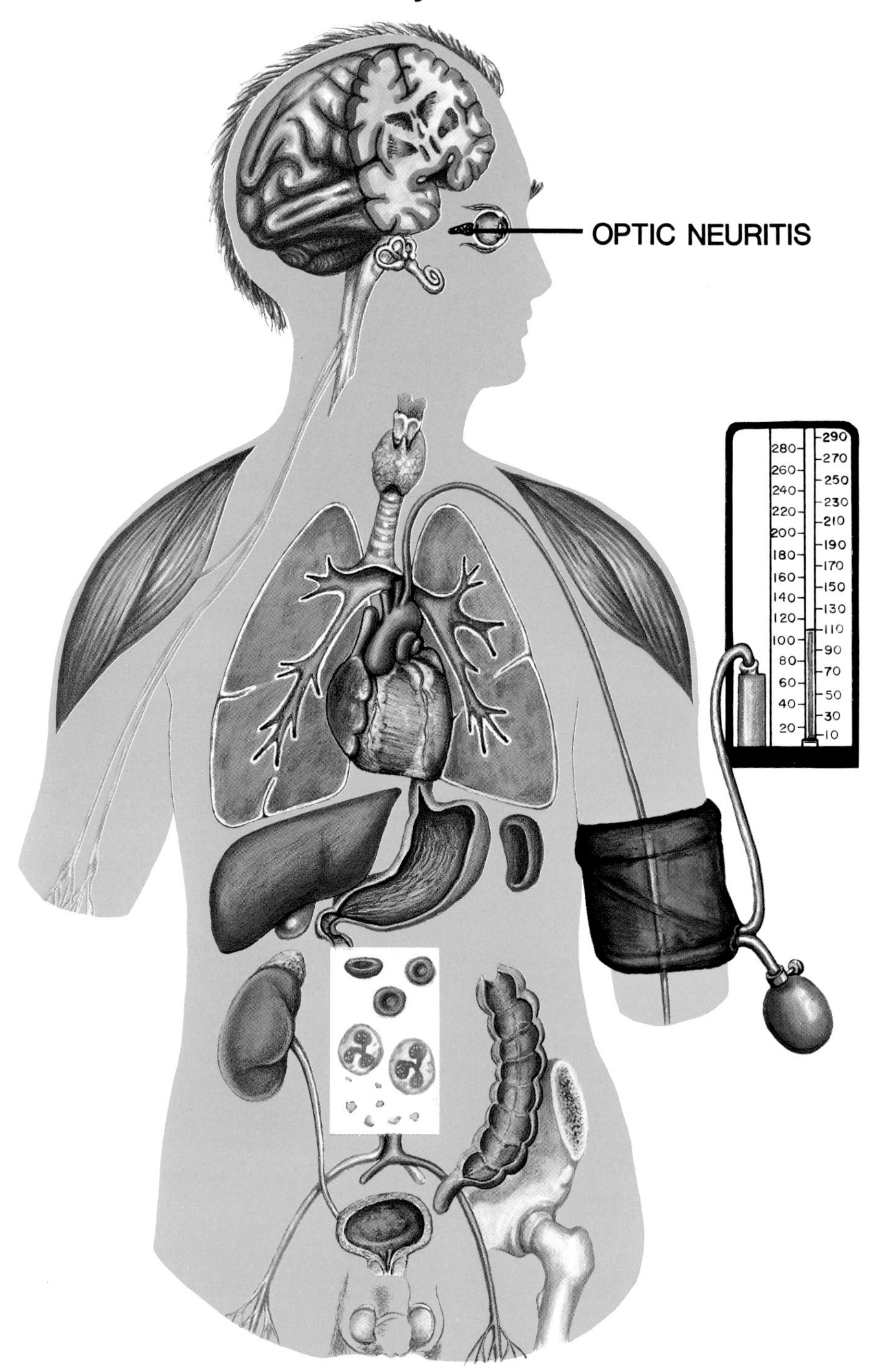

Ethambutol Hydrochloride

Representative Trade Name: Myambutol

Toxicity Rating: Low

Adverse Reactions

Optic Optic neuritis is the major side effect of this drug but is infrequent with currently prescribed dosages.

Allergic Dermatitis, pruritus, anaphylaxis, and drug fever obviously occur, but are infrequent.

Other Gastrointestinal, hepatic, and neurologic symptoms are unusual but occur. Elevated uric acid levels and gout reactions are reported.

Contraindications

Ethambutol is not recommended in patients with known sensitivity or preexisting optic neuritis, and in children under 13 years old. The need for ethambutol during pregnancy must be carefully weighed against the possibility (unproven) of teratogenic effects on the fetus.

Precautions

Visual acuity and color discrimination should be tested before ethambutol therapy is begun, and monthly during therapy. Ethambutol should be used with caution in patients with impaired renal function.

Treatment

Optic neuritis is usually reversed by withdrawal of the drug.

Rifampin

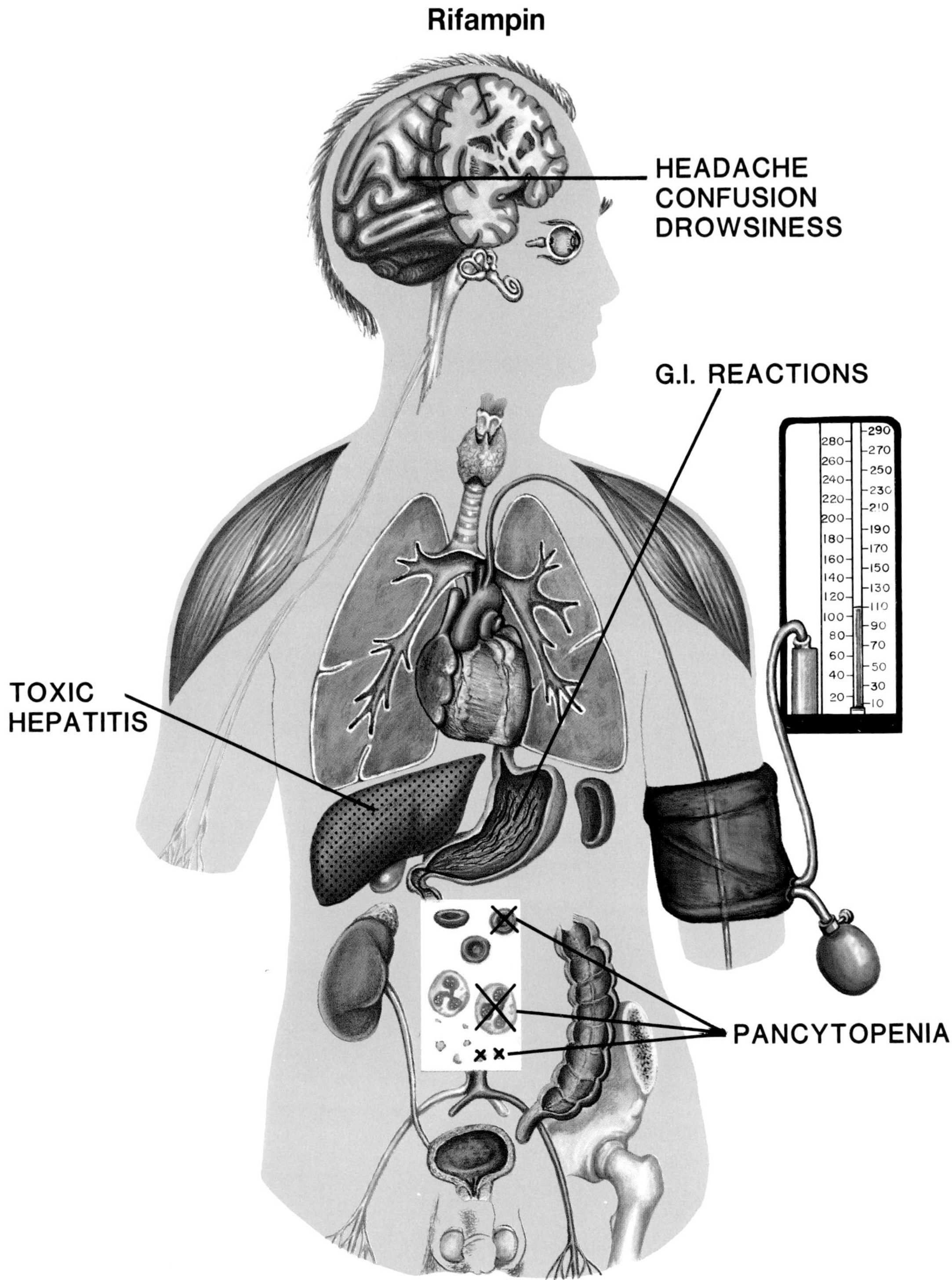
HEADACHE
CONFUSION
DROWSINESS
G.I. REACTIONS
TOXIC
HEPATITIS
PANCYTOPENIA

Rifampin

Representative Trade Names: Rifadin, Rimactane

Toxicity Rating: Medium because serious hepatotoxicity has occurred.

Adverse Reactions

Hepatic Toxic hepatitis may occur and alterations of liver function are not uncommon, especially in patients with preexisting liver disease.

Central Nervous System Headache, drowsiness, ataxia, confusion, and paresthesias are reported.

Gastrointestinal Nausea, vomiting, diarrhea, heartburn, and abdominal cramps occur.

Hematologic Thrombocytopenia, leukopenia, and anemia may occur as a result of bone marrow depession or allergic phenomena with eosinophilia.

Allergic Any type of hypersensitivity reaction may occur, including pruritus, urticaria, and a pemphigoid reaction.

Other Hemolysis and hemoglobinuria may occasionally lead to acute renal failure.

Contraindications

Known hypersensitivity to rifampin seems to be the only absolute contraindication.

Precautions

Obviously, preexisting liver disease makes rifampin hazardous, and frequent liver function studies must be done during therapy regardless. Other drugs with potential for hepatotoxicity should be withheld if possible. Frequent hematologic profiles should be done to detect hemolytic or hypoplastic anemia. Patients should be warned not to interrupt therapy once it is begun because this seems to precipitate hemolysis, hemoglobinuria, and acute renal failure.

Drug Interactions

Rifampin interacts with a variety of other drugs. It increases the catabolism of estrogen, rendering oral contraceptives less effective. It decreases the effectiveness of oral anticoagulants. When rifampin is given with other antituberculous agents, the doses of methadone, digoxin, oral hypoglycemics, quinidine, disopyramide, dapsone, and corticosteroids may have to be increased. Aminosalicylic acid may prevent rifampin absorption, so it is wise to administer these two drugs 8–12 hours apart. Probenecid, on the other hand, may increase rifampin blood levels.

Treament

Withdrawal of the drug and careful monitoring of liver function and blood counts is usually all that is necessary to treat most reactions.

Miscellaneous Antimycobacterial Agents

Aminosalicylic Acid

Representative Trade Names: Parasal Sodium, P.A.S.

Toxicity Rating: Medium because of the high percentage of gastrointestinal reactions.

Adverse Reactions

As many as 15 percent of patients taking aminosalicylic acid suffer severe nausea, vomiting, and diarrhea. Hypertensive reactions—sometimes fatal—have been reported in 4 percent of patients. Hepatitis, bone marrow depression, and hemolytic anemia may occur. An infectious mononucleosis-like syndrome has been noted.

Contraindications

Known hypersensitivity is the most significant contraindication. Pregnancy is also a contraindication.

Precautions

Patients with known liver or renal disease or gastric ulcer should probably not receive aminosalicylic acid unless there are no alternative drugs. It is best to give the drug with meals or an antacid to prevent gastric irritation.

Drug Interactions

Ascorbic acid and ammonium chloride may acidify the urine and precipitate aminosalicylic acid stones. Probenecid increases blood levels of aminosalicylic acid. Rifampin may interfere with aminosalicylic acid absorption, so these drugs should be given 8 – 12 hours apart. Diphenhydramine may inhibit the absorption of aminosalicylic acid.

Treatment

Withdrawal of the drug is usually sufficient to remedy the side effects. The patient will frequently have already done this for you.

Cycloserine

Representative Trade Name: Seromycin

Toxicity Rating: Medium because of neurologic toxicity.

Adverse Reactions

Neurologic reactions include muscle twitching, convulsions, behavioral changes, and frank psychosis. Psychotic episodes may occur in as many as 20 percent of patients, and suicide has occurred. Fortunately other reactions including allergic ones are rare.

Contraindications

This drug is contraindicated in patients with a history of epilepsy or psychosis. Known hypersensitivity is a rare contraindication.

Precautions

Caution must be exercised in giving cycloserine to anyone with a history of emotional or neurologic illnesses. The safety in pregnancy has not been established. The patient should be advised not to drink alcohol during therapy.

Drug Interactions

Concomitant administration of isoniazid or ethionamide may enhance the central nervous system toxicity of cycloserine.

Treatment

Acute convulsions are treated with intravenous diazepam or amobarbital sodium. Psychotic reactions will respond to large doses of chlorpromazine. Hospitalization for careful observation is wise.

Capreomycin Sulfate

Representative Trade Name: Capastat Sulfate

Toxicity Rating: Medium because of nephrotoxicity.

Adverse Reactions

Nephrotoxicity is the major side effect of capreomycin, but occurs in less than 15 percent of patients and is almost always reversible. Fatal toxicity has occured when the drug was given with aminosalicylic acid. Ototoxicity may occur with capreomycin as with the aminoglycosides, but is infrequent. Hypersensitivity reactions occur but are uncommon.

Contraindications

Known hypersensitivity to the drug and preexisting severe renal disease are the most significant contraindications.

Precautions

Capreomycin must be used cautiously in patients with previous renal or otic disorders, and if possible should not be given concurrently with other drugs affecting these organs. Neuromuscular blocking agents can also potentiate the renal toxicity and ototoxicity of capreomycin, and must be given with caution.

Treatment

Withdrawal of the drug and monitoring of renal function is usually all that is necessary. Of course, dialysis may be required in cases of severe renal failure.

Ethionamide

Representative Trade Name: Trecator-SC

Toxicity Rating: Low to medium because of frequent gastrointestinal reactions and jaundice in 1 – 3 percent of cases.

Adverse Reactions

Patients frequently experience nausea, vomiting, and loss of appetite. Many patients have altered liver function but only a small number get frank hepatitis. Recovery after the drug is stopped is usual. Other reactions include peripheral neuropathy, mental depression, and hypothyroidism. Hypersensitivity is rare.

Contraindications

Known hypersensitivity is the only contraindication.

Drug Interactions

Ethionamide may aggravate the seizures associated with cycloserine therapy.

Treatment

Simple withdrawal of the drug is usually all that is necessary.

Amphotericin B

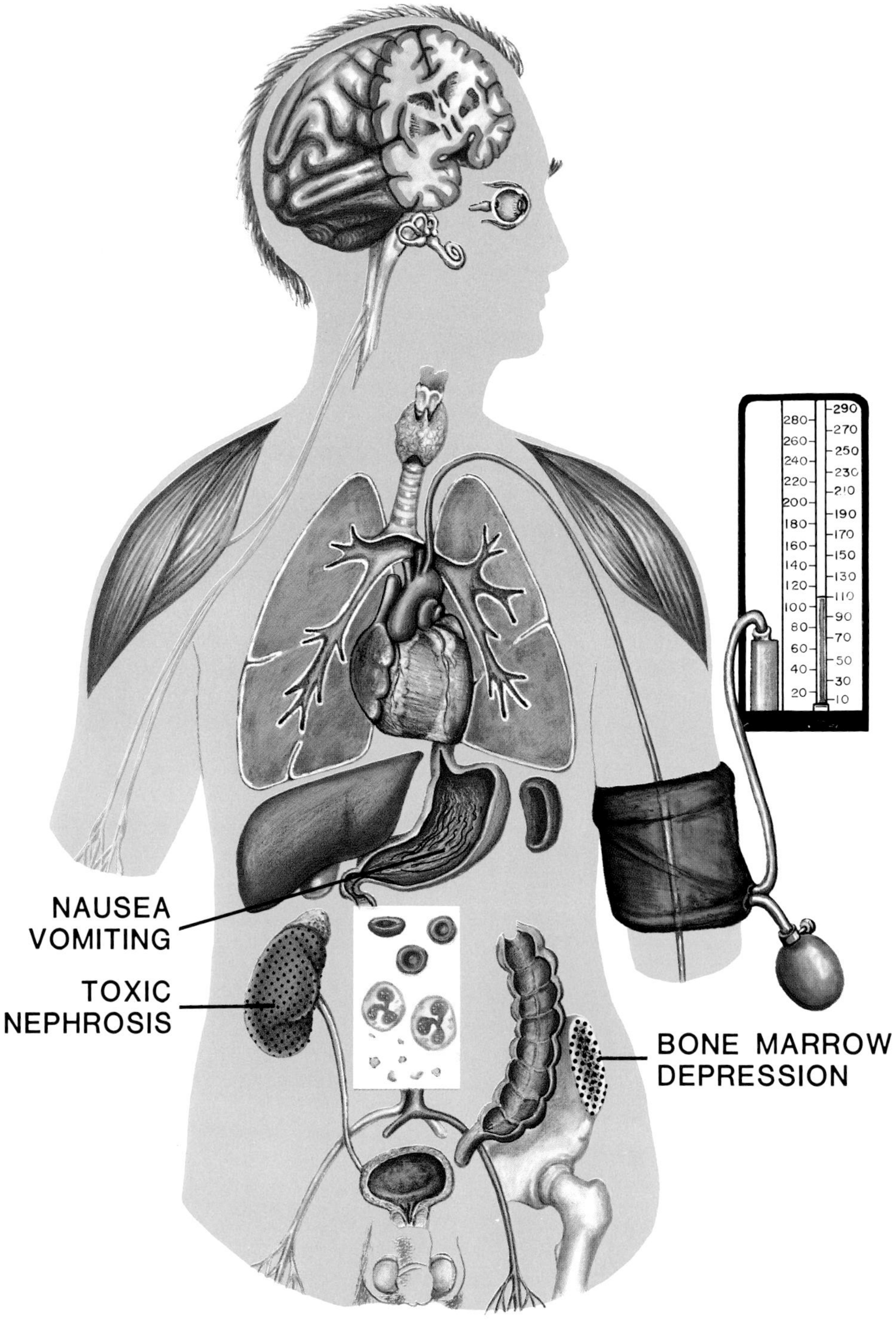

NAUSEA
VOMITING

TOXIC
NEPHROSIS

BONE MARROW
DEPRESSION

SYSTEMIC ANTIFUNGAL AGENTS

Amphotericin B

Representative Trade Name: Fungizone

Toxicity Rating: High because of nephrotoxicity.

Adverse Reactions

Renal Renal tubular damage may lead to hypokalemia, hypocalcemia, and hypomagnesemia. Amphotericin B decreases the glomerular filtration rate and creatinine clearance, and there is often an associated rise in blood urea nitrogen and creatinine. Transient azotemia is observed in nearly all patients.

Gastrointestinal Nausea, vomiting, and abdominal cramps are common.

Hepatic Liver failure is a rare but serious reaction.

Hematologic Bone marrow depression manifested by a normocytic, normochromic anemia is common.

Other Fever, chills, and headache are common, especially early in the course of therapy. In 90 percent of cases phlebitis develops within hours at the site of administration. Anaphylaxis and skin rashes are rare but bronchospasm may occur.

Contraindications

Severe renal failure and known hypersensitivity are the major contraindications.

Precautions

Mannitol 25 g intravenously in a 10 – 20 percent solution may prevent nephrotoxicity by increasing glomerular filtration. Steroids may help reduce fever, nausea, and vomiting. Heparin does not usually prevent phlebitis but is worth trying. Blood urea nitrogen and creatinine levels must be checked on alternate days. Electrolytes should be measured and a complete blood count done twice weekly. Obviously, amphotericin B must be administered with care in pregnancy.

Treatment

Amphotericin B should be discontinued if the serum creatinine exceeds 3 mg/100 ml, but may be restarted once serum creatinine returns to normal. Administration of corticosteroids prior to intravenous amphotericin will reduce the incidence and severity of the febrile reactions. Supplemental alkali medications may decrease the occurence of renal tubular acidosis. Obviously, the drug should be withheld at least temporarily if any of the other side effects become life-threatening.

Flucytosine

Representative Trade Name: Ancobon

Toxicity Rating: Low to medium because of bone marrow depression.

Adverse Reactions

Hematologic Bone marrow depression may result in leukopenia, thrombocytopenia, or aplastic anemia either separately or together. These complications have usually occurred in patients with renal failure and are reversible.

Gastrointestinal Nausea, vomiting, and diarrhea occur. Fatal bowel perforation has been reported but is rare.

Neurologic Headache, confusion, hallucinations, sedation, and vertigo may occur.

Hepatic Toxic hepatitis is rare.

Other Unlike amphotericin B, flucytosine does not cause renal toxicity.

Contraindications

Known hypersensitivity is the only absolute contraindication, but pregnancy is a relative contraindication.

Precautions

Renal and liver functions and hematologic profiles should be determined frequently during therapy.

Griseofulvin

Representative Trade Names: Fulvicin-V/F, Grifulvin-V

Toxicity Rating: Low

Adverse Reactions

Dermatologic Maculopapular rash, urticaria, and angioneurotic edema occur.

Hematologic Leukopenia occasionally occurs but is usually reversible.

Gastrointestinal Nausea, vomiting, epigastric distress, and diarrhea occur.

Neurologic Paresthesia, dizziness, insomnia, confusion, and fatigue occur. Headache occurs in as many as 15 percent of patients.

Other Proteinuria is rare. Griseofulvin may decrease the hypoprothrombinemic effects of warfarin. Hepatotoxicity occurs infrequently.

Contraindications

Known hypersensitivity, porphyria, and hepatic failure are the major contraindications. The drug may not be safe during pregnancy.

Precautions

Griseofulvin should be given with caution to patients with penicillin allergy, as cross-reactions do occur. Frequent blood counts should be done if the drug is to be administered over a long period of time.

Drug Interactions

Barbiturates may decrease the absorption of griseofulvin.

Treatment

Simple withdrawal of the drug is usually all that is necessary.

Ketoconazole

Representative Trade Name: Nizoral

Toxicity Rating: Low

Adverse Reactions

Central Nervous System Headache, dizziness, and drowsiness or excitation may occur.

Gastrointestinal Nausea is common and may be associated with vomiting, abdominal pain, diarrhea, or constipation.

Hepatic Hepatitis does occur but is rare and usually reversible.

Endocrinologic Gynecomastia occurs in 10 percent of males on this drug.

Other Pruritus is frequent, but allergic reactions are rare.

Contraindications

Known hypersensitivity and pregnancy are the major contraindications.

Precautions

The drug is not absorbed in patients with achlorhydria. Frequent liver profiles should be done to catch hepatotoxicity early.

Drug Interactions

Since hydrochloric acid is necessary for absorption, antacids, anticholinergics, and cimetidine decrease absorption.

Treatment

Simple withdrawal of the drug is usually all that is necessary.

Miconazole

Representative Trade Name: Monistat I.V.

Toxicity Rating: Medium because of the frequency of thrombophlebitis at the injection site.

Adverse Reactions

Cardiovascular Thrombophlebitis is common and is not relieved by heparin infusion, bicarbonate, or corticosteroids. Rotation of intravenous lines is advised every 48 to 72 hours. Arrhythmias may occur during rapid infusions.

Gastrointestinal Nausea, anorexia, and vomiting are common.

Endocrinologic Inappropriate antidiuretic hormone secretion often occurs and is probably responsible for hyponatremia.

Other Pruritic rash, anemia, and thrombophlebitis occur infrequently.

Contraindications

Known hypersensitivity is the major contraindication.

Precautions

The patient should be hospitalized before treatment is begun, and initial blood studies should be performed. Electrolytes, complete blood count, and liver and renal function should be monitored frequently. Pregnant women and children should not receive miconazole unless it is considered life-saving.

Drug Interactions

The cremophor vehicle used to administer this drug may cause abnormalities of electrophoretically determined lipoproteins. Miconazole may enhance the effect of coumarin derivatives on coagulation.

Treatment

Simple withdrawal of the drug is usually all that is necessary.

Chapter 11

ANTINEOPLASTIC AGENTS

Antineoplastic Agents

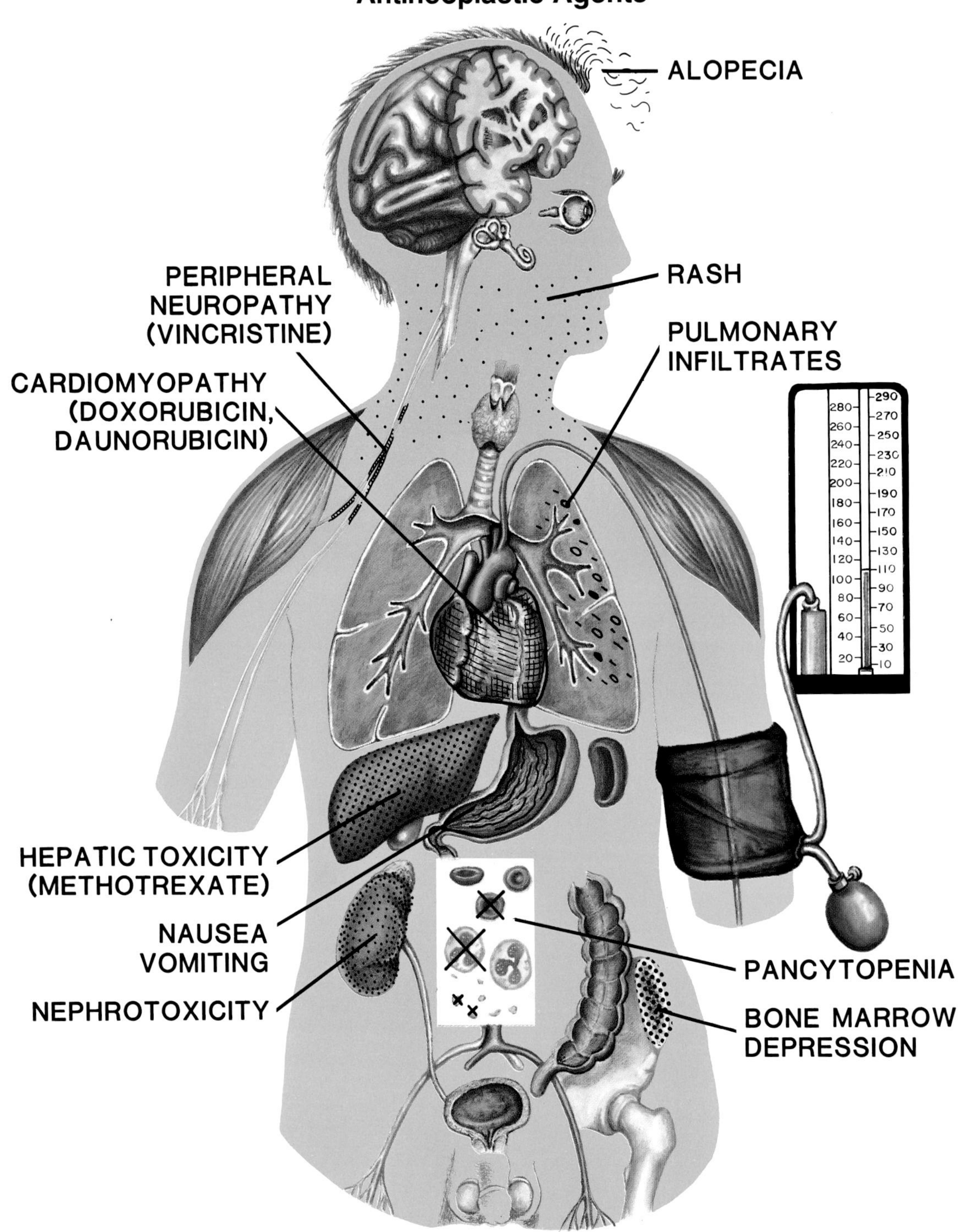

ALOPECIA
RASH
PERIPHERAL NEUROPATHY (VINCRISTINE)
PULMONARY INFILTRATES
CARDIOMYOPATHY (DOXORUBICIN, DAUNORUBICIN)
HEPATIC TOXICITY (METHOTREXATE)
NAUSEA VOMITING
PANCYTOPENIA
NEPHROTOXICITY
BONE MARROW DEPRESSION

Antineoplastic Agents

Principal Drugs

Generic Name	Representative Trade Name
Azathioprine	Imuran
Bleomycin sulfate	Blenoxane
Busulfan	Myleran
Carmustine	BiCNU
Related drugs:	
Estramustine phosphate sodium	Emcyt
Lomustine	CeeNU
Chlorambucil	Leukeran
Cyclophosphamide	Cytoxan
Cytarabine	Cytosar-U
Dactinomycin	Cosmegen
Daunorubicin hydrochloride	Cerubidine
Doxorubicin hydrochloride	Adriamycin
Fluorouracil	Adrucil
Related drug:	
Floxuridine	FUDR
Hydroxyurea	Hydrea
Mechlorethamine hydrochloride	Mustargen
Related drug:	
Thiotepa	Thiotepa
Melphalan	Alkeran
Mercaptopurine	Purinethol
Methotrexate sodium	Mexate
Mitomycin	Mutamycin
Plicamycin	Mithracin
Procarbazine hydrochloride	Matulane
Vinblastine sulfate	Velban
Vincristine sulfate	Oncovin

Toxicity Rating: High because of severe bone marrow depression and toxicity to other organs which is occasionally irreversible.

Adverse Reactions

Hematologic Bone marrow depression occurs with the use of all of these drugs except bleomycin sulfate. The depression is severe with the nitrogen mustards (mechlorethamine, etc.) and cytarabine. Leukopenia is manifested by stomatitis and sepsis. Multiple small bowel ulcers may result in severe diarrhea in patients on methotrexate.

Gastrointestinal Nausea and vomiting are the principle gastrointestinal reactions, and are prominent side effects of the nitrogen mustards and dactinomycin. Methotrexate, vinblastine, vincristine, busulfan, bleomycin, and chlorambucil rarely cause significant nausea and vomiting.

Table 11-1. Antineoplastic Agents

Drug	Bone marrow depression	Nausea and vomiting	Alopecia	Cardiac toxicity	Neuro-toxicity	Pulmonary toxicity	Skin lesions	Other
Azathioprine	+	−	+	−	−	−	+	"Serum" sickness
Bleomycin sulfate	−	−	−	−	−	++	+	Shock-like state
Busulfan	+	−	−	−	−	+	−	Adrenal insufficiency
Carmustine and related drugs estramustine phosphate sodium and lomustine	+	+	−	−	−	+	+	Hepatic and renal toxicity
Chlorambucil	+	−	−	−	−	−	−	
Cyclophosphamide	+	+	+	−	−	−	−	Cystitis, SIADH
Cytarabine	++	+	−	−	−	−	−	
Dactinomycin	+	++	+	−	−	−	+	Skin induration
Daunorubicin hydrochloride	+	−	−	+	−	−	−	Skin sloughing
Doxorubicin hydrochloride	+	+	+	+	−	−	−	
Fluorouracil and related drug floxuridine	+	+	+	−	+	−	+	
Hydroxyurea	+	+	−	−	−	−	+	
Mechlorethamine hydrochloride and related drug thiotepa	++	++	−	−	−	−	−	Skin sloughing
Melphalan	+	+	−	−	−	−	−	
Mercaptopurine	+	−	−	−	−	−	−	Cholestatic jaundice
Methotrexate sodium	+	−	+	−	+	+	−	Hepatic toxicity
Mitomycin	+	−	+	−	−	+	+	Renal toxicity
Plicamycin	+	+	−	−	−	−	−	Hemorrhagic phenomena
Procarbazine hydrochloride	+	−	−	−	+	−	−	Psychosis

Alopecia Alopecia may occur with almost any of these drugs, but is especially common with cyclophosphamide, 5-fluorouracil, methotrexate, and the antibiotics.

Cardiovascular Both doxorubicin and daunorubicin cause cardiomyopathy and congestive heart failure, especially in patients who have had previous cardiac irradiation.

Nervous System Peripheral neuropathy is not uncommon with vincristine therapy and there may also be involvement of the autonomic system and cranial nerves. Vinblastine, on the other hand, is associated with only minor neurotoxic effects. Methotrexate neurotoxicity occurs principally with intrathecal administration. 5-Fluorouracil causes cortical and cerebellar toxicity, while procarbazine may cause psychosis.

Respiratory Busulfan and bleomycin cause pulmonary infiltrates which may progress to pulmonary fibrosis. Methotrexate produces reversible pulmonary infiltrates in children with leukemia. Mitomycin infiltrates are also usually reversible.

Dermatologic Allergic skin reactions may occur with any of these drugs, but 5-fluorouracil may produce dry skin with cracking on the palms and soles. Erythema, hyperpigmentation, and lichenification of the fingertips occurs with bleomycin therapy. Stomatitis and mucocutaneous lesions occur with any of the drugs that depress the white cell count. Tissue sloughing often occurs unless care is taken to prevent extravasation.

Other Hepatic toxicity is particularly common with methotrexate, so frequent monitoring of liver function is necessary. Hepatorenal dysfunction can occur with almost any antineoplastic; consequently, frequently laboratory evaluation of liver and kidney function is needed. Inappropriate antidiuretic hormone syndrome (SIADH) may be associated with vincristine and cyclophosphamide therapy. The shock-like state produced by bleomycin in Hodgkin's patients is an unusual reaction.

Contraindications

Previous hypersensitivity and an already depressed blood count (leukopenia, thrombocytopenia, etc.) are the major contraindications.

Precautions

Hospitalization and frequent laboratory tests and roentgenograms are the most important precautions during the initial stages of therapy. An oncologist should be consulted before therapy is begun, and in many cases the oncologist should manage the therapy until the laboratory picture has stabilized. Prophylactic antibiotics may be necessary. Careful observation for sepsis is required.

Drug Interactions

Enhanced bone marrow depression can occur if drugs capable of inducing bone marrow depression are given along with antineoplastics.

Treatment

Bone marrow depression will often subside after the drug is withdrawn but transfusion of fresh blood or blood components (leukocytes, etc.) may be necessary to prevent sepsis and bleeding. Blood cultures should be done and combination antibiotic therapy (to hit both gram-negative and gram-positive organisms) begun at the first sign of sepsis. Vasopressors, steroids, and volume expansion may be necessary to prevent shock. Careful monitoring of blood volume (with Swan-Ganz catheter if necessary) is wise to prevent congestive heart failure. Most skin lesions and alopecia are reversible. An oncologist should be called upon to manage most of these reactions.

Chapter 12

ANTIPARKINSONIAN DRUGS

Levodopa

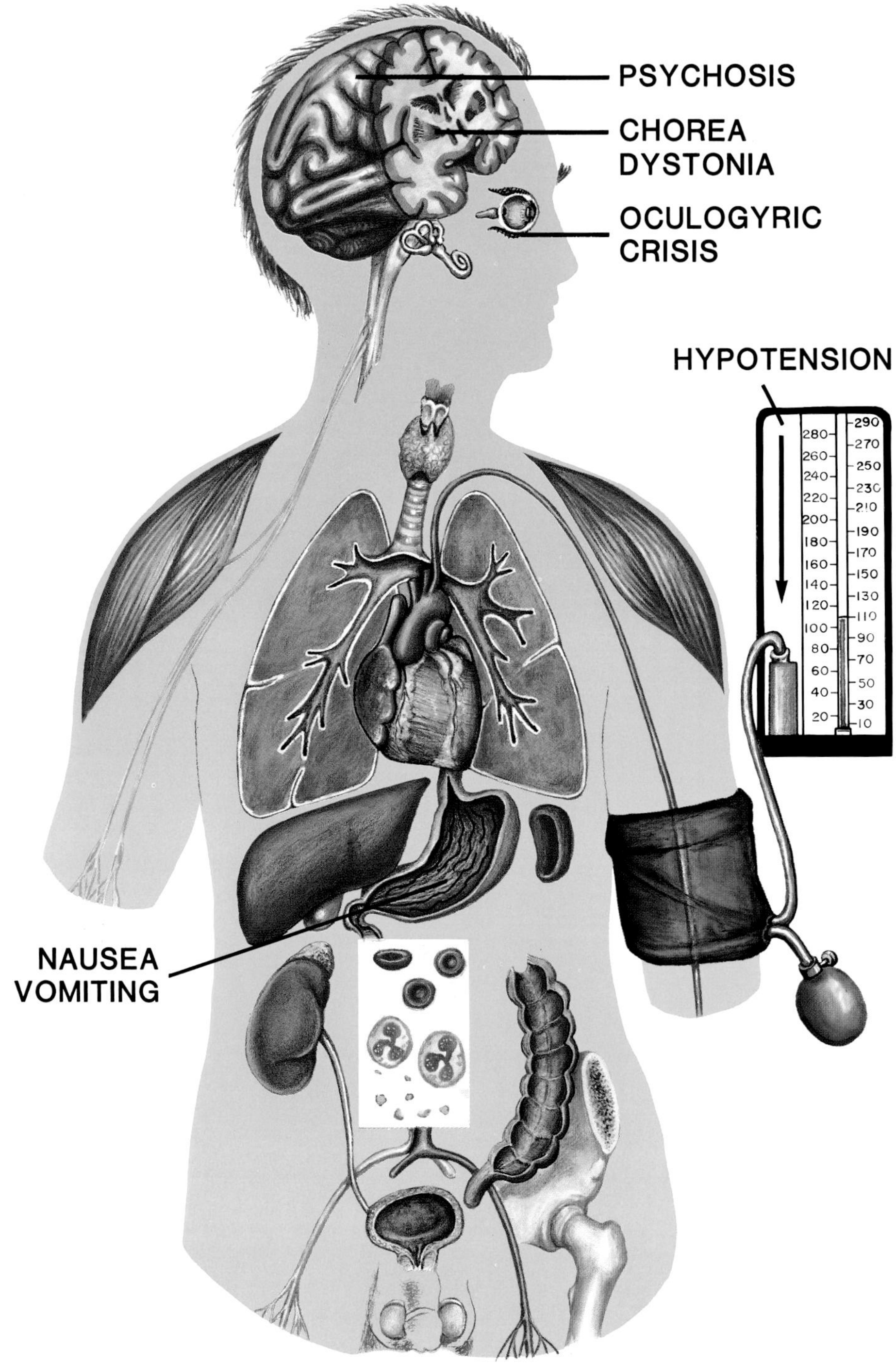

PSYCHOSIS

CHOREA
DYSTONIA

OCULOGYRIC
CRISIS

HYPOTENSION

NAUSEA
VOMITING

Introduction

Principal Antiparkinsonian Drugs

Levodopa
  Levodopa combinations:
    Levodopa – carbidopa
    Levodopa – benserazide
Bromocriptine mesylate
Amantadine hydrochloride
Anticholinergic drugs (see Chapter 4)

With the exception of the anticholinergics, all of the drugs in this group produce their side effects by increasing the body or brain levels of dopamine. The most significant systemic side effects of dopamine are hypotension and reactive tachycardia. Anorexia, nausea, and vomiting may occur. In the nervous system excessive dopamine may cause dementia, hallucinations, psychosis, and extrapyramidal reactions such as chorea and other involuntary movements. Serious pathology of the internal organs is unusual with antiparkinsonian drugs.

The side effects of the anticholinergic drugs are discussed in Chapter 4.

Levodopa and Combinations

Principal Drugs

Generic Name	Representative Trade Name
Levodopa	Dopar, Larodopa
Levodopa combinations:	
Levodopa – carbidopa	Sinemet
Levodopa – benserazide	Madopar

Toxicity Rating: Low to medium

Adverse Reactions

Central Nervous System Levodopa drugs may cause psychiatric manifestations such as dementia, hallucinations, and hypomania. Many involuntary movements including chorea, dystonia, and oculogyric crisis may occur.

Cardiovascular Hypotension is a frequent side effect — most commonly a postural hypotension with reactive tachycardia.

Gastrointestinal Anorexia, nausea, and vomiting occur. The few cases of gastrointestinal bleeding and ulcers that have been reported cannot definitely be attributed to the levodopa drug. Hiccoughs, abdominal pain, and dysphagia have occurred.

Other Levodopa may affect the results of various laboratory tests. The reader is referred to the PDR for a full discussion of these.

Contraindications

Known hypersensitivity, preexisting narrow-angle glaucoma, and skin lesions suggestive of melanoma are the principle contraindications. Levodopa drugs should not be given with MAO inhibitors or until they have been stopped for two weeks.

Precautions

A change from levodopa to a levodopa-carbidopa combination should be done gradually. Patients should be watched for suicidal ideation and depression. Levodopa drugs should be given cautiously in patients with preexisting cardiovascular, respiratory, renal, hepatic, or endocrine disorders. Periodic function testing of these organs should be determined.

Drug Interactions

Levodopa drugs interact with MAO inhibitors, antihypertensives, phenothiazines, phenytoin, papaverine, and butyrophenones.

Treatment

Withdrawal of the drug is usually all that is necessary. Pyridoxine may reverse the action of levodopa. Administration of intravenous fluids and vasopressors, and electrocardiographic monitoring for arrhythmias, may be necessary. Hypotension may be treated with oral fludrocortisone acetate 0.05–0.2 mg daily.

Amantadine Hydrochloride

Representative Trade Name: Symmetrel

Toxicity Rating: Low

Adverse Reactions

Central Nervous System The principle CNS reactions to amantadine are depression, confusion, anxiety, irritability, and even hallucinations, psychosis, or rarely convulsions. Less frequently, ataxia and dizziness have been observed.

Cardiovascular Like levodopa, amantadine HCl may cause orthostatic hypotension. Edema and congestive heart failure have also been observed.

Gastointestinal Nausea, vomiting, and constipation are the most prominent gastrointestinal symptoms, but are infrequent.

Other Leukopenia, rash, and visual disturbances may develop. Livedo reticularis is very common.

Contraindications

Known hypersensitivity is the only absolute contraindication, but it is probably unwise to use amantadine in pregnant women or nursing mothers.

Precautions

It is unwise to discontinue amantadine abruptly, because a Parkinson crisis may occasionally occur. The dosage may need to be adjusted in patients with coronary, hepatic, or renal dysfunction. Caution must be observed when giving this drug to patients with eczema, psychiatric disorders, or convulsions.

Drug Interactions

Amantadine may potentiate the action of CNS stimulants.

Treatment

Withdrawal of the drug is usually all that is necessary, but in severe central nervous system reactions, physostigmine 1 to 2 mg every 1 to 2 hours may be effective. Acidification of the urine may increase the excretion of the drug. Anticonvulsant therapy may be given for seizures and, if need be, vasopressor agents will reverse the hypotension.

Bromocriptine Mesylate

Representative Trade Name: Parlodel

Toxicity Rating: Low

Adverse Reactions

Gastrointestinal The most common side effects of bromocriptine are gastrointestinal. Nausea occurs in as many as half of patients, but is usually transient. Abdominal cramps, vomiting, constipation, and diarrhea also occur in many cases.

Respiratory Long-term therapy may cause pulmonary infiltrates and pleural reactions.

Central Nervous System As might be expected with a drug that sensitizes the postsynaptic neurons to dopamine, bromocriptine has many CNS side effects. Headache, dizziness, hallucinations, confusion, drowsiness, fatigue, ataxia, and "on-off" phenomena (in parkinsonian patients) are not infrequent. Dystonia and choreiform movements may also occur. These reactions are very similar to those occurring with levodopa.

Others Since this drug is an ergot alkaloid derivative, one or more of the side effects of ergotism (page 331) may occur. Transient hypotension occurs.

Contraindications

Known hypersensitivity to ergot alkaloids is the main contraindication.

Precautions

Before this drug is given to treat galactorrhea, a pituitary tumor should be ruled out. The drug has not been proven safe in pregnancy. Monitoring of blood pressure, particularly during the postpartum period, is especially wise since this drug may induce hypotension or aggravate the hypotension that commonly occurs postpartum. Bromocriptine should be used with caution in patients with known hepatic or renal dysfunction.

Drug Interactions

Phenothiazines should not be given with bromocriptine mesylate. Care should be taken in administering bromocriptine with other drugs that cause hypotension, as additive hypotension may occur.

Treatment

Simple withdrawal of the drug is usually effective.

Chapter 13

ANTITHYROID DRUGS

Antithyroid Drugs

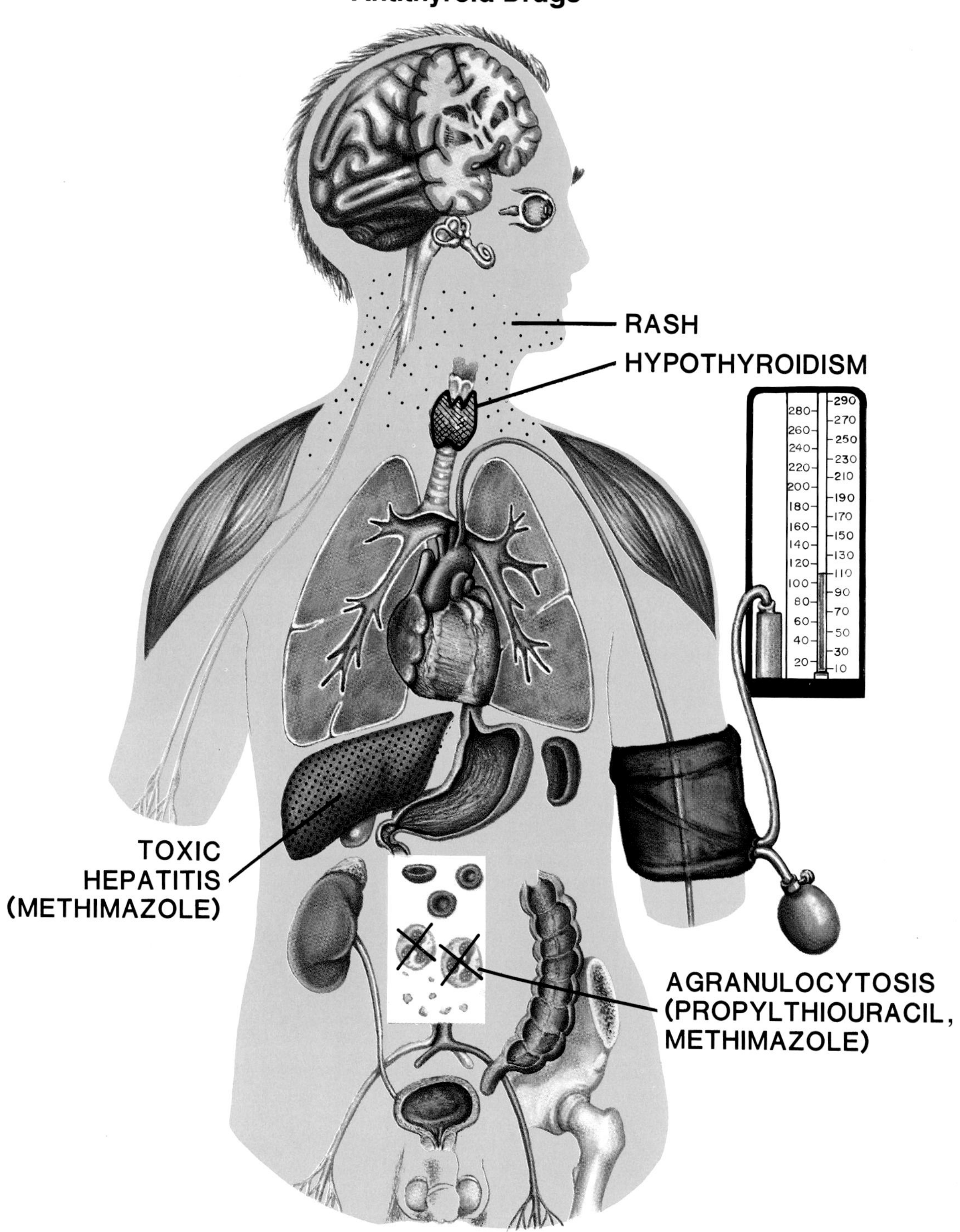

Antithyroid Drugs

Principal Drugs

Generic Name	Representative Trade Name
Propylthiouracil	Propylthiouracil
Methimazole	Tapazole
Potassium iodide	SSKI
Sodium iodide	Sodium Iodide
Sodium iodide I 131	Iodotope I-131

Toxicity Rating: Medium

Adverse Reactions

Hematologic Agranulocytosis is the most serious reaction to propylthiouracil and methimazole. It is usually reversible, but aplastic anemia may rarely develop. The iodides may produce a leukemoid eosinophilia or thrombotic thrombocytopenic purpura.

Hepatic Hepatitis may develop, especially in patients receiving methimazole.

Allergic All of these drugs produce frequent allergic reactions including skin rashes, drug fever, lupus syndrome, vasculitis, conjunctivitis, and rhinitis.

Endocrinologic As might be expected, these antithyroid drugs can induce permanent hypothyroidism. Iodine 131 does this frequently. What is not generally remembered is that the iodides may precipitate thyrotoxicosis, especially in patients with nodular goiters.

Other Radiation thyroiditis often occurs following ^{131}I administration but usually subsides. The incidence of thyroid carcinoma is not greater with ^{131}I than with other modes of therapy.

Contraindications

The only contraindication is known sensitivity to these drugs.

Precautions

Use in pregnancy may induce fetal hypothyroidism and cretinism. Frequent monitoring of the blood count is important to catch early leukopenia and other blood dyscrasias.

Treatment

Simple withdrawal of the drug is usually sufficient. However, persistent agranulocytosis should be treated with antibiotics, transfusions of fresh blood, and corticosteroids. Allergic reactions may necessitate adrenalin, vasopressors, intravenous fluids, and corticosteroids. Hypothyroidism will necessitate thyroid replacement therapy. Thyroid storm may necessitate propranolol, reserpine, and corticosteroids.

Chapter 14

ANTITUSSIVE DRUGS

Antitussive Drugs

Principal Drugs

Generic Name	Representative Trade Name
Dextromethorphan hydrobromide	Romilar
Benzonatate	Tessalon
Noscapine	Tusscapine
Levopropoxyphene	Novrad
Hydrocodone bitartrate	Dicodid
Codeine sulfate (see page 213)	

Toxicity Rating: Low

Adverse Reactions

Gastrointestinal Nausea, vomiting, and constipation are the most common side effects of these drugs.

Central Nervous System Slight drowsiness, dizziness, headache, and numbness in the chest are the principal neurologic reactions.

Other Nasal congestion or dryness, burning in the eyes, chills, skin eruptions, and tightness in the chest have been reported.

Contraindications

Known hypersensitivity is the major contraindication.

Precautions

Safety in pregnancy has not been established. Overdosage may cause respiratory depression, especially in children. Dependency is rare but can occur.

Drug Interactions

Dextromethorphan should not be used with MAO inhibitors.

Treatment

Simple withdrawal of the drug is usually all that is necessary.

Chapter 15

BRONCHODILATORS

Introduction

The principal bronchodilator drugs are the sympathomimetics (see Chapter 34) and theophylline and its analogs. The side effects of theophylline and its analogs and of the sympathomimetics are very similar. Both stimulate the cardiovascular and central nervous system and may consequently cause convulsions, tachycardia, and cardiac arrhythmias. Hypertension, both systolic and diastolic (a consistent reaction to some of the sympathomimetics) is not a side effect of theophylline. On the contrary, theophylline may occasionally produce marked hypotension. The sympathomimetics may cause significant anorexia, a side effect that is used therapeutically in obesity, but unlike theophylline they do not usually cause nausea and vomiting. Toxic nephritis has been reported with the use of theophylline. Thus theophylline and its analogs are probably overall slightly more toxic than the sympathomimetics.

Theophylline

Theophylline

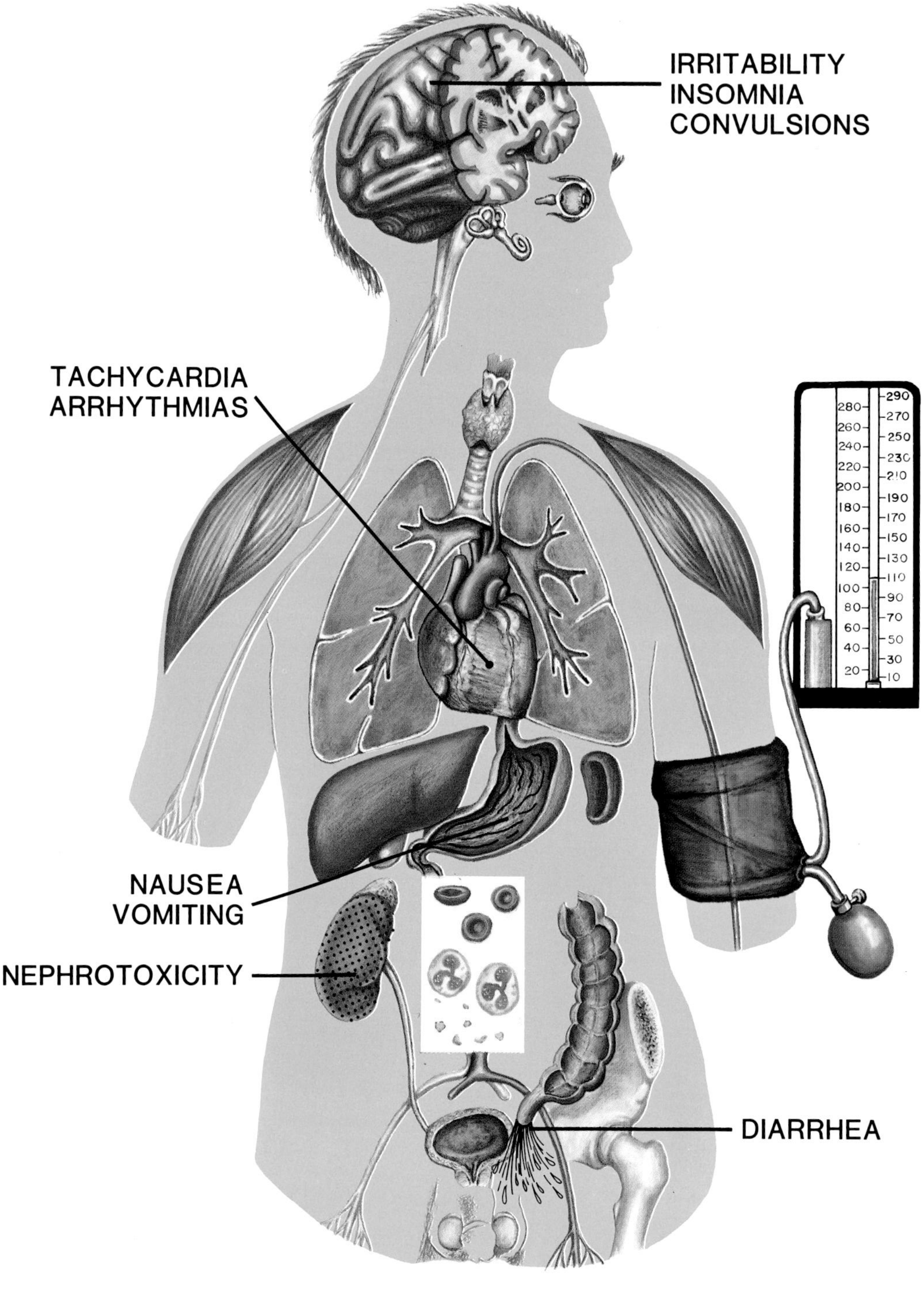

IRRITABILITY
INSOMNIA
CONVULSIONS

TACHYCARDIA
ARRHYTHMIAS

NAUSEA
VOMITING

NEPHROTOXICITY

DIARRHEA

Theophylline

Principal Drugs

Generic Name	Representative Trade Names
Theophylline	Elixophyllin, Theo-Dur, Theolair
Related drugs:	
Aminophylline (combination of theophylline and ethylenediamine)	Aminophyllin
Various other theophylline combinations	Quadrinal, Tedral
Dyphylline	Lufyllin

Toxicity Rating: Moderate because of convulsions and arrhythmias.

Adverse Reactions

Central Nervous System Like the sympathomimetics, theophylline and related drugs stimulate the central nervous system. Consequently, irritability, insomnia, muscle twitching, and even convulsions occur.

Cardiovascular Palpitations, tachycardia, and ventricular arrhythmias may occur.

Gastrointestinal Nausea, vomiting, diarrhea, epigastric pain, and hematemesis may occur.

Respiratory Hyperventilation is common.

Renal A toxic nephritis may occur, manifested by albuminuria, cellular casts, microscopic hematuria, and diuresis.

Other Allergic reactions are unusual, but hyperglycemia and inappropriate antidiuretic hormone secretion have been reported.

Contraindications

The only contraindication is known hypersensitivity to theophylline and other xanthine derivatives.

Precautions

Caution must be exercised when there is preexisting cardiac disease, hypertension, hyperthyroidism, or liver disease. Theophylline may aggravate a peptic ulcer.

Drug Interactions

Theophylline increases the diuresis induced by most diuretics. It decreases the chronotropic effect of hexamethonium. Theophylline combined with reserpine is especially likely to produce tachycardia. Various drugs — troleandomycin, erythromycin, and lincomycin — may increase theophylline blood levels.

Treatment

Careful monitoring of theophylline blood levels is advisable. Withdrawal of the drug may be all that is necessary in tachycardia, but if ventricular arrhythmias occur, hospitalization is obviously indicated for continuous cardiac monitoring and defibrillation or cardioversion as required. Seizures necessitate establishing of an airway, administering oxygen, and administering intravenous diazepam 0.1 – 0.3 mg/kg. Amobarbital and other anticonvulsants may be required.

Chapter 16

CHOLINERGIC DRUGS

Cholinergic Drugs

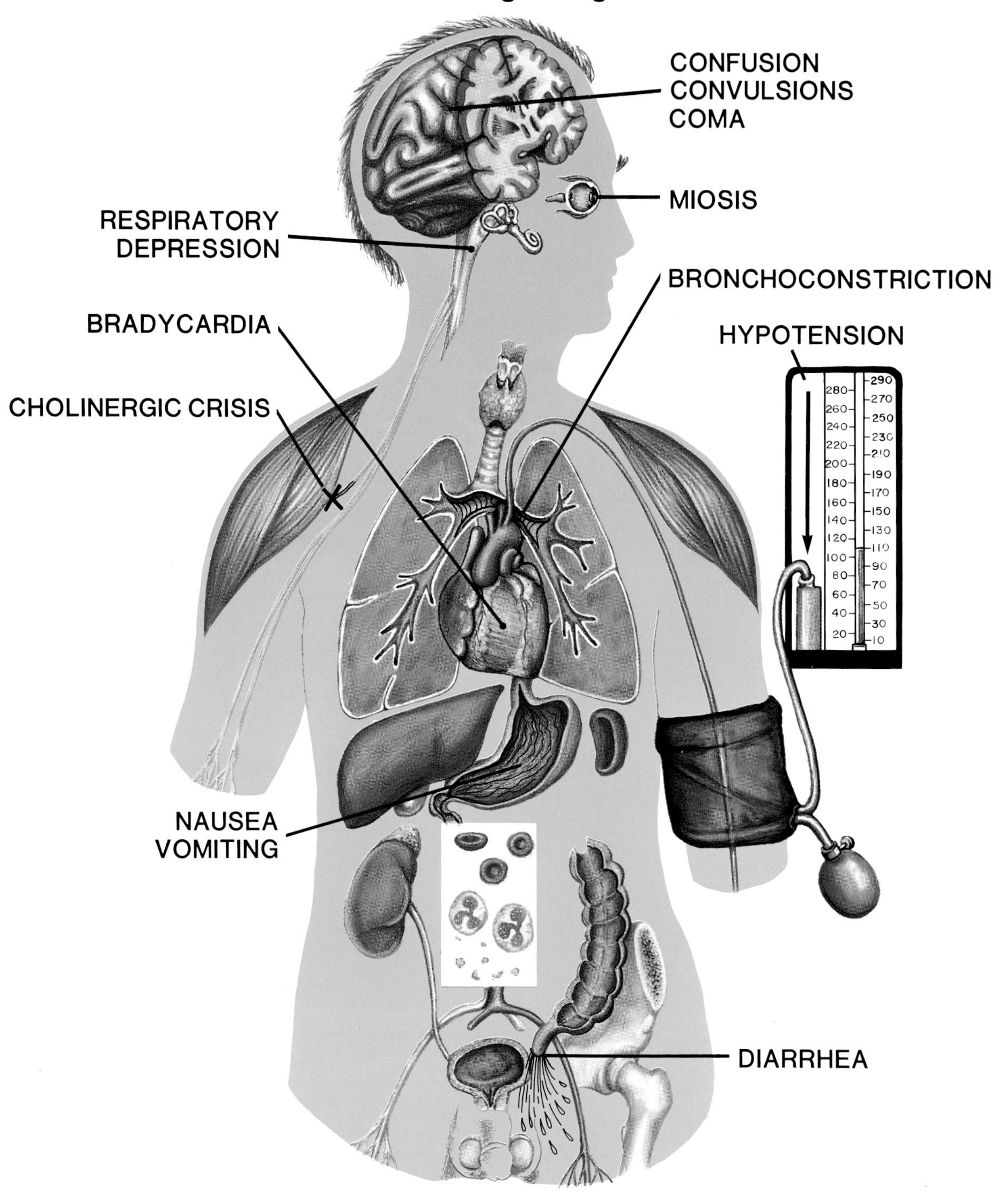

Cholinergic Drugs

Principal Drugs

Generic Name	Representative Trade Names
Neostigmine bromide	Prostigmin
Pyridostigmine bromide	Mestinon
Ambenonium chloride	Mytelase
Edrophonium chloride	Tensilon
Pilocarpine hydrochloride	Pilocar, Carpine
Physostigmine sulfate	Eserine
Bethanechol chloride	Urecholine

Toxicity Rating: Moderate because of possible neuromuscular blockade.

Adverse Reactions

Central Nervous System Confusion, slurred speech, ataxia, respiratory depression, coma, and convulsions may occur. More frequently, there is muscle weakness or paralysis ("cholinergic crisis") and fasciculations.

Gastrointestinal Nausea, vomiting, diarrhea, and abdominal cramps are frequent. There is usually excessive salivation.

Respiratory Bronchoconstriction, productive cough, and even respiratory paralysis may occur.

Cardiovascular Significant bradycardia, hypotension, and cardiac arrest have occurred.

Other Miosis, chemosis, and other local reactions occur with topical preparations.

Contraindications

Known hypersensitivity and intestinal or urinary obstruction are the major contraindications.

Precautions

Patients with bronchial asthma must be watched carefully for intensified bronchoconstriction. Dosage must be carefully monitored to prevent a cholinergic crisis. Safety in pregnancy has not been established.

Treatment

Atropine is an effective antidote: it is given in a dosage of 1 mg IV hourly until the effects are reversed. Respiratory depression must be treated with a respirator until adequate spontaneous ventilation develops. Edrophonium chloride can be used to test whether respiratory and skeletal paralysis is due to underdosage or overdosage. If there is little or no response to edrophonium chloride, a cholinergic crisis is probably present and the cholinergic drugs should be withdrawn.

Chapter 17

CENTRAL NERVOUS SYSTEM STIMULANTS

CNS Stimulants

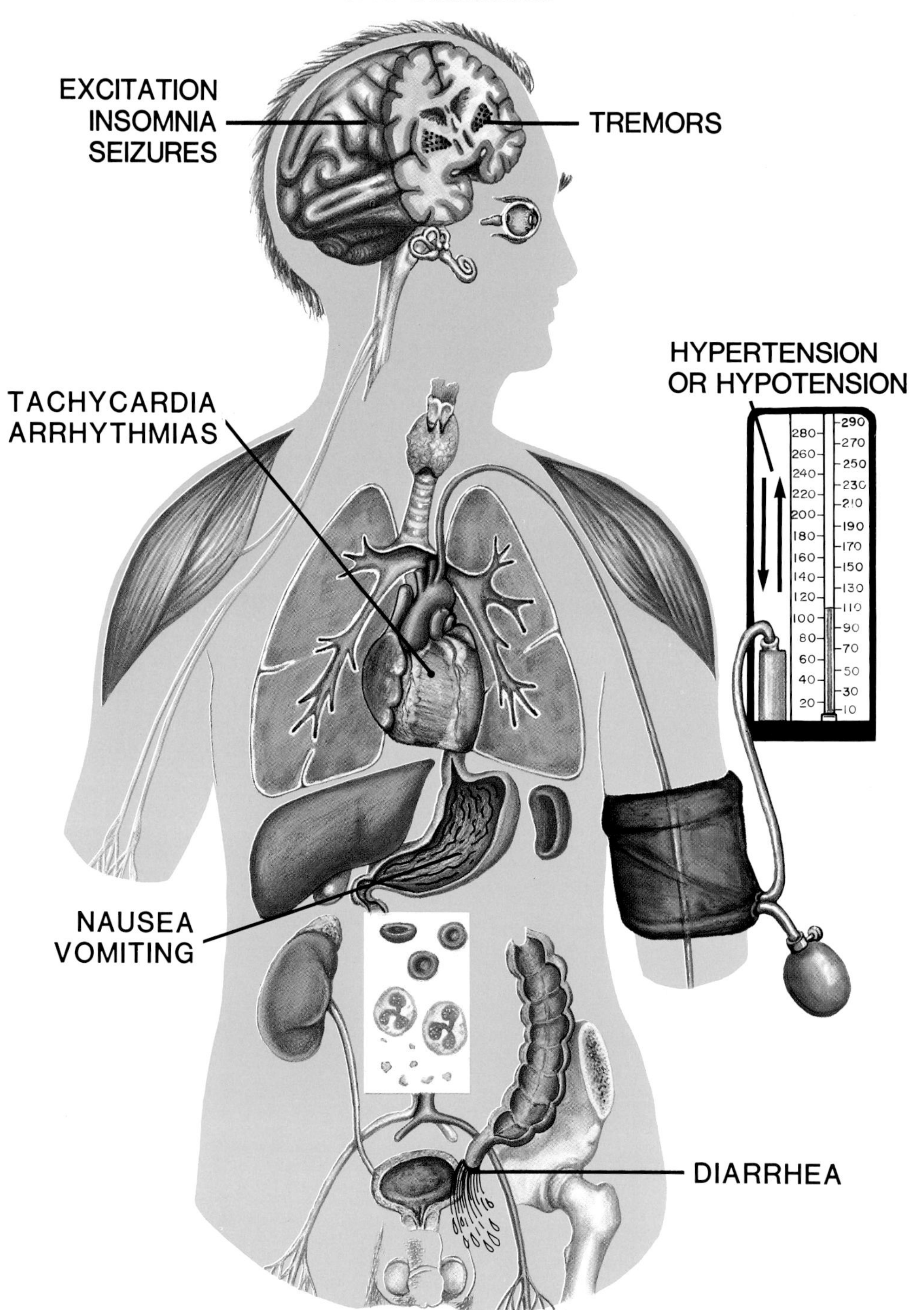

Central Nervous System Stimulants

Principal Drugs

Generic Name	Representative Trade Names
Caffeine	Nodoz
Deanol acetamidobenzoate	Deaner
Methylphenidate hydrochloride	Ritalin Hydrochloride
Pemoline	Cylert
Nikethamide	Coramine
Pentylenetetrazol	Metrazol
Doxapram hydrochloride	Dopram
Sympathomimetics (see Chapter 34)	

Toxicity Rating: Moderate because these drugs may induce seizures, arrhythmias, and hypertension.

Adverse Reactions

Central Nervous System Insomnia, nervousness, dizziness, headache, tremors, dyskinesia, fasciculations, and seizures may be encountered.

Cardiovascular Tachycardia, hypertension or hypotension, cardiac arrhythmias, angina, and occasionally bradycardia are the most significant cardiovascular reactions.

Gastrointestinal Nausea, vomiting, and diarrhea may occur.

Other Sweating, rashes, blurred vision, diuresis, and hyperesthesia may be noted. Exfoliative dermatitis has been encountered with methylphenidate HCl. These drugs, particularly the amphetamines and methylphenidate HCl, have a high potential for dependency. Alterations in liver enzymes and pancytopenia may occur with prolonged therapy.

Contraindications

Most of these drugs are contraindicated in patients with significant cardiac disease, hyperthyroidism, hypertension, coronary insufficiency, severe depression, and history of drug abuse.

Precautions

CNS stimulants should be used cautiously in patients with a history of seizure disorders. Pemoline and methylphenidate are not recommended for use in children under age 6.

Drug Interactions

MAO inhibitors potentiate the cardiovascular side effects of the sympathomimetics and doxapram; other than this there are no significant drug interactions of CNS stimulants.

Treatment

Withdrawal of the drug will alleviate most of the side effects without additional treatment. Intravenous barbiturates or diazepam may be needed to treat convulsions, and various cardiovascular reactions must be treated with appropriate agents.

Chapter 18

DIURETICS

Table 18-1. Side Effects of Diuretics

Drug	CNS	Gastrointestinal	Cardiovascular	Hematologic	Allergic	Metabolic	Endocrine	Electrolyte
Thiazides	+	+	+	+	+	+	+	↓ K, ↓ Na
Furosemide	+	+	+	+	+	+	+	↓ K, ↓ Na
Ethacrynic acid	+	+	+	+	+	+	+	↓ K, ↓ Na
Spironolactone	+	+	−	−	+	−	+	↑ K, ↓ Na
Triamterene	+	+	−	−	+	−	−	↑ K, ↓ Na
Acetazolamide	+	+	−	−	+	−	−	↓ K, ↓ Na

Introduction

Principal Types of Diuretics Still in Use

Thiazides
Furosemide
Ethacrynic acid
Triamterene
Spironolactone
Acetazolamide
Bumetanide

As Table 18-1 shows, the side effects of all the diuretics are remarkably similar. All produce central nervous system effects, usually related to the electrolyte change. The thiazides, furosemide, and ethacrynic acid lower potassium, while spironolactone and triamterene elevate potassium. While the thiazides frequently cause hypercalcemia, furosemide and ethacrynic acid usually cause hypocalcemia. Hyperglycemia and hyperuricemia accompany thiazide, furosemide, and ethacrynic acid administration. Spironolactone is the only drug with significant endocrine effects (gynecomastia, amenorrhea, etc.).

Thiazides

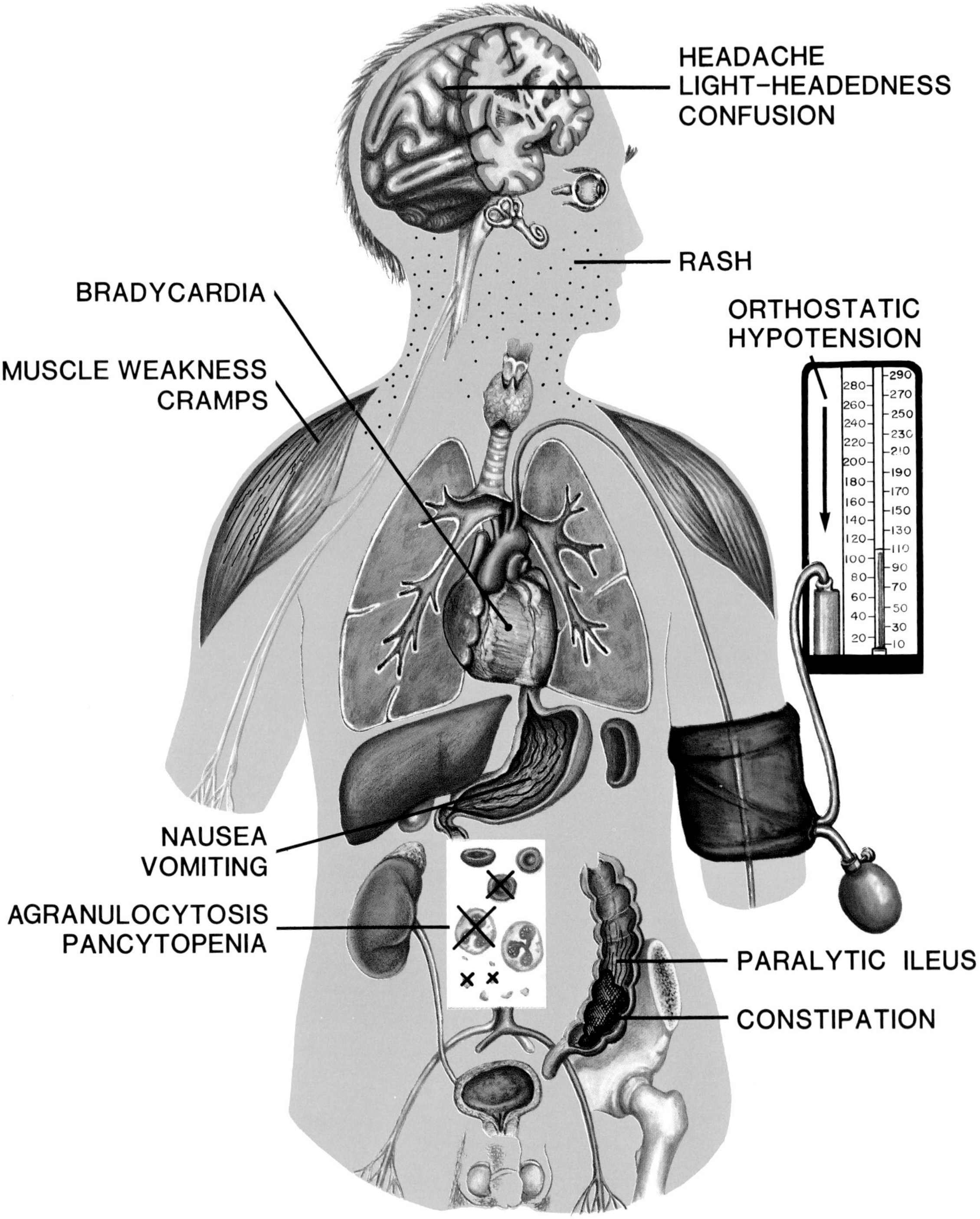

HEADACHE
LIGHT-HEADEDNESS
CONFUSION

RASH

BRADYCARDIA

ORTHOSTATIC
HYPOTENSION

MUSCLE WEAKNESS
CRAMPS

NAUSEA
VOMITING

AGRANULOCYTOSIS
PANCYTOPENIA

PARALYTIC ILEUS

CONSTIPATION

Thiazides

Principal Drugs

Generic Name	Representative Trade Name
Chlorothiazide	Diuril
Hydrochlorothiazide	HydroDIURIL, Esidrix
Chlorthalidone	Hygroton
Methyclothiazide	Enduron
Bendroflumethiazide	Naturetin
Polythiazide	Renese

Toxicity Rating: Low

Adverse Reactions

Electrolyte Balance Hypokalemia is the most common reaction, and results in weakness, lethargy, paralytic ileus, muscle cramps, and occasional nausea or vomiting. Marked sodium depletion may develop and may also cause many of the above symptoms. Metabolic alkalosis and chloride depletion may occur.

Gastrointestinal Nausea, vomiting, diarrhea, and constipation may be primary effects or secondary to the electrolyte changes.

Central Nervous System Paresthesias, vertigo, lightheadedness, and headache have been observed.

Cardiovascular Orthostatic hypotension as a result of the fluid and electrolyte depletion is not uncommon in the early stage of therapy.

Hematologic One or more of the cellular elements of the blood may be decreased in number, or there may be pancytopenia due to bone marrow depression. Pancytopenia is usually reversible.

Metabolic In addition to electrolyte alterations, there may be hyperglycemia, elevated uric acid, and hypercalcemia.

Allergic All types of skin reactions (urticaria, erythema multiforme, etc.) may occur. In addition, anaphylaxis, necrotizing angiitis, and photosensitivity may be seen.

Other Cholestatic jaundice, interstitial nephritis, and pancreatitis are the more serious—but fortunately rare—reactions.

Contraindications

Contraindications include anuria and known hypersensitivity to thiazides and other sulfonamide-like drugs.

Precautions

Patients with known renal or hepatic disease (e.g., cirrhosis) must be observed carefully. Thiazides may precipitate azotemia or hepatic coma. Lupus erythematosus may be aggravated by thiazides. Use of thiazides in pregnancy and nursing mothers is potentially risky to the fetus. Frequent determinations of serum electrolytes may be wise during the early stages of therapy.

Drug Interactions

The thiazides potentiate the hypotensive effects of other antihypertensives. Thiazides may potentiate neuromuscular blockade with tubocurarine. Thiazide diuretics decrease the renal clearance of lithium. Because of their hypokalemic effects, the thiazides may produce digitalis toxicity in patients taking digitalis.

Treatment

Withdrawal of the drug and replacement of potassium and other electrolytes, according to serum electrolyte determinations, is usually all that is necessary.

Furosemide and Ethacrynic Acid

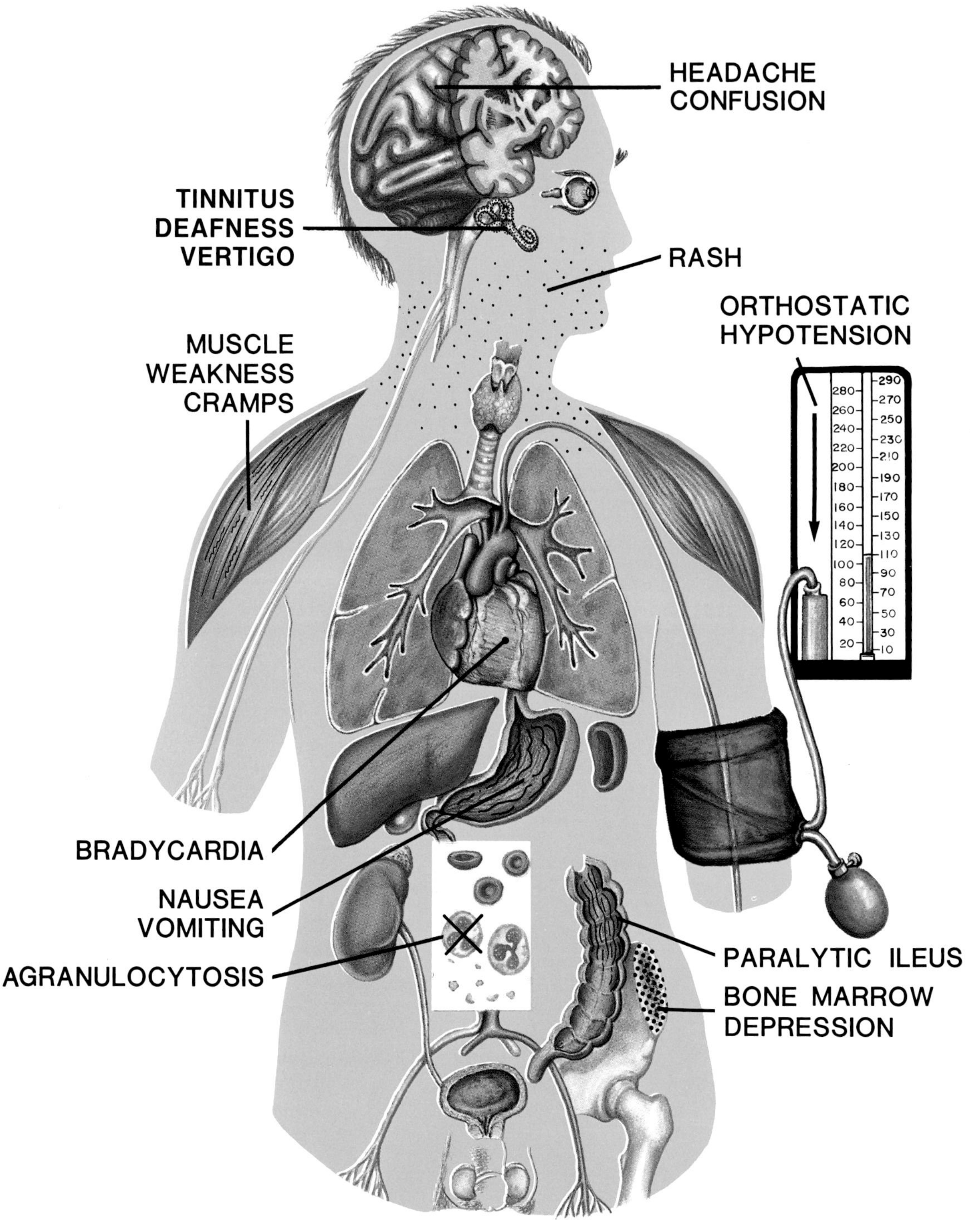

Furosemide and Ethacrynic Acid

Representative Trade Names: Lasix (furosemide), Edecrin (ethacrynic acid)

Toxicity Rating: Low

Furosemide and ethacrynic acid are chemically unrelated, but generally produce the same side effects.

Adverse Reactions

The side effects of furosemide and ethacrynic acid are usually similar to those of the thiazide diuretics, and are often secondary to electrolyte alterations.

Electrolyte Balance Hypokalemia, hyponatremia, and hypochloremic alkalosis are frequently observed, but hypokalemia is not usually as severe as with thiazide diuretics. Hyponatremia is more common than with thiazides, however, and severe volume depletion may result.

Gastrointestinal Nausea, vomiting, diarrhea, and constipation occur, usually as a result of depletion of one or more electrolyte.

Central Nervous System Symptoms similar to those of Menière's disease, such as tinnitus, deafness, and vertigo, may occur. Headache and paresthesias have also been observed.

Hematologic Bone marrow depression occurs, and results in decrease in one or more of the cellular elements of the blood.

Allergic Allergic reactions to furosemide and ethacrynic acid are similar to those to thiazide diuretics. Skin reactions — urticaria, erythema multiforme, etc. — may occur. Anaphylaxis, necrotizing angiitis, and photosensitivity may also be seen.

Metabolic As with the thiazides, hyperglycemia and hyperuricemia may occur during therapy. However, the hyperglycemia induced by furosemide and ethacrynic acid is not as frequent nor as severe as with thiazides. Unlike thiazides, furosemide and ethacrynic acid may cause not hypercalcemia but rather a lowering of serum calcium as a result of severe chloride depletion.

Other Orthostatic hypotension, cholestatic jaundice, pancreatitis, and interstitial nephritis have been noted.

Contraindications

Furosemide and ethacrynic acid are generally contraindicated in cases of anuria: however, if prerenal azotemia is suspected, a test dose of 80 mg or more of furosemide may be given provided that venous pressure is monitored and IV fluids given concomitantly.

Precautions

Caution must be observed when administering these diuretics to patients with known hepatitis or renal disease. Administration of furosemide or ethacrynic acid to patients with cirrhotic disease may induce hepatic coma.

Drug Interactions

Furosemide and ethacrynic acid may induce digitalis toxicity by reducing serum potassium. Ototoxicity has been precipitated when these drugs are given with the aminoglycosides (kanamycin, gentamicin, etc.). Like the thiazides, furosemide and ethacrynic acid decrease the renal clearance of lithium and may induce lithium toxicity. They may also enhance the hypotensive effects of many antihypertensive agents.

Treatment

Withdrawal of the drugs and correction of electrolyte imbalances are the most important elements of therapy.

Spironolactone and Triamterene

Representative Trade Names: Aldactone (spironolactone), Dyrenium (triamterene)

Toxicity Rating: Low

Adverse Reactions

Electrolyte Balance The major side effects of both spironolactone and triamterene are secondary to hyperkalemia. Thus diarrhea, cramping, headache, and lethargy may be noted.

Allergic Urticaria, maculopapular rash, and drug fever have been observed.

Other Gynecomastia, amenorrhea, irregular menses, and impotence may be found with spironolactone administration. Rare instances of interstitial nephritis have been noted with triamterene.

Precautions

These drugs are more likely to induce hyperkalemia in the elderly, in diabetics, and in patients with renal disease. Triamterene should be used with caution in patients with a history of renal stones. Triamterene may induce megaloblastic anemia in cirrhotics who already have reduced folic acid stores.

Treatment

Withdrawal of the drug is usually sufficient but enemas with ion-exchange resins (such as Kexalate) or dialysis may be necessary in rare instances.

Acetazolamide

Representative Trade Name: Diamox

Toxicity Rating: Low

Adverse Reactions

Central Nervous System Paresthesias, drowsiness, and confusion are occasionally noted.

Gastrointestinal Loss of appetite and rarely melena occur.

Other Hyperchloremic acidosis is a frequent sequel to long-term therapy. Myopia, urticaria, hematuria, glycosuria, hepatic insufficiency, flaccid paralysis, and seizures have occasionally been observed. Other reactions peculiar to sulfonamides may occur.

Contraindications

Acetazolamide is contraindicated in severe renal and hepatic insufficiency. It is also unwise to prescribe this drug in preexisting hyperchloremic acidosis and adrenal insufficiency. The drug is contraindicated for long-term use with chronic noncongestive angle-closure glaucoma.

Precautions

Increasing the dose adds to the side effects (paresthesias, etc.) but often does not increase diuresis.

Treatment

Withdrawal of the drug is usually sufficient.

Chapter 19

ENZYMES

Enzymes

Principal Drugs

Generic Name	Representative Trade Name
Bromelains	Ananase
Chymotrypsin	Avazyme
Fibrinolysin and desoxyribonuclease	Elase
Hyaluronidase	Wydase
Papain	Papase
Streptokinase–streptodornase	Varidase
Trypsin	Orenzyme
Streptokinase, parenteral	Streptase
Urokinase, parenteral	Abbokinase

Toxicity Rating: Low overall, but because some of these drugs are given intravenously serious anaphylaxis can occur.

Adverse Reactions

Allergic Allergic reactions are the most common and serious side effects of enzyme drugs. With topical preparations (e.g., Wydase, Elase, Varidase) these are the only significant side effects. Allergic reactions include hyperemia, pruritus, urticaria, other types of rashes, serum sickness, and anaphylaxis.

Gastrointestinal Oral preparations (such as Papase, Orenzyme, and Ananase) are particularly likely to cause nausea, vomiting, and diarrhea.

Hematologic Most of these drugs cause an increased tendency to bruising or hemorrhage if given orally or parenterally.

Genitourinary Trypsin and chymotrypsin may cause hematuria and albuminuria.

Contraindication

Known hypersensitivity to these enzymes or their sources (e.g. papaya fruit for papain) is the major contraindication. Anticoagulants should not be given concomitantly with oral or parenteral preparations of these enzymes.

Precautions

Patients with known renal or hepatic disease should be observed carefully.

Drug Interactions

Antacids and alkaline solutions should not be given simultaneously with the oral preparations as they will interfere with absorption. There are no significant interactions of other drugs with streptokinase–streptodornase and the components of Elase ointment (fibrinolysin and desoxyribonuclease). Topical use of papain and trypsin detergents and antiseptic solutions may decrease the enzyme activity of these preparations.

Treatment

Withdrawal of the drug will alleviate most reactions. Anaphylaxis must be treated aggressively (page 96).

Chapter 20

EXPECTORANTS

Introduction

Principal Expectorants

Guaifenesin (glyceryl guaiacolate)
Iodides
Ammonium chlorides

These drugs are extremely low in toxicity. As might be expected from any oral preparation, nausea, vomiting, and occasional diarrhea or other gastrointestinal reactions may occur. Most expectorants contain an antihistamine, so drowsiness may also occur. On the other hand, those expectorants that contain a decongestant (sympathomimetic) may be expected to cause nervousness, irritability, and cardiovascular stimulation. Obviously, all of these drugs may cause allergic reactions despite the fact that they often contain two of the drugs most useful in combating allergic reactions (antihistaminics and sympathomimetics). Reactions peculiar to specific expectorants include hypothyroidism (caused by iodides) and bronchospasm (associated with acetylcysteine).

Guaifenesin

Representative Trade Names: Robitussin, Ambenyl-D, Bronkotabs, Entex capsules and liquid, Naldecon-CX, Quibron, Novahistine, Triaminic. Many other cough syrups contain this drug.

Toxicity Rating: Low

Adverse Reactions

Nausea and drowsiness are the most frequent side effects and are reversible. Guaifenesin may decrease platelet adhesiveness, but does not alter coagulation parameters.

Drug Interactions

Guaifenesin may produce false positive reaction in urine tests for 5-hydroxyindoleacetic acid and vanillylmandelic acid.

Treatment

Withholding the drug is the only treatment necessary.

Iodides

Representative Trade Names: SSKI, Sodium Iodide

Toxicity Rating: Medium in view of potentially fatal allergic reactions and the capacity of iodides to produce hypothyroidism, goiter, and thyrotoxicosis.

Adverse Reactions

Endocrinologic Chronic iodide administration may produce hypothyroidism and goiter. Thyrotoxicosis has occasionally been precipitated and may persist after withdrawal of therapy.

Respiratory Patients on chronic iodide therapy may suffer congestion of the respiratory tract — the very condition the iodide was prescribed for. Iodides may also cause sore throat, gingivitis, conjunctivitis, and frontal sinus headache.

Dermatologic Acne, ioderma, hair loss, and various other allergic skin reactions may occur. Anaphylactoid reactions are known and are potentially fatal.

Gastrointestinal Diarrhea, nausea, and vomiting are not uncommon.

Contraindications

Iodides are contraindicated in patients with known hypersensitivity to them and in pregnant women. Cases of neonatal death have occurred when pregnant women have taken these drugs.

Drug Interactions

Iodides may produce false positive results to benzidine and guaiac tests for occult blood. Quite logically, they cause an elevated serum protein-bound iodine and radioactive iodine uptake. The urine 17-hydroxycorticosteroid levels may also be altered.

Treatment

Withdrawal of the drug will suffice for most reactions. Anaphylactoid shock can be treated with epinephrine, antihistamines, and corticosteroids. Thyroid replacement therapy may be necessary if thyroid function fails to return to normal after withdrawal of the drug.

Ammonium Chloride

Representative Trade Names: Contained in Ambenyl and Ru-Tuss Expectorant

Toxicity Rating: Low

Adverse Reactions

Gastrointestinal Nausea and vomiting are frequent.

Other Systemic acidosis may occur with large doses.

Contraindications

Systemic acidosis and known hypersensitivity are contraindications for ammonium chloride.

Precautions

This drug should be used with extreme caution in patients with liver and kidney diseases.

Drug Interactions

Ammonium chloride causes acidification of the urine and may precipitate crystalluria when given concomitantly with sulfonamides. Ammonium chloride also potentiates the action of methenamine and mercurial diuretics. The action of carbonic anhydrase inhibitors is occasionally delayed. Serum amylase and chloride may be elevated whereas serum potassium and total protein may be decreased in patients on this drug.

Treatment

Withdrawal of the drug is all that is usually necessary.

Chapter 21

HORMONES

Table 21-1. Side Effects of the Major Hormones

Drug	Psychological Disturbances	Hypertension	Tachycardia	Congestive Heart Failure	Hyperglycemia	Hypoglycemia	Muscle Hypertrophy	Muscle Atrophy	Thrombo-embolic Phenomena
Corticosteroids	+	+	−	+	+	−	−	+	−
Thyroid hormones	+	+	+	+	+	−	−	+	−
Estrogens	+	−	−	−	+ (?)	−	−	−	+
Progestins	+	−	−	−	−	−	−	−	+
Androgens	+	−	−	−	−	−	+	−	−
Insulin	+	−	+	−	−	+	−	−	−
Growth hormones	+	−	−	−	+	−	−	−	−

Introduction

Principal Types of Hormones Used Therapeutically

- Corticosteroids and ACTH
- Androgens and anabolic steroids
- Estrogens
- Progestins
- Oral contraceptives (discussed under estrogens and progestins)
- Thyroid hormones
- Insulin preparations
- Gonadotropins
- Menotropins
- Growth hormone (somatropin)
- Vasopressins
- Glucagon

As might be expected, most side effects of hormones are due to a relative or absolute overdose and consequently mimic endogenous hypersecretion. For example, the side effects of the corticosteroids are hypertension, hyperglycemia, depression, etc. — the signs of Cushing's syndrome.

Table 21-1 compares the side effects of the hormones. All of them may cause psychological disturbances. The corticosteroids and thyroid hormones may both produce hyperglycemia, hypertension, and congestive heart failure. These hormones also produce muscle atrophy. Thyroid hormones and insulin in excessive doses both produce tachycardia. It should be noted that excessive doses of one hormone may cause side effects by creating a relative deficiency of another. For example, excessive doses of exogenous corticosteroids may cause hyperglycemia because of a relative deficiency of insulin.

Corticosteroids and ACTH

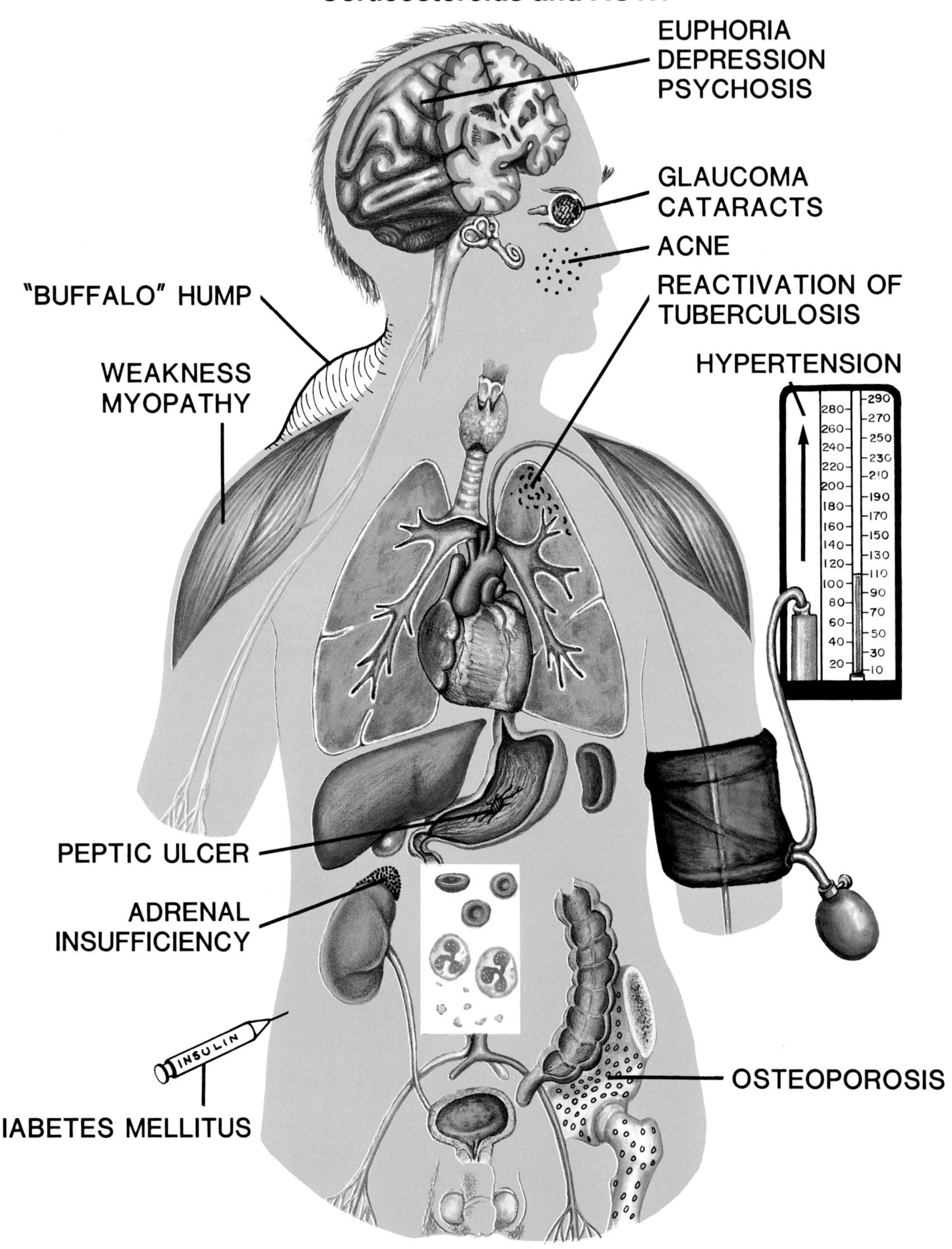

EUPHORIA
DEPRESSION
PSYCHOSIS
GLAUCOMA
CATARACTS
ACNE
REACTIVATION OF
TUBERCULOSIS
"BUFFALO" HUMP
WEAKNESS
MYOPATHY
HYPERTENSION
280 260 240 220 200 180 160 140 120 100 80 60 40 20
290 270 250 230 210 190 170 150 130 110 90 70 50 30 10
PEPTIC ULCER
ADRENAL
INSUFFICIENCY
INSULIN
DIABETES MELLITUS
OSTEOPOROSIS

Corticosteroids and ACTH

Principal Drugs

Generic Name	Representative Trade Name
Prednisone	Deltasone
Prednisolone	Prednisolone tablets, Hydeltra-T.B.A.
Methylprednisolone	Medrol, Depo-Medrol
Triamcinolone	Aristocort, Kenalog
Dexamethasone	Decadron, Hexadrol
Beclomethasone dipropionate	Beclovent
Betamethasone	Celestone
ACTH	Acthar gel

Toxicity Rating: Low to high depending upon the duration and method of therapy.

Adverse Reactions

Central Nervous System There may be euphoria or depression during initial administration. A frank organic psychosis has been reported. Convulsions, increased intracranial pressure (pseudotumor cerebri), vertigo, and headache have been reported.

Cardiovascular Hypertension, sodium retention with edema, and occasional congestive heart failure have occurred after prolonged use.

Gastrointestinal Gastritis, esophagitis, peptic ulcer, pancreatitis, and abdominal distention may occur.

Dermatologic Cushingoid face, buffalo hump, centripetal obesity, facial erythema, acne, petechiae, and ecchymoses have been noted. Atrophy of the skin after local injection may occur.

Endocrinologic Acute or chronic adrenal insufficiency may occur after the drug is withdrawn. Hyperglycemia may occur, and latent diabetes mellitus may be precipitated. Growth suppression and menstrual irregularities may occur.

Musculoskeletal Muscle weakness, myopathy, osteoporosis, aseptic necrosis of bone, and predisposition to fractures of all types are not uncommon after prolonged use.

Special senses Glaucoma, subcapsular cataracts, and exophthalmos have been observed.

Other While it may seem strange, allergic reactions including anaphylactic shock have occurred, especially after parenteral use. Charcot's arthritis-like joints may develop after repeated intraarticular injections, and arachnoiditis has been observed following intrathecal administration. There is increased susceptibility to infections of all types (including tuberculosis) after prolonged use. A withdrawal syndrome may occur.

Contraindications

Systemic fungal infection or known active tuberculosis are important contraindications. Known hypersensitivity to corticosteroids, although rare, is also a contraindication.

Precautions

The action of corticosteroids may be enhanced by hypothyroidism and cirrhosis. The drugs may predispose to corneal perforation in ocular herpes simplex. Preexisting peptic ulcer, infections, hypertension, congestive heart failure, osteoporosis, psychosis, and myasthenia gravis may be aggravated by corticosteroids.

Drug Interactions

Concurrent use of aspirin may be unwise when there is preexisting ulcer or hypoprothrombinemia. Serum salicylate activity may be reduced by steroids. The clearance of steroids is enhanced by phenytoin, phenobarbital, ephedrine, and rifampin, so when these drugs are used the steroid dosage may have to be increased to get the same effect. Steroids may decrease the effect of coumarin drugs. Steroids may enhance potassium loss in patients on thiazides or other potassium-depleting diuretics.

Treatment

Withdrawal of the drug will alleviate most reactions that occur during the early stages of treatment, but the drug must be withdrawn gradually if it has been used for more than a week. Gastritis, ulcers, and other gastrointestinal reactions may be prevented or alleviated by administering the steroids with meals or an antacid. Prophylactic antibiotics or antituberculous drugs may be indicated in susceptible individuals. Anabolic steroids may decrease a negative nitrogen balance. Patients who have been on long-term steroid therapy will need an increased dosage of steroid to prevent adrenal insufficiency during and immediately following an operation. This recommendation also applies to an operation up to 18 months after steroid therapy has been discontinued. Coadministration of a potassium supplement may prevent the muscle weakness and fatigue associated with corticosteroid therapy.

Androgens and Anabolic Steroids

Principal Drugs

Generic Name	Representative Trade Name
Methyltestosterone	Android, Metandren, Oreton
Oxymetholone	Anadrol-50
Testosterone enanthate	Delatestryl
Fluoxymesterone	Halotestin
Oxandrolone	Anavar
Nandrolone phenpropionate	Durabolin
Testolactone	Teslac
Stanozolol	Winstrol
Danazol	Danocrine

Toxicity Rating: Moderate because of rare reports of hepatitis and hepatocellular neoplasms.

Adverse Reactions

Central Nervous System Excitation, insomnia, and increased or decreased libido occur.

Endocrinologic Oligospermia and gynecomastia occur in adult men, whereas virilism may be seen in women and prepubertal boys. Priapism may also occur.

Gastrointestinal Nausea, vomiting, hepatitis, and hepatocellular neoplasms have occurred.

Other Allergic reactions, including anaphylactic reactions, have occurred. There may also be edema, hypercalcemia, acne, alopecia, menstrual irregularities, and premature closure of the epiphyses in children. Patients on anticoagulant therapy may develop bleeding. Results of several laboratory tests including glucose tolerance, thyroid function, electrolytes, liver function, and the metyrapone test may be altered.

Contraindications

These drugs should not be given to men with carcinoma of the prostate or breast or to some women with breast cancer. Pregnancy and nephrosis are also contraindications.

Precautions

Patients should be observed for the development of hypercalcemia, amenorrhea, bleeding (in patients already on anticoagulants), and alterations in results of various laboratory tests. Diabetics may need their insulin dosage adjusted. Men with prostatic hypertrophy may develop bladder neck obstruction. Fluid retention may be significant in patients with cardiac, hepatic, or renal disease.

Treatment

In most cases withdrawal of the drug will be sufficient. Diuretics may be required in patients who develop significant edema. Virilism may be irreversible in women and children.

Drugs that Are Exceptions to the Above

Testolactone

Alopecia, nail growth disturbance, edema, rash, and gastrointestinal disturbances are rarely reported. Most of the reactions associated with the other anabolic steroids are so rarely associated with testolactone that their cause-and-effect relationship with it is doubtful.

Danazol

Hepatic dysfunction has developed with danazol therapy, but hepatic neoplasms have not. However, muscle cramps, joint swelling, hematuria, and a wider variety of central nervous system reactions have been noted with danazol than with other androgens.

Estrogens

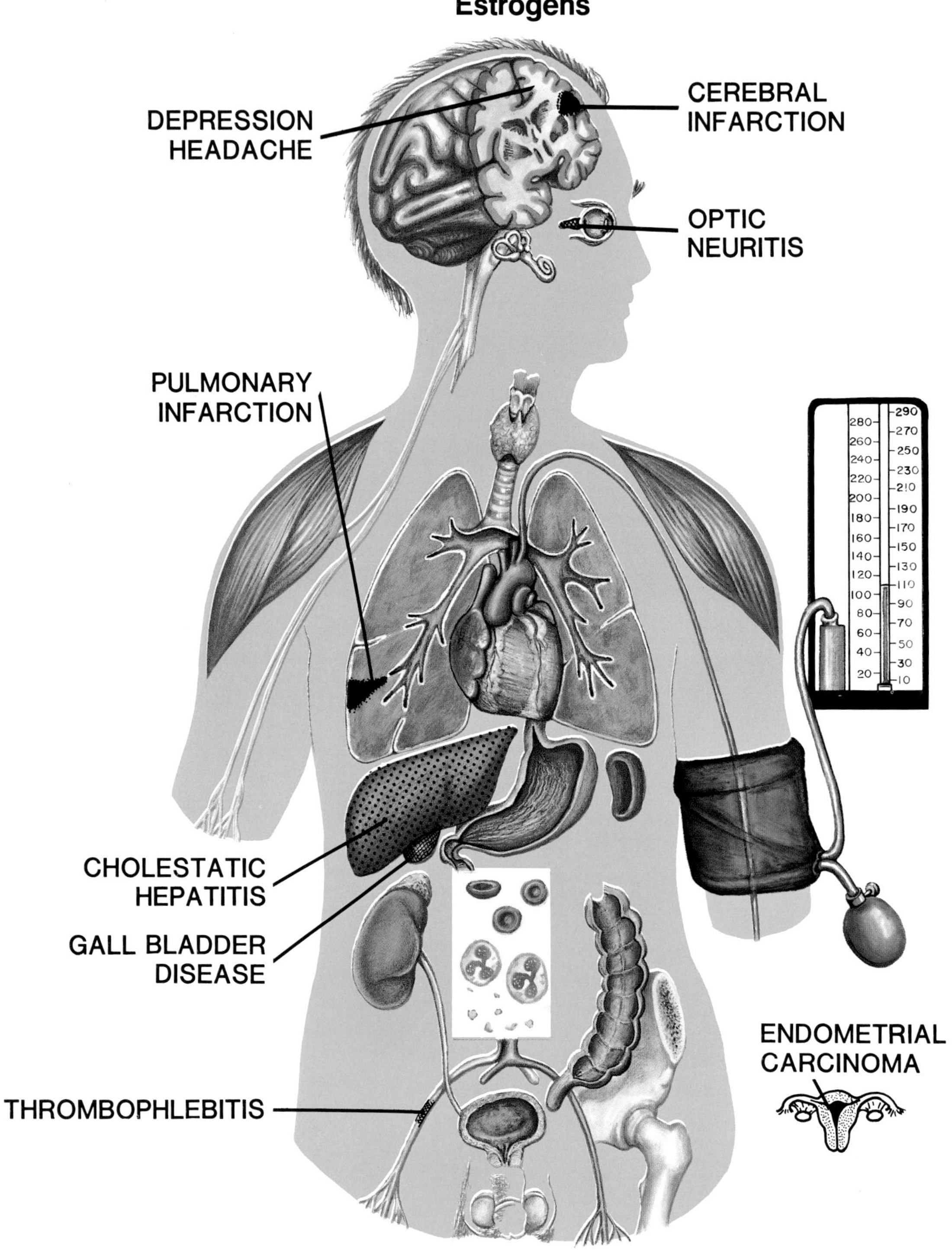
DEPRESSION
HEADACHE
CEREBRAL
INFARCTION
OPTIC
NEURITIS
PULMONARY
INFARCTION
CHOLESTATIC
HEPATITIS
GALL BLADDER
DISEASE
ENDOMETRIAL
CARCINOMA
THROMBOPHLEBITIS

Estrogens

Principal Drugs

Generic Name	Representative Trade Name
Conjugated estrogens	Premarin
Estropipate	Ogen
Ethinyl estradiol	Estinyl
Diethylstilbestrol	Diethylstilbestrol VSP
Estradiol	Estrace
Polyestradiol phosphate	Estradurin
Quinestrol	Estrovis
Esterified estrogens	Evex, Menrium
Chlorotrianisene	TACE
Estrogens in combination with progestins in various contraceptives	

Toxicity Rating: Medium because of reports of thromboembolic phenomena and various neoplasms.

Adverse Reactions

Central Nervous System Depression, headache (particularly migraine), chorea, and dizziness have been observed. Occasional cases of cerebral thrombosis or emboli have been reported; optic neuritis and retinal thrombosis are also known to occur.

Genitourinary Some controversial studies suggest an increased incidence of endometrial carcinoma and carcinomas of other female organs including the breast. Women taking these hormones may experience an increase or decrease of libido. Amenorrhea, spotting, or other menstrual irregularities may occur, as well as premenstrual tension and dysmenorrhea. Uterine fibroids are reported to increase in size.

Cardiovascular Thrombophlebitis, pulmonary emboli, and myocardial infarction are thought to occur, especially in individuals otherwise predisposed to these conditions. The incidence of other thromboembolic phenomena seems also to be increased.

Gastrointestinal Nausea, vomiting, bloating, cholestatic hepatitis, and hepatic adenomas may result from the use of estrogens. Estrogens also predispose to gallbladder disease.

Dermatologic Estrogens may cause erythema nodosum and erythema multiforme. Hair loss as well as its opposite (hirsutism) may occur. Chloasma, petechiae, and other skin reactions have been reported.

Other Estrogens may increase weight, cause fluid retention, and result in steepening of the corneal curvature. Results of various laboratory tests may be altered. For example, glucose tolerance may be decreased, T_3 resin uptake may be decreased, and hypercalcemia and porphyria may be aggravated.

Contraindications

Estrogen hormones are contraindicated in patients with known or suspected estrogen-dependent neoplasms, whether in the breast or elsewhere. They should not be used in the presence of known or suspected thromboembolic disease or in persons with a history of such phenomena. Pregnancy and undiagnosed genital bleeding are additional contraindications.

Precautions

A thorough physical examination including a Papanicolaou test should be done before prescribing estrogens and estrogen-containing contraceptives. Careful observation is advisable when administering estrogens to patients with epilepsy, migraine, asthma, or preexisting cardiac, hepatic, or renal disease. Depression may be increased. Uterine fibroids may increase in size. Patients with a history of jaundice during pregnancy may have a recurrence during estrogen administration.

Treatment

Withdrawal of the drug is important, but when there are thromboembolic phenomena it is not enough. Anticoagulants should probably be given after appropriate laboratory and x-ray studies are done.

Progestins

Principal Drugs

Generic Name	Representative Trade Name
Megestrol acetate	Pallace
Medroxyprogesterone acetate	Amen, Depo-Provera, Provera
Norethindrone	Aygestin, in Micronor, Norlutin
Norgestrel	Ovrette
Progestins in combination with estrogens in oral contraceptives	

Toxicity Rating: Moderate because of the reports of increased risk of thromboembolic phenomena and the association of progestins with various neoplasms.

Adverse Reactions

It may surprise the reader to learn that virtually all the reactions listed for estrogens are suspected to be associated also with progestins, alone or in combination with estrogens. A possible exception is megestrol (see below).

Precautions

The precautions for progestins are the same as for estrogens.

Treatment

Progestin reactions are treated by withdrawal of the drug and institution of anticoagulant therapy when indicated after appropriate laboratory and x-ray studies.

Reactions Peculiar to Megestrol

Other than a few reports of carpal tunnel syndrome, deep vein thrombophlebitis, and alopecia, no untoward side effects have been associated with this drug. However, megestrol has been used only in the palliative treatment of patients with advanced carcinoma of the breast or endometrium.

Thyroid Hormones

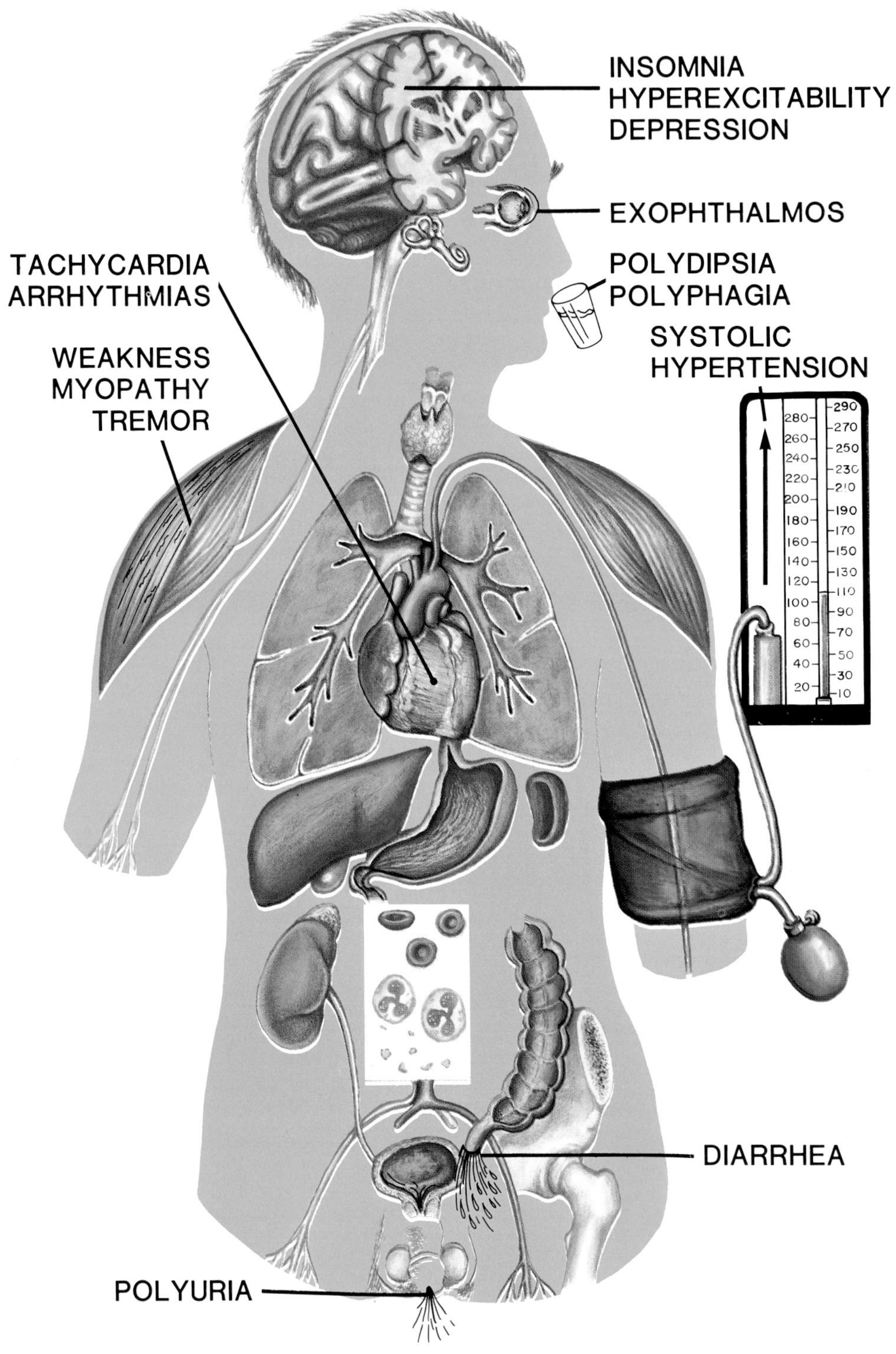
INSOMNIA
HYPEREXCITABILITY
DEPRESSION
EXOPHTHALMOS
TACHYCARDIA
ARRHYTHMIAS
POLYDIPSIA
POLYPHAGIA
WEAKNESS
MYOPATHY
TREMOR
SYSTOLIC
HYPERTENSION
DIARRHEA
POLYURIA

Thyroid Hormones

Principal Drugs

Generic Name	Representative Trade Name
Dessicated thyroid	Armour Thyroid
Thyroglobulin	Proloid
Levothyroxine sodium	Synthroid, Levothroid
Liothyronine sodium (L-triiodothyronine)	Cytomel; in Euthroid

Toxicity Rating: Low when recommended dosages are used.

Adverse Reactions

Adverse reactions to thyroid hormones mimic the clinical picture of hyperthyroidism.

Central Nervous System Thyroid hormones may cause hyperexcitability, insomnia, hypomania or depression, tremor, fatigue, muscle wasting, exophthalmos, and increased psychomotor activity.

Cardiovascular Tachycardia, systolic hypertension, arrhythmias, and palpitations may occur.

Gastrointestinal Polyphagia or diarrhea may occur. Polydipsia is common. Less commonly there may be anorexia, nausea, and vomiting.

Genitourinary Polyuria is common.

Dermatologic Diaphoresis, smooth skin, alopecia, and oily hair and skin may be noted.

Metabolic Weakness and weight loss are common. Heat intolerance may also be noted.

Miscellaneous Menstrual irregularities and amenorrhea may be noted.

Contraindications

Adrenal insufficiency is a contraindication.

Precautions

Administration of thyroid preparations must be undertaken with caution in patients with known cardiovascular disease, especially coronary insufficiency. Frequent laboratory evaluation of thyroid function may be necessary.

Drug Interactions

Thyroid hormones may increase the prothrombin time in patients on coumarin derivatives. Cholestyramine resin prevents the absorption of thyroid hormone. Diabetic patients who are given thyroid hormones will occasionally require more insulin. Digitalis requirements are sometimes increased when thyroid hormone therapy is begun in digitalized subjects.

Treatment

Withdrawal of the drug is usually all that is necessary to treat the reactions. When there has been an overdose (iatrogenic thyroid storm), administration of propranolol, steroids, sodium iodide, or other antithyroid drugs may be necessary. The reader is referred to Conn's Current Therapy* (page 494) for a detailed discussion of the management of this condition.

* Rakel, R. E. (ed): Current Therapy 1984. Philadelphia: Saunders, 1984.

Insulin

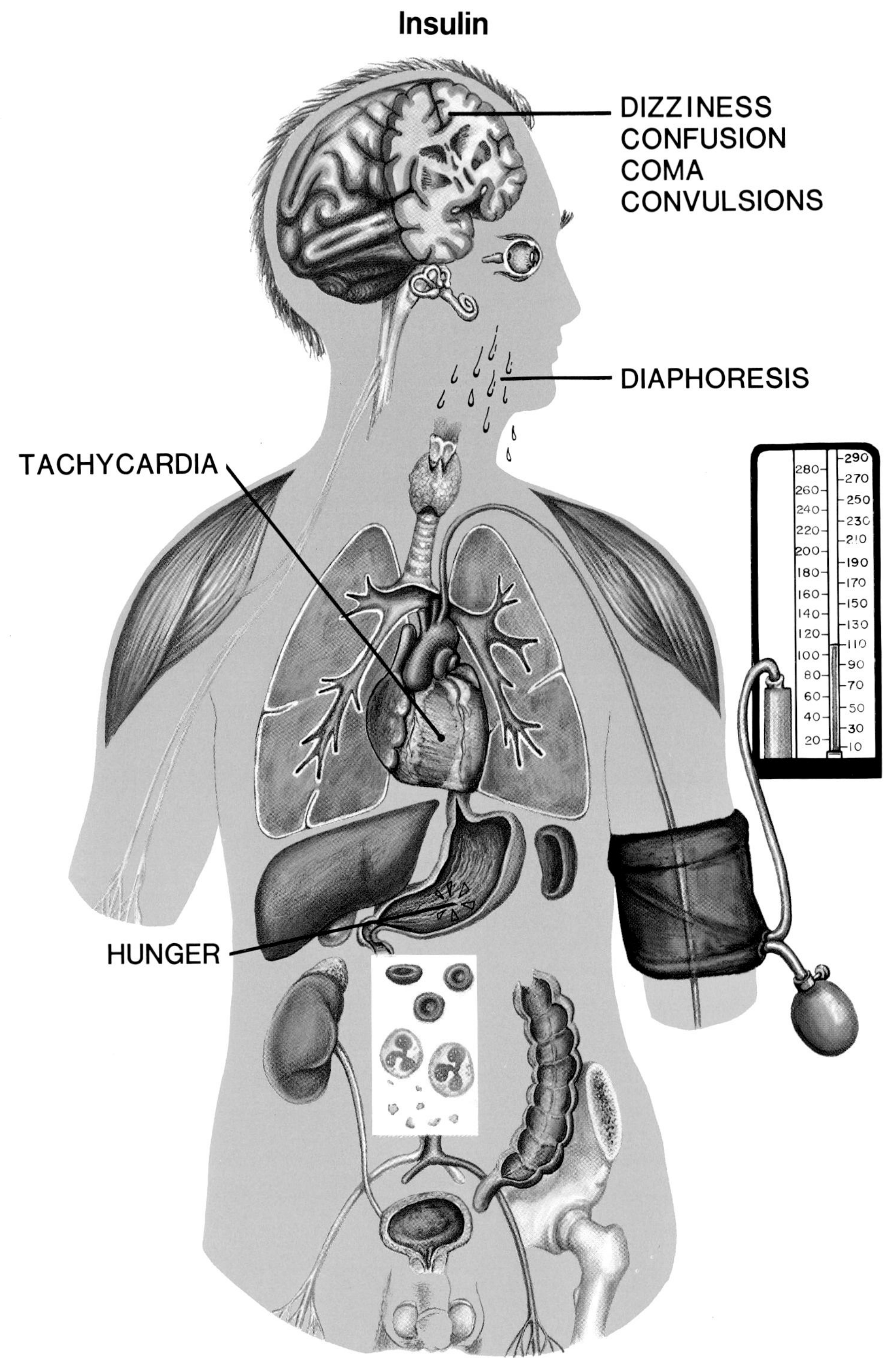
DIZZINESS
CONFUSION
COMA
CONVULSIONS
DIAPHORESIS
TACHYCARDIA
HUNGER

Insulin Preparations

Toxicity Rating: Low if used in therapeutic doses.

Adverse Reactions

Most of the reactions to insulin are due to hypoglycemia.

Central Nervous System Dizziness, weakness, irritability, confusion, and coma may occur. Convulsions have also been noted.

Cardiovascular Epinephrine release can cause tachycardia. Serious anaphylaxis occurs rarely.

Dermatologic Sweating is an important manifestation, although it is occasionally absent. Allergic skin rashes have been noted occasionally with almost all insulin preparations.

Contraindications

Known hypersensitivity to insulin preparations is the major contraindication.

Precautions

The diagnosis of insulin-dependent diabetes should be well established before giving insulin.

Treatment

Intravenous administration of 50% glucose solution is adequate to treat most reactions, but when a long-acting preparation has been given, hospitalization, continuous administration of 5 – 10 percent glucose solution, and careful monitoring of blood glucose levels may be necessary.

Gonadotropins

Principal Drug

Generic Name	Representative Trade Names
Chorionic gonadotropin	A.P.L., Profasi HP

Toxicity Rating: Low

Adverse Reactions

Central Nervous System Headache, irritability, depression, weakness, and nervousness are the principle CNS reactions.

Endocrinologic Precocious puberty and gynecomastia occur.

Other Rare allergic reactions and pain at the injection site have been noted.

Contraindications

Contraindications are precocious puberty, prostatic carcinoma, seminoma, and known hypersensitivity to gonadotropins.

Precautions

Therapy should be discontinued if signs of precocious puberty appear. Because androgens have been known to cause increased fluid retention, the gonadotropins, which stimulate androgen production, may cause edema in patients with preexisting cardiac, hepatic, or renal disease.

Treatment

Withdrawal of the drug should be sufficient treatment for most reactions.

Menotropins

Representative Trade Name: Pergonal

Toxicity Rating: Low to moderate due to the hyperstimulation syndrome (see below).

Adverse Reactions

Cardiovascular Rare cases of arterial thromboembolism have been reported.

Endocrinologic Ovarian enlargement with occasional hemoperitoneum may occur. If ovarian enlargement is sudden, there may be severe abdominal pain, ascites, and even pleural effusion (reminiscent of Meigs' syndrome).

Other Allergic reactions, including a febrile reaction, occur. Five cases of birth defects have been reported. Erythrocytosis and gynecomastia may occur in men given this hormone preparation.

Contraindications

Women with high levels of LH and FSH in the urine do not need this hormone preparation. Also, women with overt thyroid or adrenal disorders, intracranial neoplasms, abnormal menstrual bleeding, infertility not due to anovulation, ovarian cysts, and pregnancy should not be given this drug. Men should not take this drug if they have elevated LH or FSH levels in the urine, or if their infertility is considered to be due to primary gonadal failure.

Precautions

A thorough workup by a physician experienced in infertility should be performed prior to instituting menotropin therapy. The dosage must be carefully controlled, particularly in women, and the patient closely observed for ovarian enlargement and other signs of the hyperstimulation syndrome.

Treatment

If evidence of the hyperstimulation syndrome is seen, the patient must be hospitalized and the fluid and electrolyte balance carefully controlled. Sexual intercourse must be prohibited until ovarian size diminishes. Surgery may be required if rupture of an ovarian cyst occurs.

Growth Hormone (Somatropin)

Representative Trade Name: Asellacrin

Toxicity Rating: Low

Adverse Reactions

The only significant reaction to somatropin is the formation in 50 percent of patients of sufficient neutralizing antibodies to inhibit the action of the hormone. These antibodies should be tested for if clinical evidence indicates an inadequate response to therapy.

Contraindications

Patients with closed epiphyses will not benefit from this hormone. Progressive intracranial neoplasms (pituitary tumors) are another important contraindication.

Precautions

A slight risk of hepatitis transmission when the hormone is extracted from human serum is expected. Since the drug may cause hyperglycemia, caution must be exercised when giving it to diabetics. Local lipodystrophy may result from subcutaneous administration. Bone maturation must be monitored during therapy.

Treatment

Withdrawal of somatropin and treatment of allergic or anaphylactic reactions are the principle methods of management.

Vasopressin

Principal Drugs

Generic Name	Representative Trade Name
Vasopressin	Pitressin
Related drugs:	
Lypressin	Diapid
Desmopressin acetate	DDAVP

Toxicity Rating: Low

Adverse Reactions

The major reactions are local and systemic hypersensitivity, including anaphylactic shock. There may be tremor, sweating, vertigo, pounding in the head, abdominal distention, cramps, and gas, as well as nausea or vomiting.

Contraindications

Known hypersensitivity to the hormone is the only contraindication.

Precautions

Vasopressin and related drugs should be used with caution in patients with known coronary insufficiency, as myocardial infarction may occur. Since water intoxication may occur, the patient should be watched for such symptoms as drowsiness, listlessness, coma, and convulsions. Uremia should be corrected before these drugs are given.

Treatment

Withdrawal of the drug is sufficient for most reactions; allergic and anaphylactic shock must be treated if they develop.

Glucagon

Representative Trade Name: Glucagon

Toxicity Rating: Low

Adverse Reactions

The main adverse reactions reported are nausea and vomiting, and these symptoms may be due to preexisting hypoglycemia. Hypersensitivity is known but is fortunately rare.

Contraindications

The main contraindications are known hypersensitivity and preexisting insulinoma or pheochromocytoma (because glucagon may induce severe hypoglycemia or hypertensive crisis)

Precautions

Adequate liver glycogen must be available if glucagon is to be effective in the treatment of hypoglycemia.

Treatment

Withdrawal of the drug is sufficient.

Chapter 22

HYPNOTICS

Hypnotics

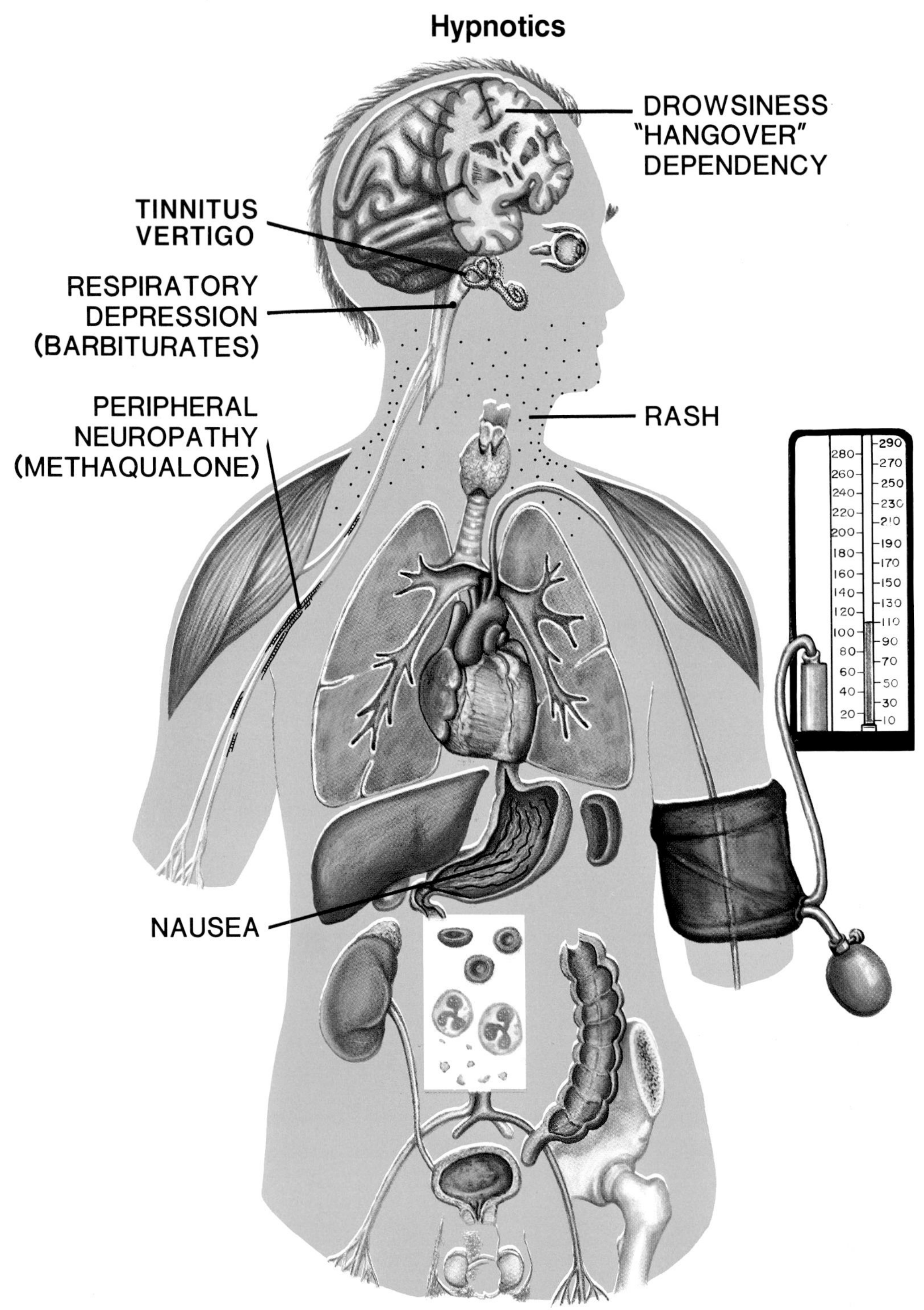
DROWSINESS
"HANGOVER"
DEPENDENCY
TINNITUS
VERTIGO
RESPIRATORY
DEPRESSION
(BARBITURATES)
PERIPHERAL
NEUROPATHY
(METHAQUALONE)
RASH
NAUSEA
280 260 240 220 200 180 160 140 120 100 80 60 40 20
290 270 250 230 210 190 170 150 130 110 90 70 50 30 10

Introduction

Principal Hypnotics

Flurazepam hydrochloride
Barbiturates
 Sodium pentobarbital
 Secobarbital sodium
Chloral hydrate
Glutethimide
Methyprylon
Methaqualone
Paraldehyde
Ethchlorvynol

The hypnotics are for the most part only mildly toxic. The search for a hypnotic without a hangover continues; so far flurazepam and temazepam seem to be the least likely to produce this side effect. All hypnotics produce drowsiness—their main therapeutic action. All of them can produce *physical* and *psychological dependency,* but flurazepam seems to have very little addictive potential. Because of the drowsiness, there is an additive effect when hypnotics are used with alcohol and other CNS depressants. Suicidal individuals should probably not receive these drugs except in a controlled environment. Most hypnotics produce a withdrawal reaction similar to delirium tremens, and close hospital supervision may be necessary during withdrawal. Despite all these disadvantages, the hypnotics remain a useful addition to the wise physician's armamentarium.

Flurazepam Hydrochloride

Representative Trade Name: Dalmane

Toxicity Rating: Low

Adverse Reactions

Central Nervous System Obviously, oversedation is the major side effect. Oversedation is followed by a significant hangover in up to 10 percent of patients. Respiratory and circulatory depression is unusual. Dependency can develop, and dizziness, ataxia, and even coma have occurred.

Other Rare cases of neutropenia, gastrointestinal distress, hypotension, skin rashes, and paradoxical excitation have occurred, as with other benzodiazepines.

Contraindications

Patients with known hypersensitivity to benzodiazepines or known addiction and drug dependency should not receive these drugs.

Treatment

Withdrawal of the drug is usually sufficient treatment.

Table 22-1. Side Effects of Hypnotics

Drug	Drowsiness	Hangover	Significant respiratory depression	Nausea, vomiting	Hematologic effects	Paradoxical excitation	Dependency	Other
Flurazepam hydrochloride	+	+	−	−	+	−	+	−
Barbiturates	+	++	+	−	−	+	++	−
Chloral hydrate	+	+	−	+	+	+	+	Somnambulism
Glutethimide	+	+	−	+	+	−	+	−
Methyprylon	+	+	−	+	+	+	+	−
Methaqualone	+	+	−	+	−	−	++	Peripheral neuropathy
Ethchlorvynol	+	+	−	−	+	++	++	Facial numbness
Paraldehyde	+	+	−	+	−	−	+	−

Barbiturates

Principal Drugs

Generic Name	Representative Trade Name
Sodium pentobarbital	Nembutal Sodium
Secobarbital sodium	Seconal Sodium

Toxicity Rating: Low

Adverse Reactions

Central Nervous System Oversedation, hangover, slurred speech, and ataxia are the major side effects.

Respiratory System Slowing of respirations and even apnea may occur.

Cardiovascular Hypotension and even shock are unusual but may occur.

Gastrointestinal Nausea, vomiting, and constipation occur rarely.

Allergic Any barbiturate may cause urticaria, angioneurotic edema, and various skin rashes.

Dependency These drugs are class II narcotics because both psychic and physical dependence do occur. Withdrawal reactions include convulsions and delirium.

Contraindications

Porphyria, known hypersensitivity, liver failure, severe emphysema, and a history of known addiction to barbiturates or other drugs are important contraindications.

Precautions

Paradoxical reactions are more frequent in the elderly and in children.

Drug Interactions

Barbiturates may decrease the potency of coumarin derivatives and cortisone preparations. They may potentiate the action of other CNS depressants.

Treatment

Withdrawal of the drug is usually sufficient. Careful observation and prophylaxis for seizures (with phenytoin, etc.) may be necessary during withdrawal after prolonged use.

Chloral Hydrate

Representative Trade Name: Noctec

Toxicity Rating: Low

Adverse Reactions

Central Nervous System Oversedation or hangover may occur but the most significant CNS side effect is somnambulism. Patients also may experience disorientation, paranoid behavior, hallucinations, and vertigo.

Gastrointestinal Nausea, vomiting, and diarrhea may occur.

Hematologic Neutropenia and eosinophilia have been noted.

Other Allergic reactions, headache, ketonuria, and a paradoxical excitability are occasionally reported. Chloral hydrate may be habit forming.

Contraindications

Patients with impaired renal, hepatic, or cardiac function should not take this drug. Obviously patients with known hypersensitivity should not be given the drug either. Preexisting gastric irritation is another contraindication. Known drug dependency to other sedatives is also a contraindication. Like the barbiturates, chloral hydrate may precipitate porphyria. Pregnancy is a relative contraindication.

Drug Interactions

Chloral hydrate may decrease the effect of coumarin drugs. Many side effects including change in blood pressure may occur when furosemide is given intravenously to someone who has just taken chloral hydrate. Like most sedatives, chloral hydrate can increase the effects of other CNS depressants.

Treatment

Withdrawal of the drug is usually all that is necessary.

Glutethimide

Representative Trade Name: Doriden

Toxicity Rating: Low

Adverse Reactions

Central Nervous System Drowsiness and hangover are not uncommon, and of course are only extensions of the therapeutic action of the drug. Less commonly, there may be vertigo, ataxia, headache, confusion, slurred speech, and tinnitus. Paradoxical excitation is rare.

Gastrointestinal Nausea is common but other gastrointestinal reactions are unusual.

Dermatologic A skin rash is observed in nearly 10 percent of patients, but it disappears when the drug is discontinued. Glutethimide, like barbiturates, may occasionally provoke porphyria.

Hemotologic Blood dyscrasias (thrombocytopenia, leukopenia, and anemia) occur but are rare.

Dependency Glutethimide may cause physical as well as psychological dependency, and withdrawal reactions such as nausea, tremors, convulsions, and delirium occur.

Contraindications

Porphyria and known hypersensitivity to the drug are the major contraindications. Obviously, patients prone to addiction or suicide should not be given this drug.

Precautions

Patients should be warned about the additive effects of glutethimide and other CNS depressants and about the risk of addiction. They should be warned to avoid driving an automobile or working around dangerous machinery while on glutethimide. Glutethimide should be administered to pregnant women only if clearly necessary.

Drug Interactions

Like other hypnotics, glutethimide enhances hepatic degradation of coumarin derivatives, and may thus shorten the prothrombin time in patients on this type of anticoagulant.

Treatment

Simple withdrawal of the drug is sufficient for mild side effects. However, when severe dependency is suspected, hospitalization with careful monitoring of vital signs, gradual withdrawal, and administration of anticonvulsants may be wise. Phenobarbital is occasionally substituted during the withdrawal phase. Hemodialysis may be necessary in acute overdosage.

Methyprylon

Representative Trade Name: Noludar

Toxicity Rating: Low to moderate in view of some of the central nervous system side effects, particularly in the elderly.

Adverse Reactions

Central Nervous System Convulsions, hallucinations, ataxia, and true vertigo occur. Like other hypnotics, methyprylon can cause morning drowsiness and hangover. More distressing is the organic psychosis encountered in the elderly. Paradoxical excitation (such as occurs with barbiturates) is also seen.

Gastrointestinal Nausea, vomiting, diarrhea, and constipation have all been observed.

Hematologic Bone marrow depression of one or more of the cellular elements of the blood is infrequent but has been encountered.

Allergic Rash, urticaria, and pruritus have been noted.

Dependency Physical and psychological dependency do occur. As with glutethimide, withdrawal from methyprylon can involve tremor, delirium, and convulsions.

Contraindications

Contraindications include known hypersensitivity, known addiction, and suicidal ideation.

Precautions

Patients with liver and kidney damage should be warned that they are more likely to accumulate the drug. Patients with porphyria may suffer an acute exacerbation while on the drug. The drug should not be given to patients who work around dangerous machinery.

Drug Interactions

Other CNS depressants (alcohol, etc.) enhance the effect of methyprylon.

Treatment

Simple withdrawal of the drug is usually sufficient, but in patients with a history of chronic usage, hospitalization for management of withdrawal symptoms may be indicated. Gradual withdrawal on an outpatient basis may be attempted if anticonvulsants are given concomitantly.

Methaqualone

Representative Trade Name: Quāālude

Toxicity Rating Low to medium primarily because of the potential for drug abuse.

Adverse Reactions

Central Nervous System The effects are similar to those of the other hypnotics. Acroparesthesias are more common and several cases of peripheral neuropathy have been reported. The major side effect of this drug is dependency. Tolerance to the drug is frequent in abusers and withdrawal reactions are not uncommon.

Treatment

Treatment is similar to that for adverse reactions to other hypnotics.

Paraldehyde

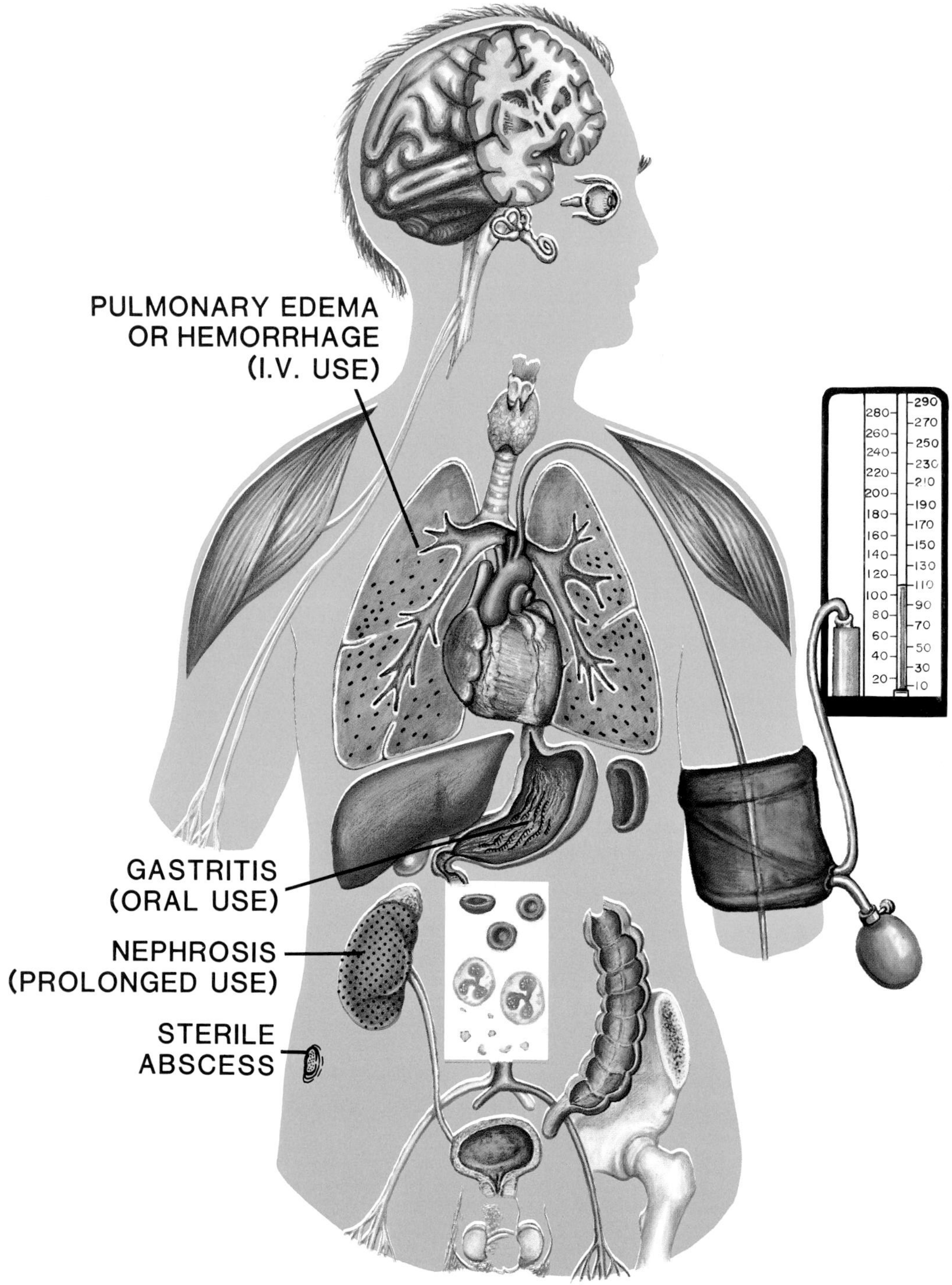

PULMONARY EDEMA
OR HEMORRHAGE
(I.V. USE)

GASTRITIS
(ORAL USE)

NEPHROSIS
(PROLONGED USE)

STERILE
ABSCESS

Paraldehyde

Representative Trade Name: Paraldehyde

Toxicity Rating: Low except when given intravenously.

Adverse Reactions

Central Nervous System Drowsiness and hangover are frequent side effects.

Gastrointestinal Oral administration may cause gastric irritation.

Respiratory Pulmonary edema and/or hemorrhage may occur with intravenous administration.

Genitourinary Nephrosis may occur with prolonged use.

Dermatologic An erythematous rash and other allergic reactions may occur.

Other Sterile abscesses, pain, and even sloughing of the skin at the site of the injection occur. A sweetish acetone-like breath results from the paraldehyde fumes.

Contraindications

This drug is contraindicated in patients with bronchopulmonary disease, gastroenteritis with ulceration, and known hypersensitivity to the drug.

Precautions

Paraldehyde should be used with caution in patients with hepatic dysfunction — the very patients who sometimes need it most.

Drug Interactions

Paraldehyde compounds the CNS depressant effects of alcohol. Disulfiram may increase blood concentrations of paraldehyde and acetaldehyde to toxic levels.

Treatment

Withdrawal of the drug is the major treatment as there is no antidote.

Ethchlorvynol

Representative Trade Name: Placidyl

Toxicity Rating: Low to moderate because of the tendency for physical and psychological dependency.

Adverse Reactions

Central Nervous System Drowsiness and hangover occur as with other hypnotics, but not quite as often. Paradoxical excitation seems to be more frequent and is manifested by excitement and hysteria. Facial numbness, weakness, fatigue, hypotension, and syncope have occurred.

Hematologic Thrombocytopenia has occurred.

Other Hypersensitivity reactions include urticaria, rash, and cholestatic jaundice, but are infrequent. Dependency, as mentioned above, is a very real hazard.

Contraindications

Like all hypnotics, ethchlorvynol should not be given to known addicts, suicidal patients, or patients with a history of dependency on other drugs or substances. Known hypersensitivity is another contraindication. Patients on ethchlorvynol should not work around dangerous machinery. The safety in pregnancy has not been established.

Drug Interactions

Simultaneous use of ethchlorvynol and alcohol, barbiturates, MAO inhibitors, or other CNS depressants is forbidden. The combined use of ethchlorvynol and a tricyclic antidepressant may cause delirium. Ethchlorvynol inhibits the anticoagulant activity of coumarin drugs.

Treatment

Treatment of side effects of ethchlorvynol is similar to that for other hypnotics.

Chapter 23

LAXATIVES

Laxatives

Principal Drugs

Generic Name	Representative Trade Name
Bulk laxatives	
Calcium polycarbophil	Mitrolan
Methylcellulose	Methylcellulose
Psyllium hydrocolloid	Effersyllium
Psyllium hydrophilic mucilloids	Metamucil
Mucosal irritants	
Bisacodyl	Dulcolax
Cascara sagrada	Cascara Sagrada
Castor oil	Castor Oil
Danthron	Modane
Phenolphthalein	Phenolax
Senna	Senokot
Stool softeners	
Docusate calcium (dioctyl calcium sulfosuccinate)	Surfak
Docusate potassium (dioctyl potassium sulfosuccinate)	Dialose
Docusate sodium (dioctyl sodium sulfosuccinate)	Colace
Lactulose	Chronulac
Lubricant laxatives	
Mineral oil	Mineral Oil
Saline laxatives	
Glycerin suppositories	Glycerine Suppositories
Magnesium citrate	Citrate of Magnesia
Magnesium sulfate	Epsom Salts
Milk of magnesia (magnesium hydroxide)	Milk of Magnesia
Enemas	
Sodium phosphate and sodium biphosphate	Fleet Enema

Toxicity Rating: Very low as most of these drugs are not absorbed and thus cause only local effects.

Adverse Reactions

Dependency This is perhaps the most frequent and important reaction to laxatives. Prolonged use of mucosal irritants (e.g. bisacodyl) can even produce radiographic changes ("cathartic colon").

Gastrointestinal Any laxative may cause severe diarrhea, which is merely an extension of its therapeutic effect. However, most laxatives also cause nausea, vomiting, and abdominal cramps. In cases of intestinal obstruction, severe abdominal pain may occur. Many laxatives cause decreased absorption of drugs (e.g., tetracycline) and vitamins. Prolonged ingestion of cascara and senna may give a picture on sigmoidoscopy identical to melanosis coli. Mineral oil may cause pruritus ani.

Metabolic Osmotically active laxatives (magnesium salts, etc.) may cause severe intravascular volume depletion in some cases. Magnesium absorption may be harmful in patients with renal disease who cannot excrete it.

Respiratory Lipoid pneumonia is possible if mineral oil is aspirated.

Allergic Phenolphthalein may produce skin rashes, nonthrombocytopenic purpura, and even anaphylaxis. Allergic reactions also occur to the color additive FD & C Yellow No. 5.

Contraindications

Magnesium salts (citrate of magnesia, etc.) are contraindicated in patients with renal disease, while sodium phosphates are contraindicated in congestive heart failure. Lactulose should be used with caution in diabetics as it contains lactose and galactose. Intestinal obstruction is an obvious contraindication.

Drug Interactions

Mineral oil may potentiate the action of coumarin drugs by inhibiting the absorption of vitamin K. Enemas and contact laxatives (castor oil, etc.) may cause potassium depletion and are potentially hazardous in patients on potassium-depleting diuretics or with preexisting hypokalemia.

Treatment

Simple withdrawal of the drug is usually sufficient therapy for most reactions. It is important to question any patients with chronic diarrhea and other gastrointestinal symptoms about chronic laxative abuse!

Chapter 24

LOCAL ANESTHETICS

Local Anesthetics

Principal Drugs

Generic Name	Representative Trade Name
Lidocaine hydrochloride	Xylocaine
Procaine hydrochloride	Novocain Hydrochloride
Bupivacaine hydrochloride	Marcaine Hydrochloride
Chloroprocaine hydrochloride	Nesacaine
Etidocaine hydrochloride	Duranest
Mepivacaine hydrochloride	Carbocaine Hydrochloride

Toxicity Rating: Low

Adverse Reactions

Allergic Reactions Allergic dermatitis of many varieties may result from either the anesthetic itself or the preservatives in the preparation (e.g., methylparaben). These reactions may be local or generalized. Systemic allergic reactions include edema, status asthmaticus, and anaphylactic shock.

Central Nervous System Excitation manifested by nervousness, tremor, or convulsions may occur. Depression manifested by drowsiness and unconsciousness is infrequent but has been observed. There may be respiratory arrest.

Cardiovascular Arrhythmias, hypotension, and cardiac arrest have occurred.

Other Blurred vision, nausea, and vomiting are reported.

Contraindications

The only absolute contraindications is known hypersensitivity to the anesthetics or other ingredients in the solution.

Precautions

The lowest dose possible for the particular local anesthesia required must be used to prevent adverse reactions. Elderly or malnourished patients require appropriately reduced dosage.

Drug Interactions

Echothiophate iodide may enhance the action of procaine. Bupivacaine, etidocaine, and lidocaine may cause cardiac arrhythmias when administered concomitantly with epinephrine and certain general anesthetics (halothane, cyclopropane, etc.). Local anesthetic preparations with epinephrine should not be used in patients on MAO inhibitors, tricyclic antidepressants, or phenothiazines.

Treatment

Severe allergic reactions, respiratory depression, and cardiac arrhythmias must be treated with epinephrine (0.2–1 ml of 1 : 1000 solution subcutaneously or 5–10 ml of 1 : 10,000 solution intravenously), ventilatory assistance, and antiarrhythmic drugs. Cardiopulmonary resuscitation equipment should be available if large doses of local anesthetics are going to be given. Convulsions can be controlled by intravenous barbiturates or diazepam and oxygen.

Chapter 25

NARCOTIC ANALGESICS

Narcotic Analgesics

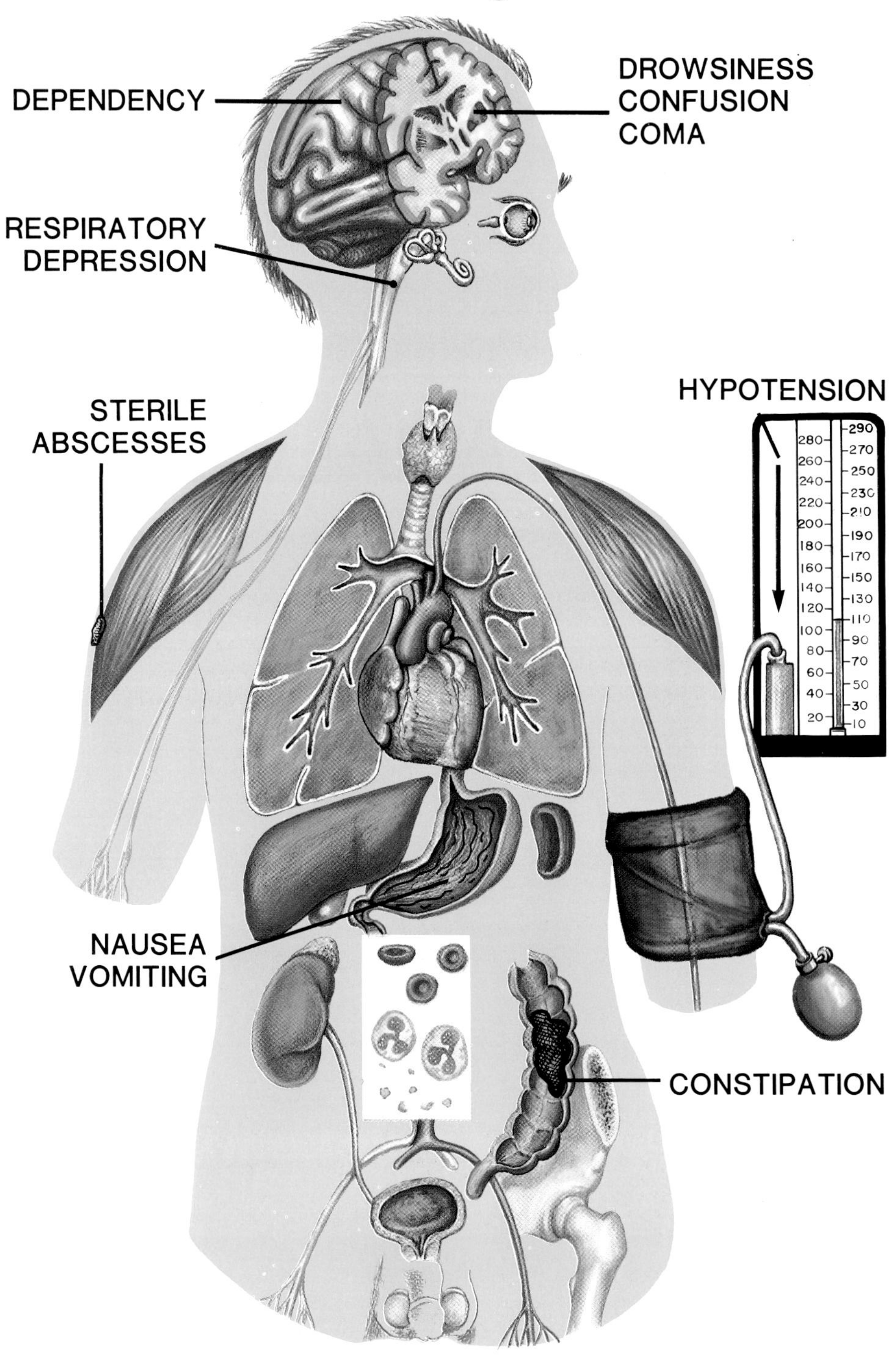
DEPENDENCY
DROWSINESS
CONFUSION
COMA
RESPIRATORY
DEPRESSION
STERILE
ABSCESSES
HYPOTENSION
280
260
240
220
200
180
160
140
120
100
80
60
40
20
290
270
250
230
210
190
170
150
130
110
90
70
50
30
10
NAUSEA
VOMITING
CONSTIPATION

Narcotic Analgesics

Principal Drugs

Generic Name	Representative Trade Name
Morphine sulfate	Morphine Sulfate
Codeine sulfate	Codeine Sulfate (and combinations with other narcotic analgesics)
Meperidine hydrochloride	Demerol Hydrochloride
Hydromorphone hydrochloride	Dilaudid Hydrochloride
Hydrochlorides of opium alkaloids	Pantopon
Oxymorphone hydrochloride	Numorphan
Levorphanol tartrate	Levo-Dromoran
Methadone hydrochloride	Dolophine Hydrochloride
Alphaprodine hydrochloride	Nisentil
Propoxyphene	Darvon and related compounds
Pentazocine hydrochloride	Talwin
Butorphanol tartrate	Stadol
Nalbuphine hydrochloride	Nubain
Buprenorphine	Buprenex
Oxycodone	In Percodan

Toxicity Rating: Medium primarily because of dependency—both physiological (addiction) and psychological.

Adverse Reactions

The adverse reactions to all the narcotic analgesics are very similar; they are compared in Table 25-1.

Central Nervous System Drowsiness, confusion, and occasional coma are the most common central nervous system reactions. These "adverse reactions" are merely an extension of the therapeutic effects of narcotic analgesics, because sedation raises the pain threshold. Vertigo, hallucinations, dizziness, disorientation, and even convulsions have occurred.

Respiratory Depression of respiration is a major side effect of narcotic analgesics and is more readily induced in elderly and debilitated patients. It has caused fatalities.

Gastrointestinal Gastrointestinal reactions are probably the most common side effects of the group as a whole. They include nausea, vomiting, colicky pain, and constipation.

Cardiovascular Hypotension and even vascular collapse may occur on parenteral administration of narcotic analgesics, but are unusual when they are given orally.

Dependency Dependency, of course, is a major side effect of narcotic analgesics.

Withdrawal Reactions All narcotic analgesics can cause withdrawal reactions, but as shown in Table 25-1, the severity of withdrawal symptoms differs greatly from drug to drug.

Other Sterile abscesses are not uncommon with intramuscular injections of narcotic analgesics, perhaps because injections are usually repeated frequently. Allergic reactions occur, but considering the

Table 25-1. Side Effects of Narcotic Analgesics

Drug	Sedation	Respiratory Depression	Hypotension	Gastro-intestinal Effects	Withdrawal Reactions	Hallucinations	Potential for Dependency	Other
Morphine	++	++	+	++	++	−	High	−
Codeine	+	−	−	+	+	−	High	−
Meperidine	+	++	++	+	++	−	High	−
Hydromorphone	+	+	+	+	+	−	High	−
Oxymorphone	++	++	+	++	+	−	High	−
Levorphanol	++	++	+	+	++	−	High	−
Methadone	+	−	−	++	+	−	Low	−
Alphaprodine	+	+	+	+	+	−	Medium	−
Propoxyphene	+	+	−	+	+	−	Low	−
Pentazocine	+	+	+	+	+	+	Low	Disorientation
Butorphanol	+	+	−	+	+	−	Low	−
Nalbuphine	+	+	+	+	+	+	Low	−
Buprenorphine	+	+	+	+	+	+	Medium	−
Oxycodone	+	+	−	+	+	++	High	−

widespread use of these drugs, they are very infrequent indeed.

Precautions

Narcotic analgesics should be used with caution in patients with myxedema, hepatic insufficiency, renal insufficiency, or adrenal insufficiency. Patients in shock from whatever cause may develop further hypotension with these drugs.

Drug Interactions

The CNS depression from other sedative drugs may be potentiated by narcotic analgesics. Meperidine may cause severe adverse reactions when used with MAO inhibitors. These include convulsions, hypertension, hypotension, hallucination, and respiratory depression.

Treatment

Most side effects can be treated by withdrawing the drug and awaiting metabolic detoxification. Sometimes hospitalization and careful attention to vital signs is necessary. The administration of naloxone may be necessary in severe respiratory and central nervous system depression.

Chapter 26

NARCOTIC ANTAGONISTS

Narcotic Antagonists

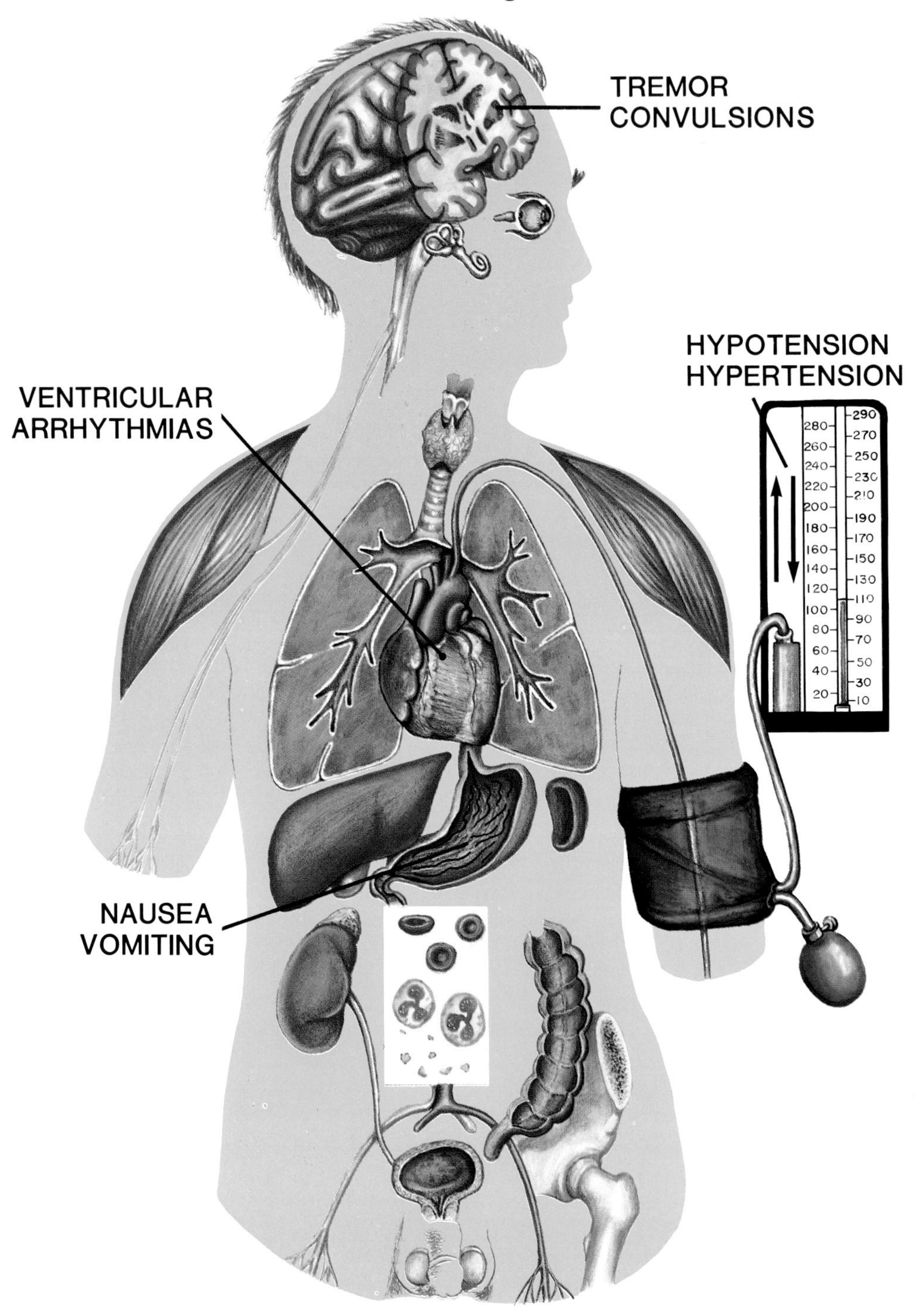

Narcotic Antagonists

Principal Drugs

Generic Name	Representative Trade Name
Naloxone hydrochloride	Narcan
Nalorphine hydrochloride	Nalline Hydrochloride
Levallorphan tartrate	Lorfan

Toxicity Rating: Low

Adverse Reactions

Central Nervous System Excitation of the nervous system may result in convulsions and tremor.

Cardiovascular Hypotension, hypertension, ventricular tachycardia, and fibrillation have been reported. There may be acute postoperative pulmonary edema.

Other Nausea, vomiting, and sweating may occur but allergic reactions are rare. Some sedation and analgesia may occur. An acute drug withdrawal reaction may occur.

Contraindications

Known hypersensitivity is the major contraindication.

Precautions

The dosage should be carefully adjusted to the patient's degree of sedation and respiratory depression, because an overdose may cause respiratory and CNS depression.

Treatment

Simple withdrawal of the drug is effective. However, if an acute withdrawal syndrome occurs, administration of mild sedatives may be necessary.

Chapter 27

NARCOTIC ANTIDIARRHEAL AGENTS

Narcotic Antidiarrheal Agents

Principal Drugs

Generic Name	Representative Trade Name
Diphenoxylate hydrochloride	in Lomotil (combination with atropine)
Loperamide hydrochloride	Imodium
Tincture of opium	Parepectolin
Paregoric (camphorated opium tincture)	Paregoric

Toxicity Rating: Low

Adverse Reactions

The side effects of these drugs are similar to those of the narcotic analgesics (Chapter 25). Consequently they may affect the central nervous system with sedation and confusion; the gastrointestinal system with nausea, vomiting, and constipation; and they are capable of causing physical dependence. However, definite physical dependence has not been a significant problem. Allergic reactions are unusual but may occur with all of these drugs. Respiratory depression is rare.

Contraindications

These drugs are prohibited in patients with known hypersensitivity and toxic megacolon. The safety in pregnancy and nursing mothers has not been established. These drugs are contraindicated in children under 2 years old.

Precautions

These drugs should be used with caution in inflammatory bowel disease, advanced liver disease, and amebic colitis. The use in children under age 12 is not recommended.

Treatment

Simple withdrawal of the drug is sufficient for the therapy of most reactions.

Chapter 28

NONSTEROIDAL ANTIINFLAMMATORY DRUGS

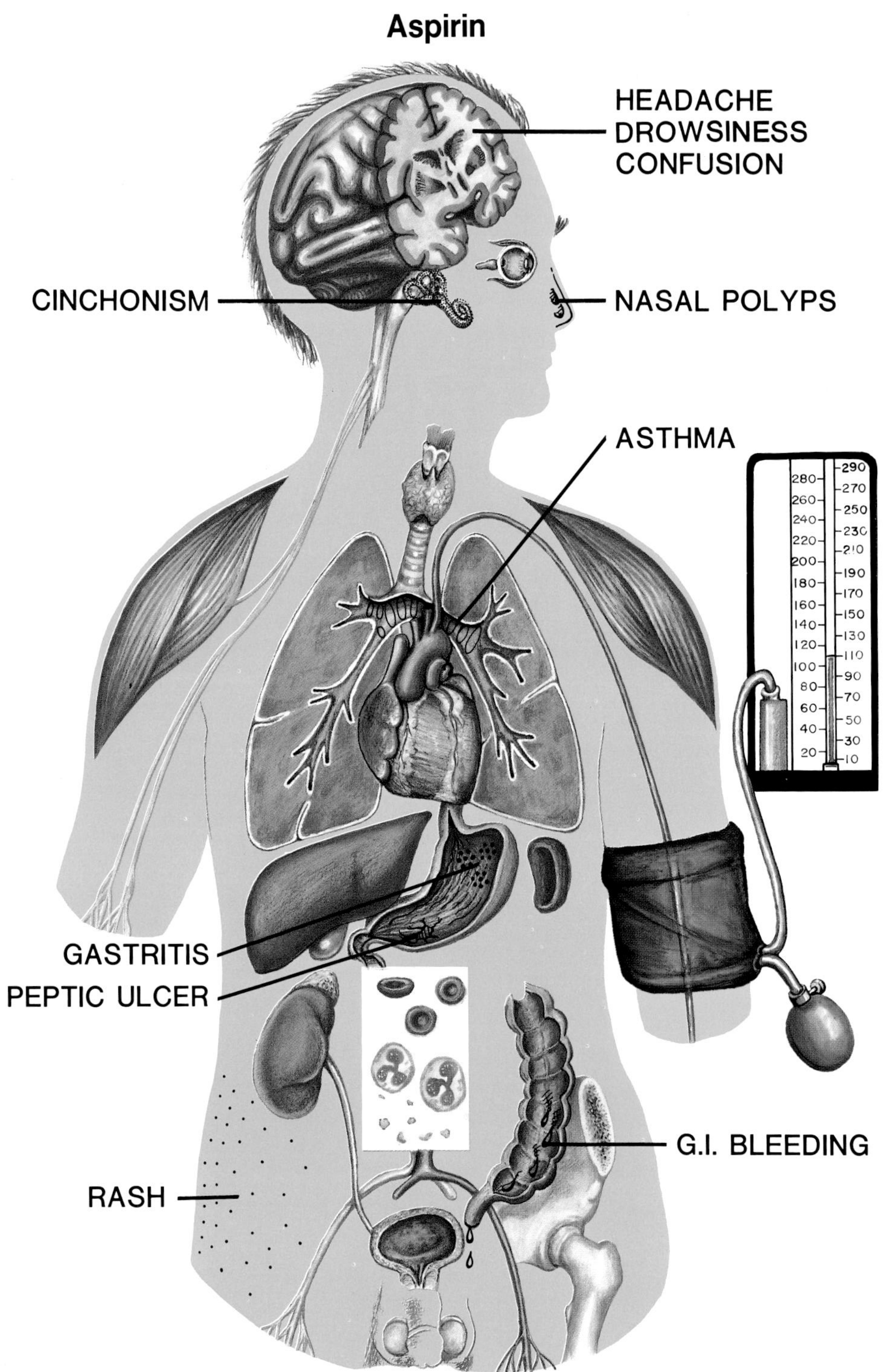
Aspirin
HEADACHE
DROWSINESS
CONFUSION
CINCHONISM
NASAL POLYPS
ASTHMA
GASTRITIS
PEPTIC ULCER
G.I. BLEEDING
RASH

Introduction

All of these drugs cause gastric irritation, peptic ulceration, and gastrointestinal bleeding. Some authorities hold that of the newer nonsteroidal antiinflammatory drugs, tolmetin sodium seems to have a greater tendency to cause peptic ulceration; this remains to be proven. These drugs are also hepatotoxic and nephrotoxic in a small percentage of cases. Phenylbutazone is the real sleeper in this group of drugs. It still remains among the top 200 drugs prescribed (according to the 1979 National Prescription Index) despite its ability to produce agranulocytosis and even fatal aplastic anemia. In the author's opinion, there is no justification for the popularity of this drug.

Aspirin

Principal Drugs

Generic Name	Representative Trade Name
Aspirin	Empirin
Related drugs:	
Sodium salicylate	Bayer Aspirin
Choline salicylate	
Salsalate	

Toxicity Rating: Low

Adverse Reactions

Central Nervous System Headache, drowsiness, and confusion occur, particularly in chronic intoxication.

Special Senses Tinnitus, hearing impairment, and occasional vertigo — a triad of symptoms that resembles cinchonism — occur. There may also be visual impairment.

Gastrointestinal Nausea, vomiting, heartburn, gastritis, and frank peptic ulceration, particularly of the gastric mucosa, are not uncommon. Prolonged aspirin administration can produce chronic ulceration of the gastric mucosa with mild or occasionally severe gastrointestinal bleeding.

Hematologic Because aspirin produces hypoprothrombinemia and interferes with platelet function, frequent bruising and excessive bleeding from lacerations or puncture wounds occur. Bone marrow depression has been reported, and rare hemolytic anemia may occur in patients with glucose-6-phosphate dehydrogenase deficiency.

Allergic Allergic reactions include urticaria, maculopapular rash, rhinorrhea, asthma, and gastroenteritis. Some patients develop a combination of nasal polyposis and asthma on chronic aspirin ingestion. Anaphylactic shock has been reported.

Other Hepatotoxicity has been reported.

Contraindications

Known hypersensitivity, severe coagulation disorders, and known peptic ulceration are the major contraindications.

Precautions

Aspirin should be administered with care in patients with a history of peptic ulcer or gastrointestinal bleeding. Patients with allergic rhinitis or asthma are

Phenylbutazone

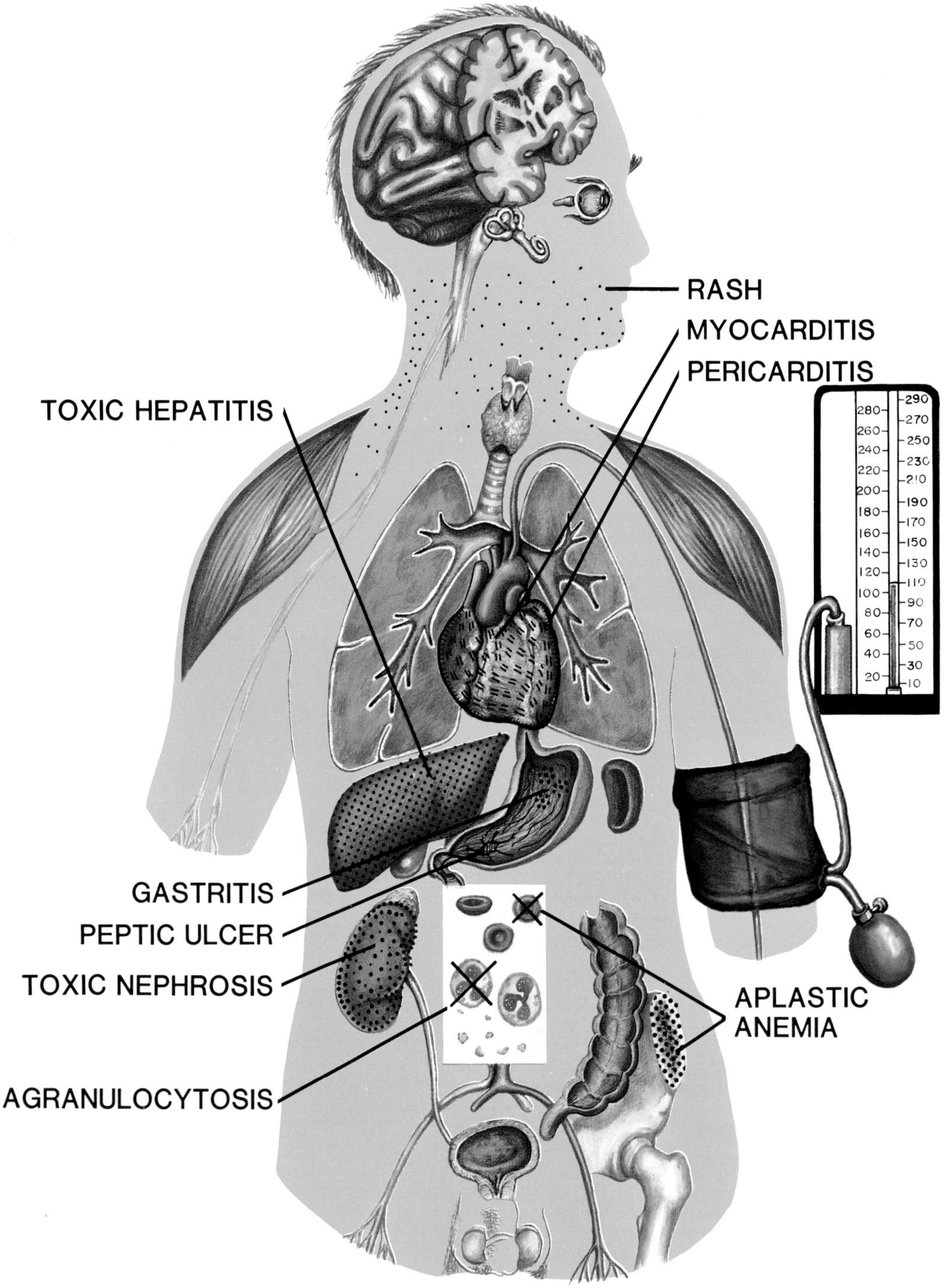

RASH
MYOCARDITIS
PERICARDITIS
TOXIC HEPATITIS
GASTRITIS
PEPTIC ULCER
TOXIC NEPHROSIS
APLASTIC
ANEMIA
AGRANULOCYTOSIS

more prone to aspirin hypersensitivity. Aspirin should also be given cautiously in patients with hepatic, renal, or cardiac insufficiency and a history of blood dyscrasias or coagulation disorders. Frequent monitoring of liver, renal, or coagulation function may be indicated under these circumstances. Monitoring of serum salicylate levels makes good sense in chronic therapy.

Drug Interactions

Aspirin enhances the anticoagulant effects of coumarin drugs. Aspirin may also increase the hypoglycemic effect of oral antidiabetic agents and insulin. The effects of MAO inhibitors, pencillin, sulfonamides, and certain cancer chemotherapeutic agents are enhanced by aspirin. Aspirin may potentiate the action of corticosteroids by displacing them from their protein binding sites. The effect of uricosuric agents (e.g., probenecid) is reduced by salicylates. Furosemide, vitamin C, and aminosalicyclic acid may cause the accumulation of toxic levels of aspirin. There are also numerous laboratory tests (serum amylase, blood glucose, cholesterol, etc.) the results of which may be altered by aspirin therapy.

Treatment

Simple withdrawal of the drug is usually all that is necessary. In severe bleeding, vitamin K and fresh whole blood may be necessary. Large doses of aspirin may cause respiratory alkalosis and cardiac insufficiency requiring appropriate therapy.

Phenylbutazone

Principal Drugs

Generic Name	Representative Trade Name
Phenylbutazone	Butazolidin
Related drug:	
Oxyphenbutazone	Tandearil

Toxicity Rating: High because of the potential of phenylbutazone to cause bone marrow depression and renal disease.

Adverse Reactions

Gastrointestinal Like aspirin, phenylbutazone can cause nausea, vomiting, gastritis, and peptic ulceration; gastrointestinal bleeding and perforation of the intestinal tract may also occur. Fatal hepatitis has been noted.

Hematologic Unlike aspirin, phenylbutazone causes agranulocytosis and even aplastic anemia in a small but significant number of patients.

Cardiovascular Unlike aspirin, phenylbutazone may cause significant edema, congestive heart failure, pericarditis, and myocarditis.

Renal Glomerulonephritis, nephrosis, and tubular necrosis may occur.

Allergic Like aspirin, phenylbutazone can induce urticaria, drug fever, and anaphylaxis. However, phenylbutazone may also cause an allergic vasculitis and aggravate lupus erythematosus and temporal arteritis. Various other skin reactions occur (erythema nodosum, erythema multiforme, etc.).

Other Tinnitus and hearing loss may occur (as with aspirin). Drowsiness, headaches, and confusion have also been reported.

Contraindications

Contraindications to phenylbutazone are known hypersensitivity, cardiac failure, blood dyscrasias, temporal arteritis, pancreatitis, preexisting renal or he-

Newer Nonsteroidal Antiinflammatory Agents

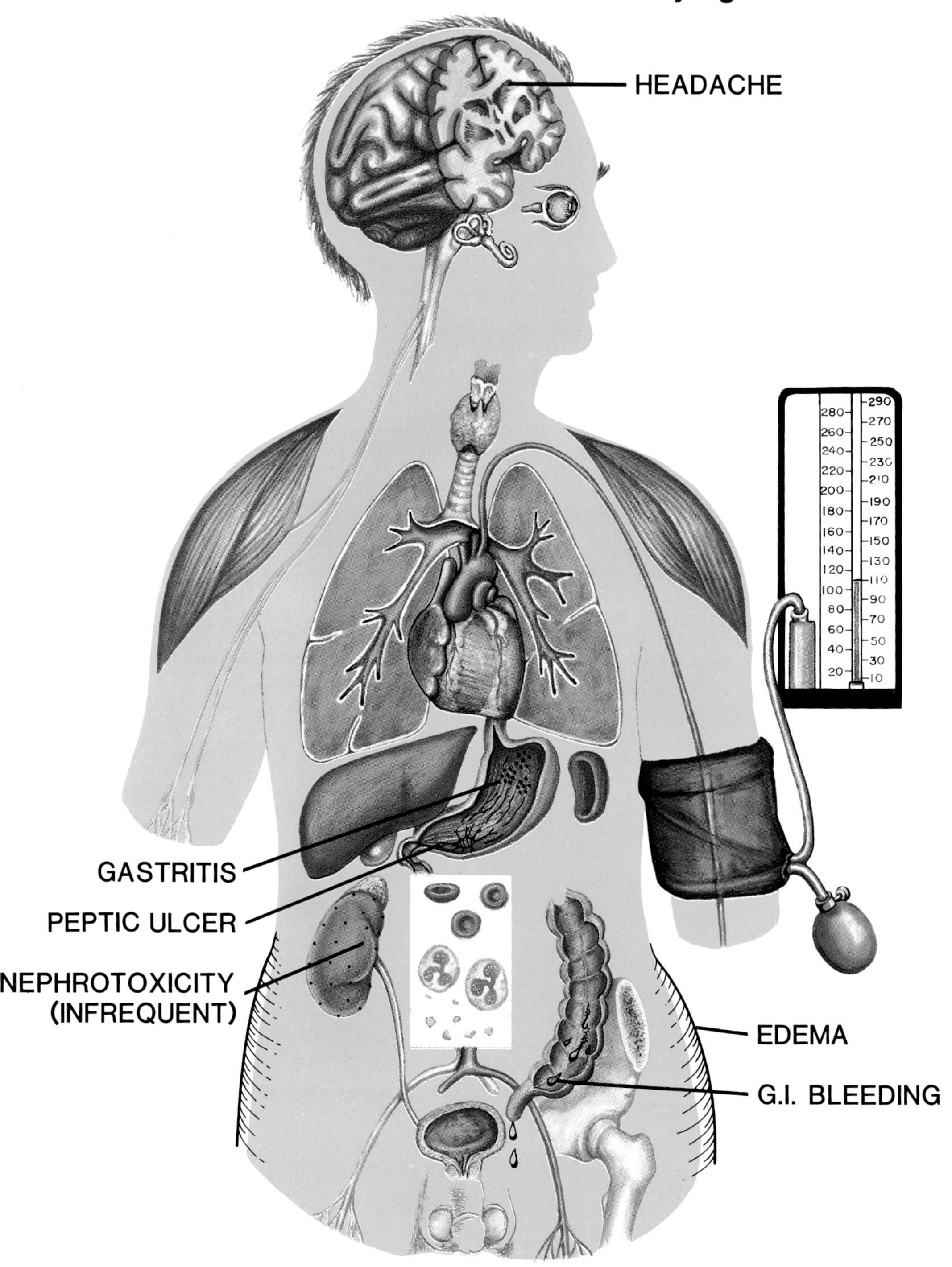

patic disease, and active or inactive peptic ulceration. Phenylbutazone should not be used with other drugs that can also produce any of its serious adverse reactions. It is also unwise to give this drug during pregnancy.

Precautions

Before receiving phenylbutazone, patients should have a complete physical examination, hemogram, urinalysis, and hepatic and renal function tests. These examinations should be repeated at regular intervals throughout the period of therapy. Elderly patients should be given only a short course of therapy. Patients taking this drug should be told to report any visual disturbances immediately!

Drug Interactions

Phenylbutazone potentiates the action of oral anticoagulants, oral antidiabetic agents, insulin, and sulfonamides. The drug may also elevate serum levels of phenytoin, producing toxicity.

Treatment

Simple withdrawal of the drug is usually all that is necessary if the patient has been carefully monitored by laboratory studies during therapy. Aplastic anemia and cardiac, renal, and liver toxicity should be treated in consultation with the appropriate specialist without delay.

Newer Nonsteroidal Antiinflammatory Drugs

Principal Drugs

Generic Name	Representative Trade Name
Diflunisal	Dolobid
Fenoprofen calcium	Nalfon
Ibuprofen	Motrin
Indomethacin	Indocin
Meclofenamate sodium	Meclomen
Mefenamic acid	Ponstel
Naproxen	Naprosyn
Piroxicam	Feldene
Sulindac	Clinoril
Tolmetin sodium	Tolectin

Adverse Reactions

Gastrointestinal The most serious pathologic reactions to these drugs are peptic ulcer and gastrointestinal bleeding. Symptoms such as nausea, dyspepsia, flatulence, diarrhea, and vomiting are also frequent.

Cardiovascular Edema is a common reaction to these drugs but is usually reversible upon discontinuing the drug.

Hematologic A few patients develop anemia and granulocytopenia.

Central Nervous System Headache occurs in as many as 1 percent of patients. Nervousness, dizziness, and lightheadedness as well as insomnia and depression are occasionally encountered.

Special Senses Tinnitus, hearing disturbance, and visual disturbances are reported.

Dermatologic Rash, pruritus, and other skin irritations may occur but are fortunately infrequent.

Other Asthenia, chest pain, and anaphylactoid reactions have been reported.

Table 28-1. Side Effects of Newer Nonsteroidal Antiinflammatory Drugs

Drug	Ulcers and Gastrointestinal Bleeding	Edema	Anemia, Thrombocytopenia, Granulocytopenia	Headache	Other CNS Reactions	Tinnitus	Visual Disturbance	Rash	Allergic Reactions	Hepatic Reactions	Renal Toxicity
Sulindac	+	+ (congestive heart failure)	+	+	+	+	+	+	+	+	−
Indomethacin	+	+	+	+	+	+	+ (corneal deposits)	+	+	+	−
Meclofenamate	+	+	+	+	+	+	+	+	+	−	+
Ibuprofen	+	+	+	+	+	+	+	+	+	+	+
Fenoprofen	+	+	+	+ (in 15%)	+	+	+	+	+	+	+
Naproxen	+	+	+	+	+	+	+	+	+	+	+
Tolmetin sodium	+ (peptic ulcers in more than 1%)	+	+	+	+	+	−	+	+	+	+
Piroxicam	+	+ (hypertension)	+	+	+	−	+	+	−	+	+

Reactions to Specific Drugs

Reactions peculiar to or more frequent with specific drugs in this group, as well as the reactions common to all of them, are shown in Table 28-1.

Sulindac

A hypersensitivity syndrome has been reported with fever, chills, skin rash, and hematologic and liver function abnormalities. True vertigo has been reported with this drug. Stomatitis and a Stevens-Johnson syndrome have recently been reported. Azotemia may occur in patients with preexisting renal disease.

Indomethacin

Headache is more common with this drug than with the other agents in this group. Indomethacin may aggravate psychiatric disorders, epilepsy, and parkinsonism. It has been known to cause convulsions and peripheral neuropathy. Cardiovascular disturbances include palpitations and arrhythmias. Metabolic disturbances include hypoglycemia and hyperkalemia. Toxic hepatitis is reported.

Meclofenamate

Renal failure occurs in less than 1 percent of patients. Peptic ulcer occurs in more than 1 percent of patients.

Ibuprofen

Renal papillary necrosis is rare, but acute renal failure in patients with preexisting renal disease may be more frequent. Gynecomastia and hypoglycemic reactions are rare, and their cause-and-effect relationship with ibuprofen has not been established. These symptoms have occasionally been reported with other drugs in this group.

Naproxen

Toxic nephritis and the nephrotic syndrome occur occasionally, but toxic hepatitis is rarely reported.

Tolmetin Sodium

Peptic ulcer occurs more frequently with this drug (in one of 50 patients) than with the others in this group. However, liver and renal toxicity seems to be less frequent with this drug.

Summary

It can be seen that all of the reactions listed in Table 28-1 can occur with any of the drugs in this group, but those that cause a higher incidence of peptic ulceration seem to cause renal or hepatic toxicity infrequently.

Precautions

1. These drugs should be used with caution in patients with known peptic ulceration, previous gastrointestinal bleeding, or other gastrointestinal disorders.
2. When there is known preexisting hepatic or renal disease, the benefits of these drugs should be weighed against the potential hazards. Close observation of hepatic and renal function should be maintained.
3. Caution should be observed in giving these drugs to patients with hypertension and heart failure because of the increased fluid retention they may cause.
4. Periodic ophthalmic examinations are recommended because of the visual disturbances that are known to occur.
5. Concurrent administration of aspirin with these drugs may decrease the net antiinflammatory action and lower the blood level of the newer nonsteroidal antiinflammatory agent.
6. Use of these drugs with aspirin and corticosteroids increases their ulcerogenic potential.
7. These drugs should not be given during pregnancy.
8. While these drugs may not prolong prothrombin times, they do increase the bleeding time by their effects on platelet agglutination, and they should

thus be used with caution when other anticoagulants are given.

Treatment

Obviously, most symptoms can be relieved by withdrawing the drug; however, this may not be necessary unless there is evidence of peptic ulceration, gastrointestinal bleeding, significant edema, or hepatic or renal toxicity. Persistent visual disturbances, especially when confirmed by ophthalmologic examination, are a clear indication for withdrawing the drug. Appropriate therapy of ulcers and gastrointestinal bleeding is required.

Contraindications

Known active peptic ulceration or gastrointestinal bleeding are the most important contraindications. Patients with known hypersensitivity to aspirin or other antiinflammatory drugs should not receive these drugs.

Chapter 29

NONNARCOTIC ANALGESICS

Acetaminophen

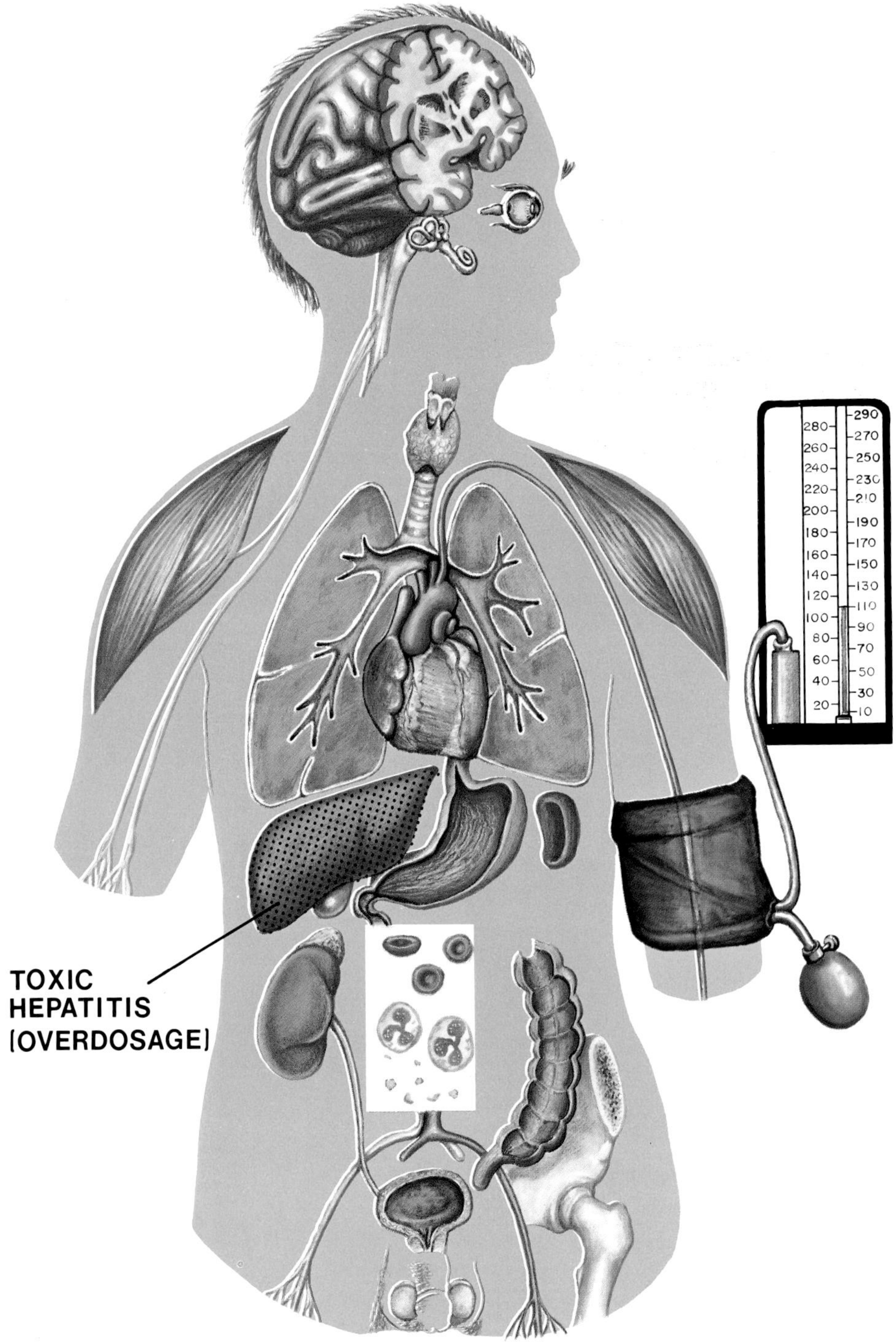

TOXIC
HEPATITIS
(OVERDOSAGE)

Nonnarcotic Analgesics

Principal Drugs

Acetaminophen
Aspirin (see page 225)
Mefenamic acid (see page 229)
Diflunisal (see page 229)

Acetaminophen

Representative Trade Name: Tylenol

Toxicity Rating: Very low since acetaminophen has rare side effects in therapeutic doses.

Adverse Reactions

Because this drug is a metabolite of phenacetin, claims of possible renal damage have been made, but they have not been adequately substantiated. There are no reports of gastric irritation, ulcers, or bleeding with acetaminophen, unlike aspirin. Hypersensitivity and drug interactions are rare. In cases of overdosage (usually deliberate) severe and fatal toxic hepatitis may occur.

Contraindications

There are no contraindications except known hypersensitivity, which is exceedingly rare.

Treatment

Withdrawal of the drug is sufficient for the minimal side effects that occur with therapeutic doses. However, with overdosage, the administration of acetylcysteine will replenish the glutathione important in detoxification of acetaminophen.

Chapter 30

ORAL ANTIDIABETIC AGENTS

Oral Antidiabetic Agents

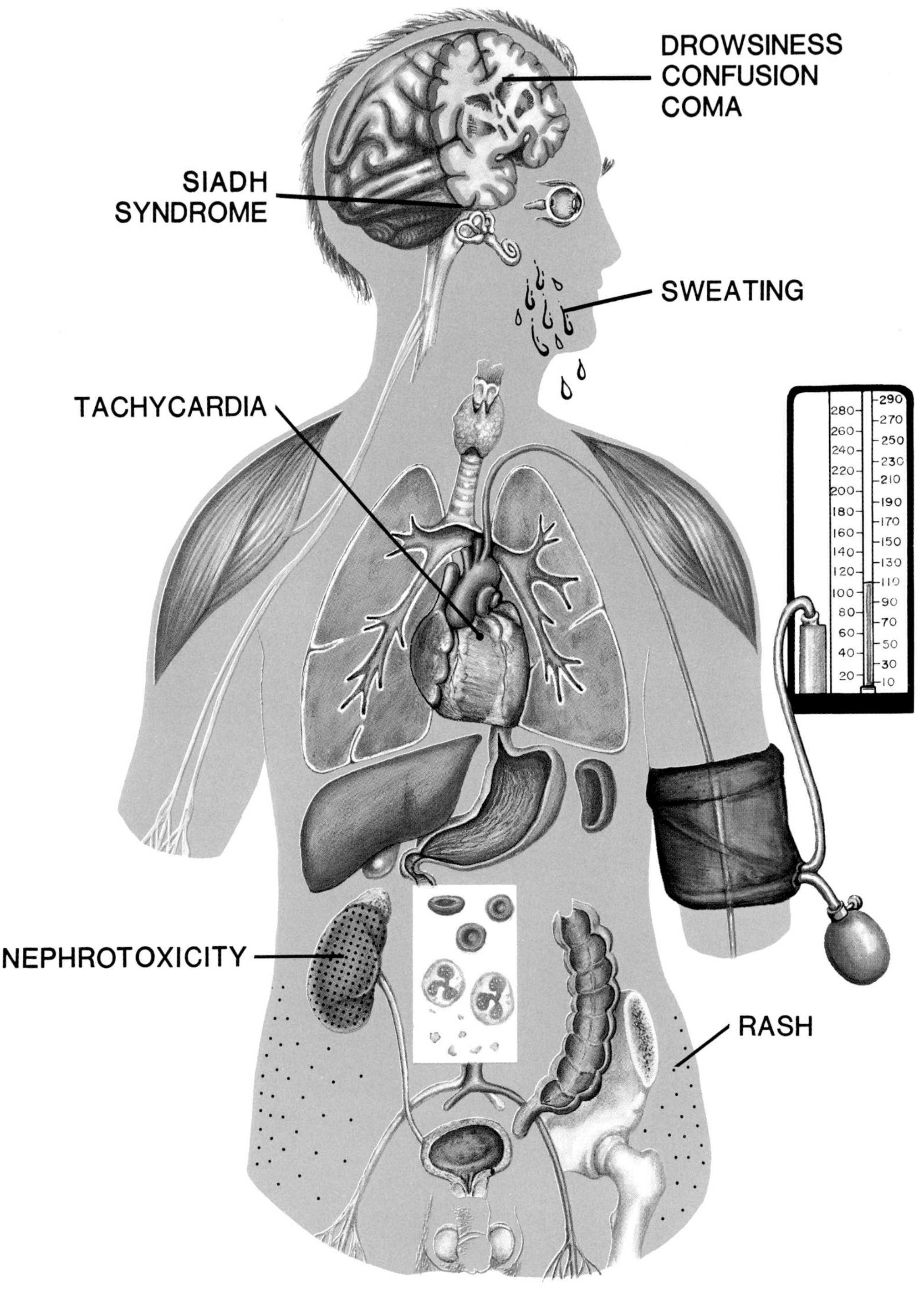

Oral Antidiabetic Agents

Principal Drugs

Generic Name	Representative Trade Name
Tolbutamide	Orinase
Chlorpropamide	Diabinese
Acetohexamide	Dymelor
Tolazamide	Tolinase
Glipizide	Glucotrol
Glyburide	Micronase

Toxicity Rating: These drugs are low to medium in toxicity since they can produce severe hypoglycemia.

Adverse Reactions

Endocrinologic Severe hypoglycemia is the most important side effect. The drugs are mildly goitrogenic in animals.

Central Nervous System The CNS reactions are secondary to hypoglycemia. There may be drowsiness, delirium, and coma, with sweating and tachycardia from catecholamine release. The neurologic signs may mimic almost any neurologic disorder including stroke.

Gastrointestinal Cholestatic hepatitis has occurred rarely.

Genitourinary The syndrome due to inappropriate ADH release (SIADH) may result from sulfonylurea therapy, causing dilutional hyponatremia.

Allergic Like all sulfa compounds these drugs may cause erythema, urticaria, and maculopapular eruptions. These reactions are frequently transient.

Other Rarely, bone marrow depression, headache, nausea and vomiting may occur. A flushing reaction may occur when glipizide is ingested with alcohol.

Contraindications

These drugs are contraindicated in juvenile diabetic coma and diabetic ketosis. These drugs should also not be used in severe renal insufficiency. The sulfonylureas should not be used during pregnancy.

Drug Interactions

Hypoglycemia may result from ingestions of alcohol, salicylates, propranolol, dicoumarol, sulfonamides, and phenylbutazone while taking the sulfonylureas. Severe nausea and vomiting may develop when chlorpropamide and alcohol are taken together.

Hyperglycemia may develop in patients trying to control their diabetes with sulfonylureas if they take oral contraceptives, glucocorticoids, or thiazide diuretics concurrently.

Treatment

Withdrawal of the drugs and administering 10–15 percent glucose intravenously or glucagon is the best treatment for hypoglycemia. With the longer-acting sulfonylureas (chlorpropamide, etc.), hospitalization for continued intravenous glucose and monitoring of the blood sugar may be necessary. Other reactions usually subside when the drug is withdrawn. Inappropriate ADH release may necessitate therapy with demeclocycline HCL or lithium to reduce the dilutional hyponatremia until the effect of the drug is removed.

Chapter 31

PARASITICIDAL AGENTS

Chloroquine Hydrochloride

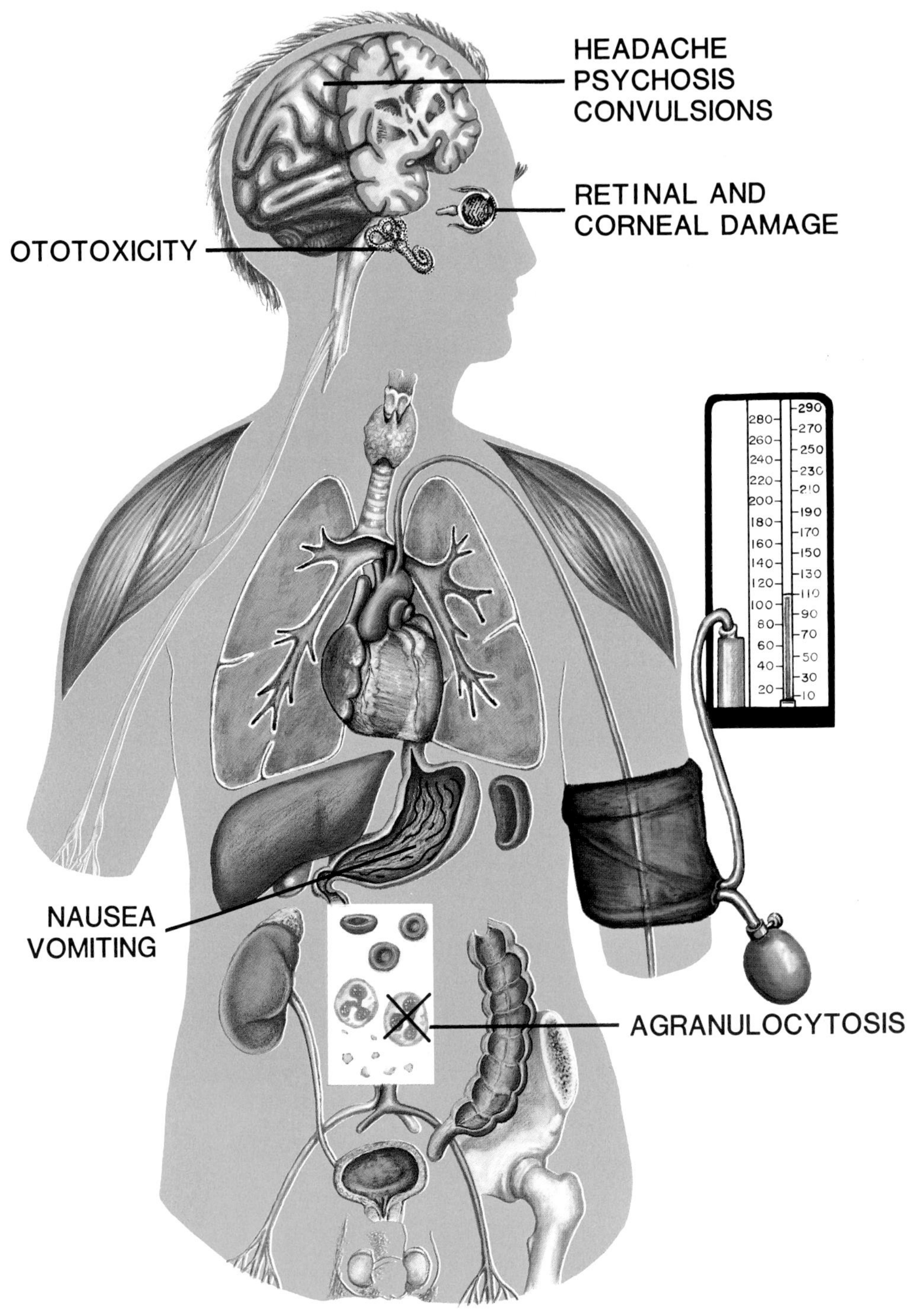

Parasiticidal Agents

Principal Drugs

ANTIMALARIAL AGENTS

- Chloroquine hydrochloride
  - Related drugs:
    - Chloroquine phosphate
    - Hydroxychloroquine sulfate
    - Amodiaquin hydrochloride
- Pyrimethamine
- Primaquine phosphate
- Quinine sulfate (see page 27)

AMEBICIDES

- Iodoquinol (diiodohydroxyquin)
- Emetine hydrochloride
- Metronidazole
  - Related drug:
    - Tinidazole
- Paromomycin sulfate
- Oxytetracycline hydrochloride (see page 101)

ANTHELMINTICS

- Bithionol
- Bephenium hydroxynaphthoate
- Dichlorophen
- Diethylcarbamazine citrate
- Mebendazole
- Niclosamide
- Niridazole
- Piperazine citrate
- Pyrantel pamoate
- Pyrvinium pamoate
- Stibocaptate
- Thiabendazole

ANTIMALARIAL AGENTS

Chloroquine Hydrochloride

Principal Drugs

Generic Name	Representative Trade Name
Chloroquine hydrochloride	Aralen Hydrochloride
Related drugs:	
Chloroquine phosphate	Aralen Phosphate
Hydroxychloroquine sulfate	Plaquenyl Sulfate
Amodiaquin hydrochloride	Camoquin

Toxicity Rating: Moderate because of rare instances of hypotension, cardiovascular collapse, and convulsions.

Adverse Reactions

Central Nervous System Headache, psychosis, and convulsions are rare but do occur.

Pyrimethamine

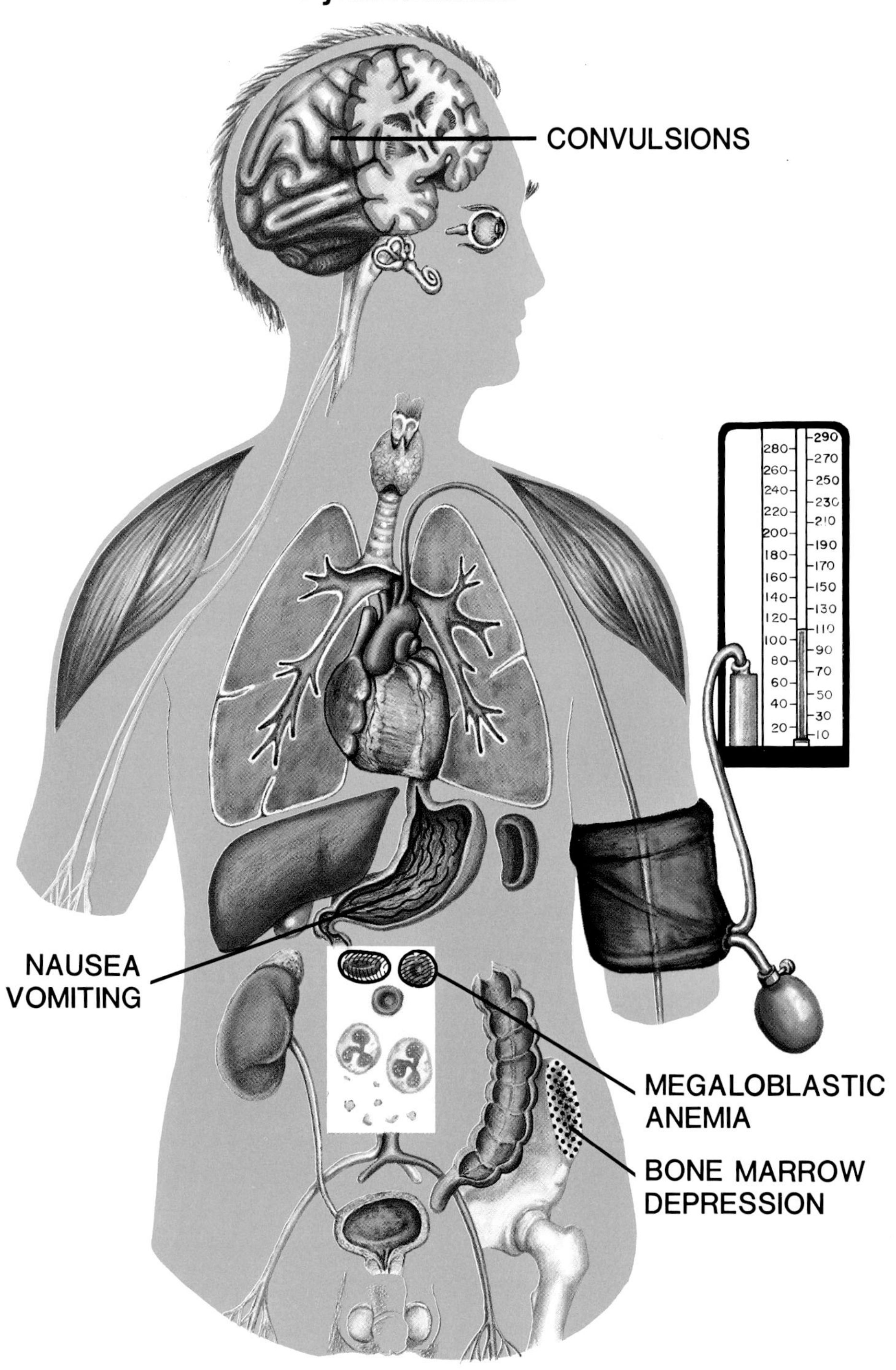

Special Senses Nerve deafness, blurred vision, scotoma, and retinal damage have occurred.

Gastrointestinal Nausea, vomiting, abdominal cramps, and diarrhea may be observed.

Other Blood dyscrasias, neuromyopathy, lichen-planus eruptions, and mucosal pigment changes occur. Overdosage may produce cardiac arrest, especially in children.

Contraindications

Known hypersensitivity and preexisting retinal or visual field impairment are good reasons for not using this drug.

Precautions

Chloroquine should be used with caution in patients with psoriasis, porphyria, or previous retinal damage. The drug should be avoided during pregnancy and in the presence of preexisting liver damage.

Treatment

Simple withdrawal of the drug may be all that is necessary, but if respiratory depression or shock has occurred, intensive treatment with oxygen, intravenous fluids, and phenylephrine HCl parenterally will be necessary.

Pyrimethamine

Representative Trade Name: Daraprim

Toxicity Rating: Low to moderate depending on the dosage.

Adverse Reactions

Gastrointestinal Anorexia, nausea, and vomiting are noted with large doses.

Hematologic Bone marrow depression with megaloblastic anemia, leukopenia, and thrombocytopenia occur, especially with the large doses needed in toxoplasmosis.

Other Excessive doses of this drug may cause convulsions.

Contraindications

Known hypersensitivity is the major contraindication.

Precautions

Since large doses produce a relative folic acid deficiency, folinic acid should be given at the first sign of bone marrow depression. A dose of 3 – 9 mg may be given intramuscularly. Pyrimethamine should be used cautiously in pregnancy since teratogenic effects have been known to occur in animals. Frequent blood and platelet counts should be done during high-dose therapy.

Treatment

Withdrawal of the drug is often all that is necessary, but if the drug must be continued despite reactions, folinic acid should be given concomitantly. A parenteral barbiturate should be given for convulsions.

Primaquine Phosphate

Representative Trade Name: Aralen Phosphate with Primaquine Phosphate

Toxicity Rating: Low

Adverse Reactions

Hematologic This drug may cause hemolytic anemia in patients with preexisting glucose-6-phosphate dehydrogenase deficiency, but the hemolysis is usually self-limited.

Gastrointestinal Mild abdominal cramps and epigastric distress may occur, but as a rule are not a reason to stop the drug.

Contraindications

Known hypersensitivity is the only significant contraindication.

Precautions

Known glucose-6-phosphate dehydrogenase deficiency should be a reason for frequent blood counts and observation for hemolysis.

Treatment

Simple withdrawal of the drug is usually all that is necessary.

AMEBICIDES

Iodoquinol (Diiodohydroxyquin)

Representative Trade Name: Yodoxin

Toxicity Rating: Low

Adverse Reactions

Dermatologic Several types of skin eruptions occur, including urticaria, acne, bullae, and tuberous iododerma.

Gastrointestinal Nausea, vomiting, abdominal distress and diarrhea may occur. Pruritus ani is also reported.

Other Fever, thyroid enlargement, elevated protein-bound iodine, optic neuritis, and peripheral neuropathy are infrequently reported.

Contraindications

Known hypersensitivity to this drug and other iodine preparations is the major contraindication. Safety in pregnancy has not been established.

Precautions

This drug should be used with caution in patients with thyroid disease. Thyroid function may be altered for up to 6 months after therapy with this drug.

Treatment

Simple withdrawal of the drug is usually all that is necessary.

Emetine Hydrochloride

Emetine Hydrochloride

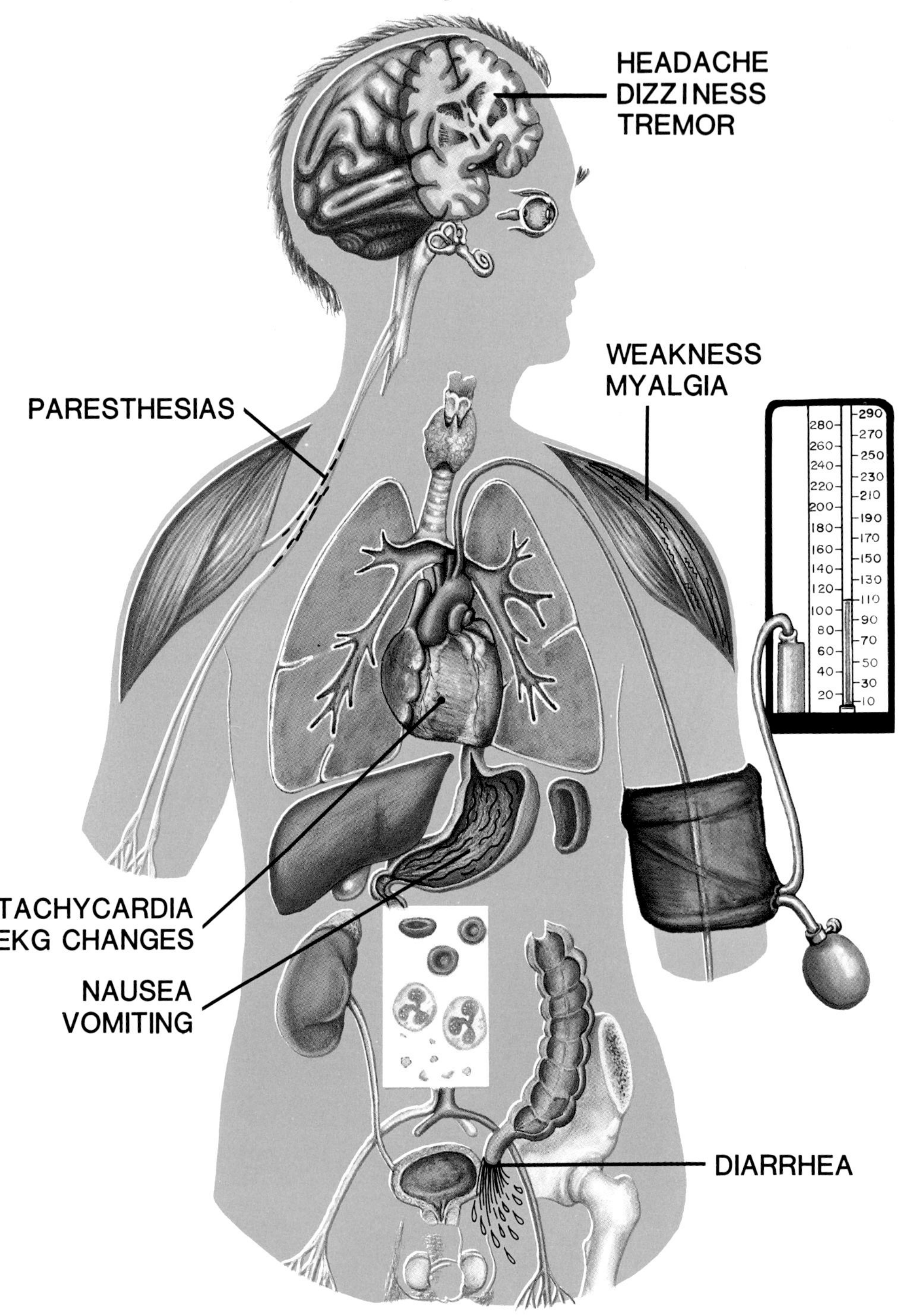

Emetine Hydrochloride

Representative Trade Name: Emetine Hydrochloride

Toxicity Rating: Low

Adverse Reactions

Nervous System Muscular weakness, pain, paresthesias, and tremors are the most frequent adverse manifestations. Occasional dizziness, fainting, and headache have been reported.

Cardiovascular Hypotension, chest pain, tachycardia, and dyspnea may develop along with EKG changes (in as many as 50 percent of patients).

Gastrointestinal Nausea, vomiting, diarrhea, and abdominal cramps occur. Feces may contain mucus and blood.

Dermatologic Urticaria, petechial rash, and eczema occur. Myositis at the injection site has been noted.

Contraindications

Known hypersensitivity to the drug is the principle contraindication.

Precautions

The drug should be avoided in patients with known cardiac and renal disease if possible. Patients should be hospitalized for treatment, with frequent monitoring of vital signs and electrocardiograms.

Treatment

Most of the above reactions are reversible upon discontinuing treatment. However, EKG changes and muscle weakness and pain may persist for months after treatment is discontinued.

Metronidazole

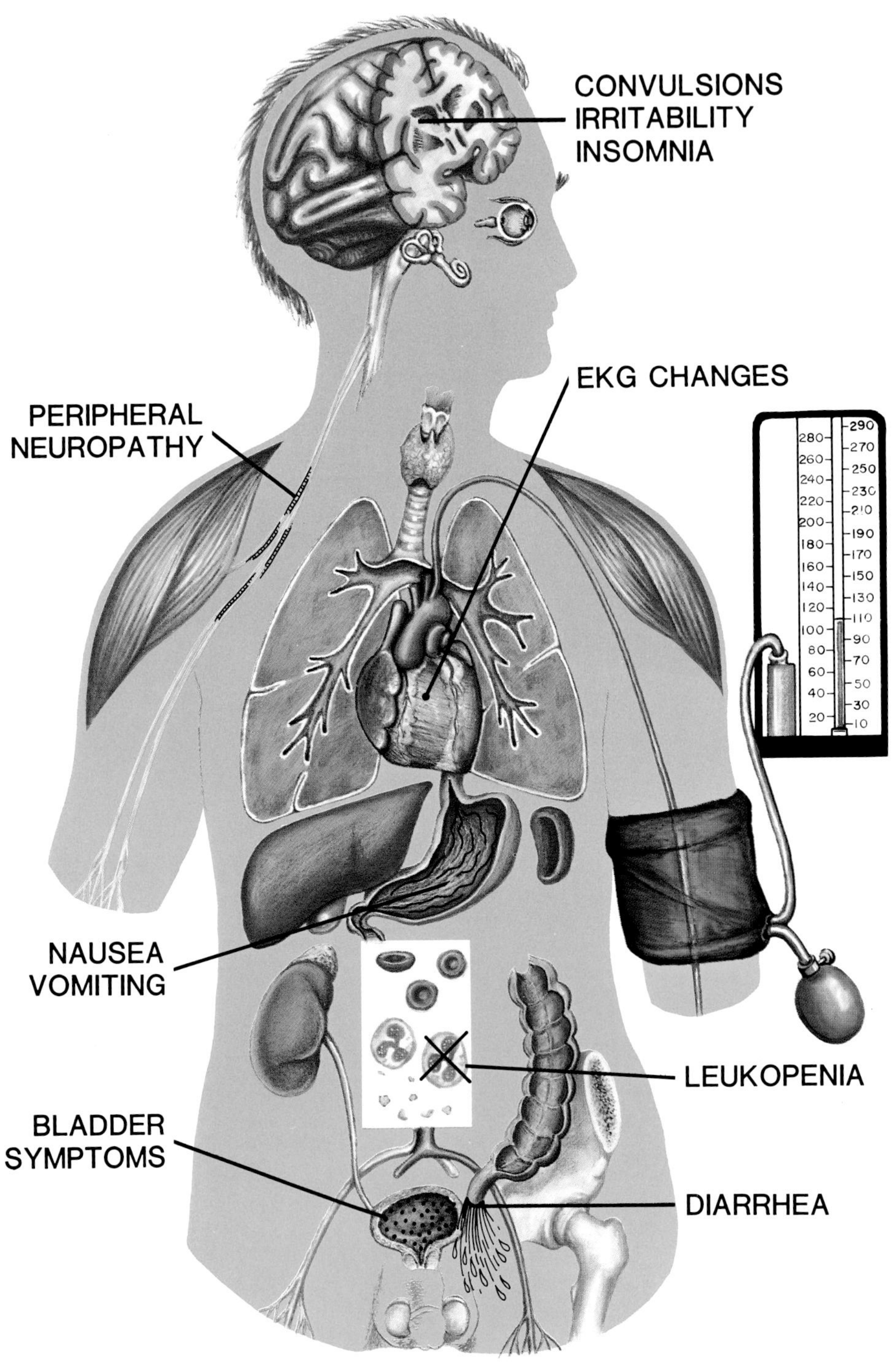

Metronidazole

Principal Drugs

Generic Name	Representative Trade Name
Metronidazole	Flagyl
Related drug:	
Tinidazole	Fasigyn

Toxicity Rating: Low to moderate because of occasional irreversible peripheral neuropathy.

Adverse Reactions

Nervous System The most serious side effects of this drug are convulsions and peripheral neuropathy, but these usually occur only after prolonged therapy. Dizziness, dyskinesia, ataxia, confusion, depression, and insomnia may occur. Headache has also been reported.

Gastrointestinal The commonest side effects of metronidazole are nausea, vomiting, diarrhea, and abdominal pain. Constipation, glossitis, and stomatitis may occur. The latter may be due to monilial overgrowth.

Cardiovascular The electrocardiograms may show flat T-waves.

Hematologic Leukopenia occurs but is reversible.

Renal Cystitis, polyuria, incontinence, and pelvic pressure occur. Dark urine due to an unidentified metabolite of metronidazole has been observed.

Other Various hypersensitivity reactions occur (urticaria, etc.) A disulfiram-like effect (flushing, abdominal distress, etc.) after drinking alcohol may occur. Dyspareunia and decreased libido are not uncommon.

Contraindications

Known hypersensitivity and pregnancy are the major contraindications.

Precautions

Lower doses should be given in patients with known liver disease. Frequent white counts should be done during treatment and alcoholic beverages should be avoided. Patients should be warned to stop the drug if paresthesia and weakness develop. If itching persists, patients should be checked for moniliasis.

Drug Interactions

The anticoagulant effects of coumarin drugs may be potentiated by metronidazole. The interaction with alcohol has already been mentioned. The laboratory values for serum glutamic-oxaloacetic transaminase (SGOT) may be decreased.

Treatment

Most reactions, including the neuropathy, will usually subside when the drug is discontinued.

Paromomycin Sulfate

Representative Trade Name: Humatin

Toxicity Rating: Low

Adverse Reactions

Adverse reactions to paromomycin are primarily gastrointestinal and include abdominal pain, diarrhea, heartburn, and pruritus ani. As with metronidazole, overgrowth by *Candida* may occur. Concomitant ingestion of alcohol may cause abdominal pain.

Treatment

Simple withdrawal of the drug is sufficient.

Anthelmintics

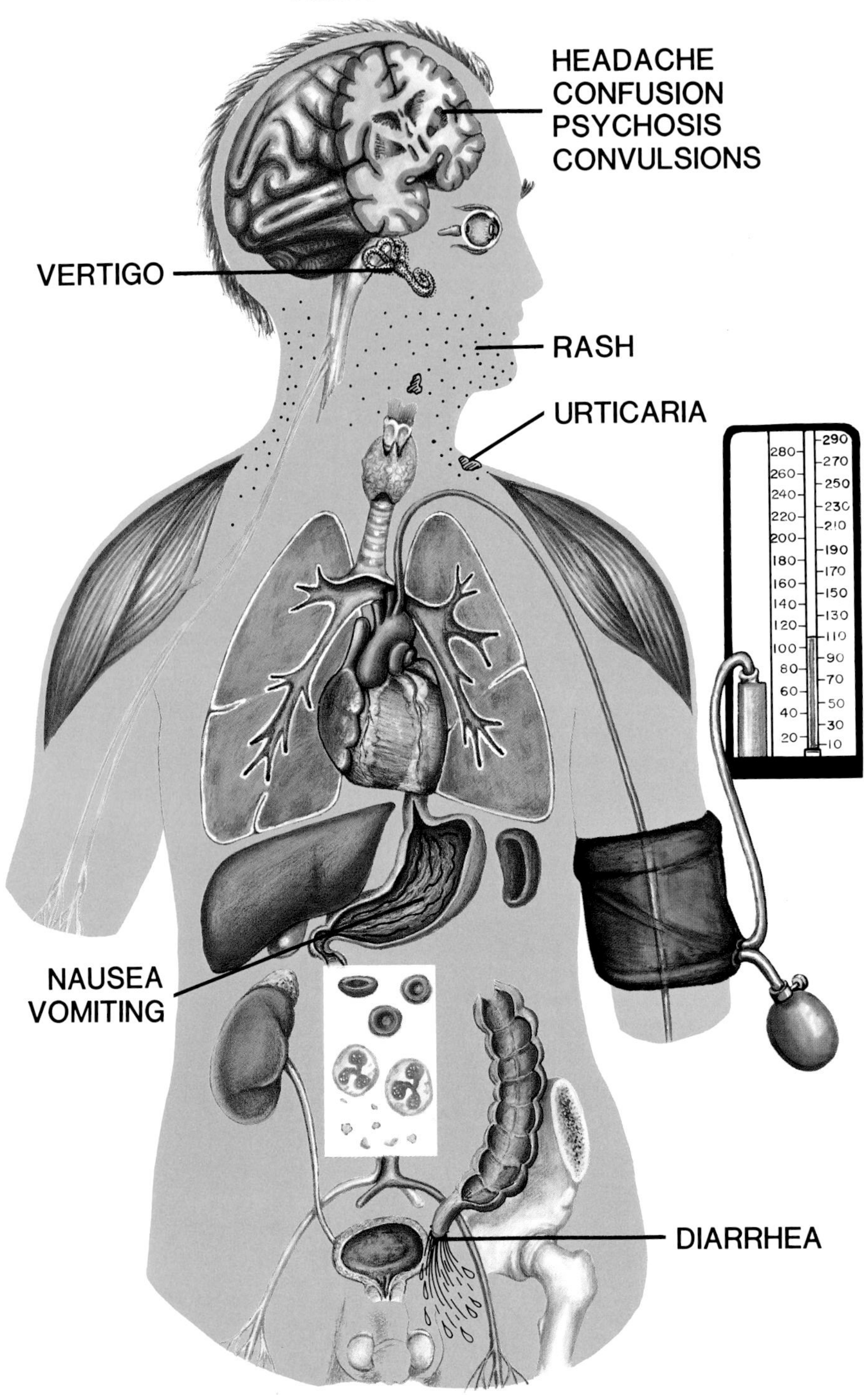
HEADACHE
CONFUSION
PSYCHOSIS
CONVULSIONS
VERTIGO
RASH
URTICARIA
280 260 240 220 200 180 160 140 120 100 80 60 40 20
290 270 250 230 210 190 170 150 130 110 90 70 50 30 10
NAUSEA
VOMITING
DIARRHEA

Anthelmintics

Principal Drugs

Generic Name	Representative Trade Name
Bithionol	Bithionol
Bephenium hydroxynaphthoate	Alcopar
Dichlorophen	Dichlorophen
Diethylcarbamazine citrate	Hetrazan
Mebendazole	Vermox
Niclosamide	Yomesan
Niridazole	Ambilhar
Piperazine citrate	Antepar
Pyrantel pamoate	Antiminth
Pyrvinium pamoate	Povan
Stibocaptate	Astiban
Thiabendazole	Mintezol

Toxicity Rating: Low to moderate because of the cerebral symptoms that may occur if there is involvement of the liver by the parasite.

Adverse Reactions

Gastrointestinal Almost all the drugs in this group produce nausea, vomiting, diarrhea, and abdominal pain.

Central Nervous System Headache and vertigo are frequently reported, but if there is associated liver disease (as in schistosomiasis, for example) there may be mental confusion, hallucinations, delirium, and convulsions.

Allergic Any of these agents may produce urticaria, maculopapular rashes, and fever. Skin eruptions develop in 63 percent of patients taking stibocaptate.

Other Isolated cases of cardiac toxicity and hepatotoxicity have been observed. Pyrvinium pamoate may cause red stools and red vomitus.

Contraindications

Known hypersensitivity to the drug and pregnancy are the major contraindications.

Precautions

Patients should be warned that pyrvinium pamoate may stain stools and vomit red, and that thiabendazole gives an asparagus odor to the urine.

Treatment

Simple withdrawal of the drug is usually all that is necessary.

Chapter 32

PSYCHOPHARMACEUTICAL DRUGS

Psychopharmaceutical Drugs

Principal Types of Psychopharmaceutical Drugs

ANTIANXIETY AGENTS

- Benzodiazepines
- Barbiturates (see page 199)
- Antihistamines (see Chapter 8)
- Propanediols

ANTIDEPRESSANTS

- Tricyclic antidepressants
- Monoamine oxidase inhibitors
- Lithium salts
- Benactyzine hydrochloride

ANTIPSYCHOTIC DRUGS

- Phenothiazines
- Haloperidol

ANTIANXIETY AGENTS

Benzodiazepines

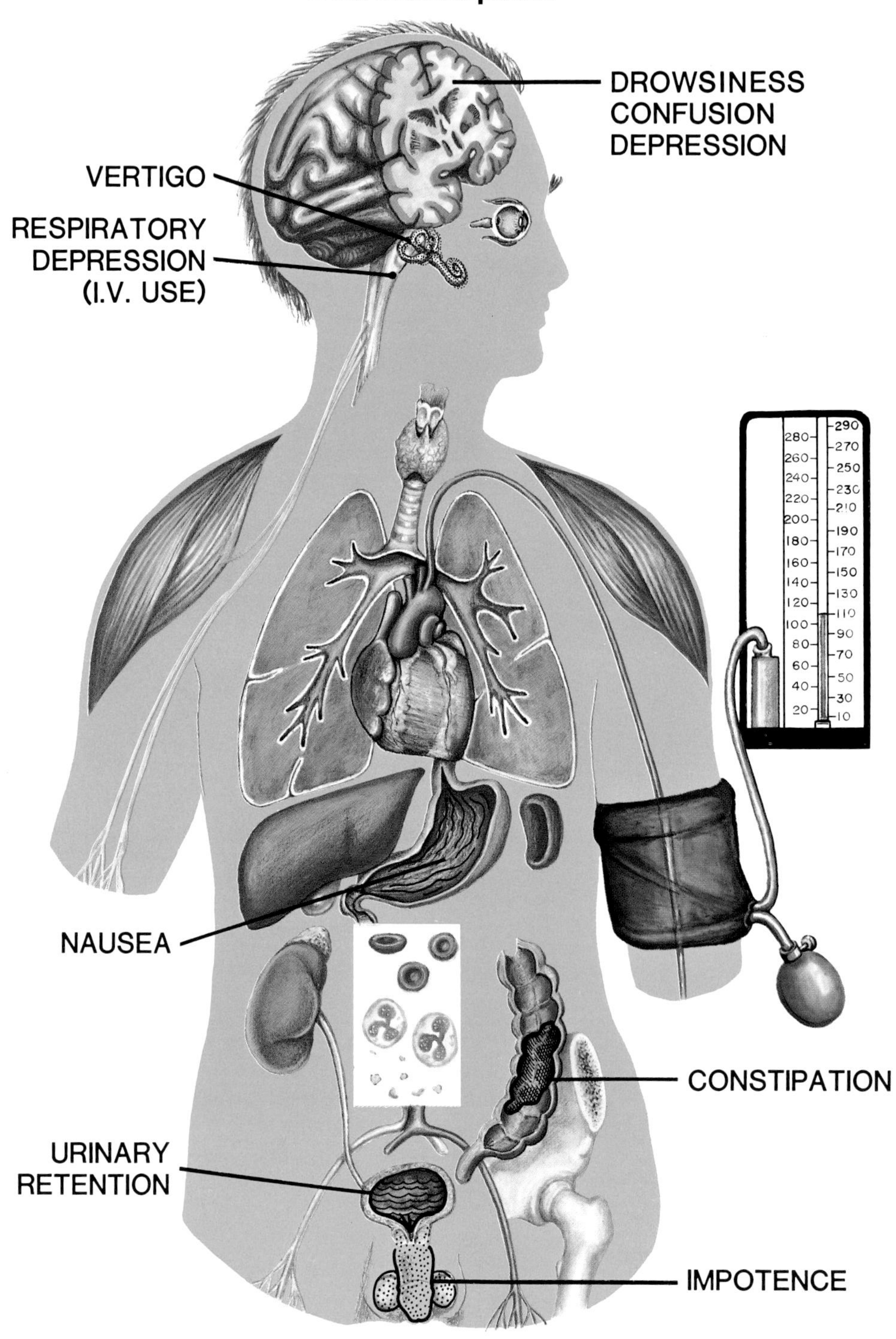

ANTIANXIETY AGENTS

Benzodiazepines

Principal Drugs

Generic Name	Representative Trade Name
Chlordiazepoxide hydrochloride	Librium
Diazepam	Valium
Clorazepate dipotassium	Tranxene
Oxazepam	Serax
Lorazepam	Ativan
Alprazolam	Xanax
Halazepam	Paxipam

Toxicity Rating: Low

Adverse Reactions

Central Nervous System Since the main therapeutic value of these drugs is sedation, it is logical that the major side effect is drowsiness. Fatigue, ataxia, confusion, depression, vertigo, and dysarthria are also not uncommon. Most of these effects wear off with continued use. It should be no surprise that paradoxical excitation occurs in a few patients.

Gastrointestinal Nausea and constipation are occasionally encountered.

Genitourinary Urinary retention, loss of libido, and occasional incontinence are encountered.

Cardiovascular Cardiovascular reactions to benzodiazepines are not common but deserve mention. They include bradycardia and hypotension (particularly postural hypertension).

Respiratory Intravenous administration may induce apnea, which must be treated promptly.

Dependency Drug dependency occurs, but much less frequently than is claimed.

Other Allergic urticaria and other rashes are rare. Occasional neutropenia and jaundice have been reported — although the author has yet to encounter these reactions in over twenty years of prescribing benzodiazepines. Venous thrombosis may occur with intravenous administration.

Contraindications

Known hypersensitivity and acute narrow-angle glaucoma are contraindications. The drug should not be used in pregnancy.

Precautions

Lower doses are advisable for the elderly and for patients already taking other sedatives. Patients with poor hepatic or renal function may also require a reduction in dosage.

Drug Interactions

The effects of benzodiazepines are potentiated by other CNS depressants such as alcohol, phenothiazines, narcotics, barbiturates, MAO inhibitors, and other antidepressants.

Treatment

Withdrawal of the drug is usually sufficient. Ventilatory assistance, blood pressure monitoring, and intravenous fluids may be required when the drugs are given intravenously.

Propanediols

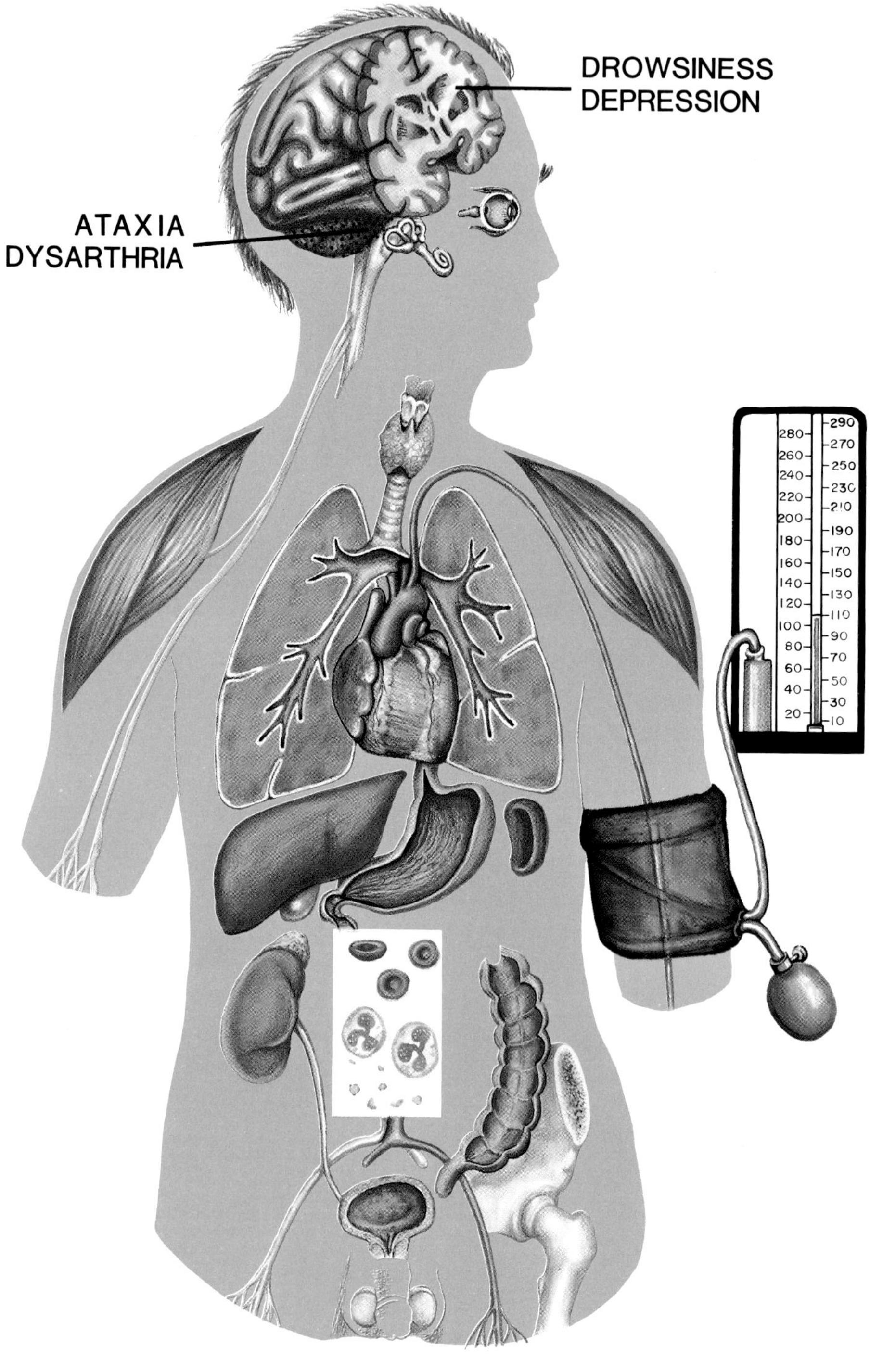

DROWSINESS
DEPRESSION

ATAXIA
DYSARTHRIA

Propanediols

Principal Drugs

Generic Name	Representative Trade Name
Meprobamate	Equanil, Miltown
Tybamate	Tybatran

Toxicity Rating: Low

Adverse Reactions

Central Nervous System The major effects of propanediols, as of benzodiazepines, are excessive drowsiness, depression, ataxia, and dysarthria. Depression may be so severe as to contribute to suicide.

Other Allergic reactions undoubtedly occur but are rare.

Dependency Dependency is an infrequent but especially serious side effect of propanediols.

Contraindications

Pregnancy, porphyria, and known hypersensitivity are the major contraindications.

Precautions

Propanediols must be used with caution in elderly patients with compromised renal or hepatic function and in patients taking other CNS depressants.

Treatment

Withdrawal of the drug is usually sufficient. Large numbers of the tablets should not be given in one prescription lest they be used for suicide.

Tricyclic Antidepressants

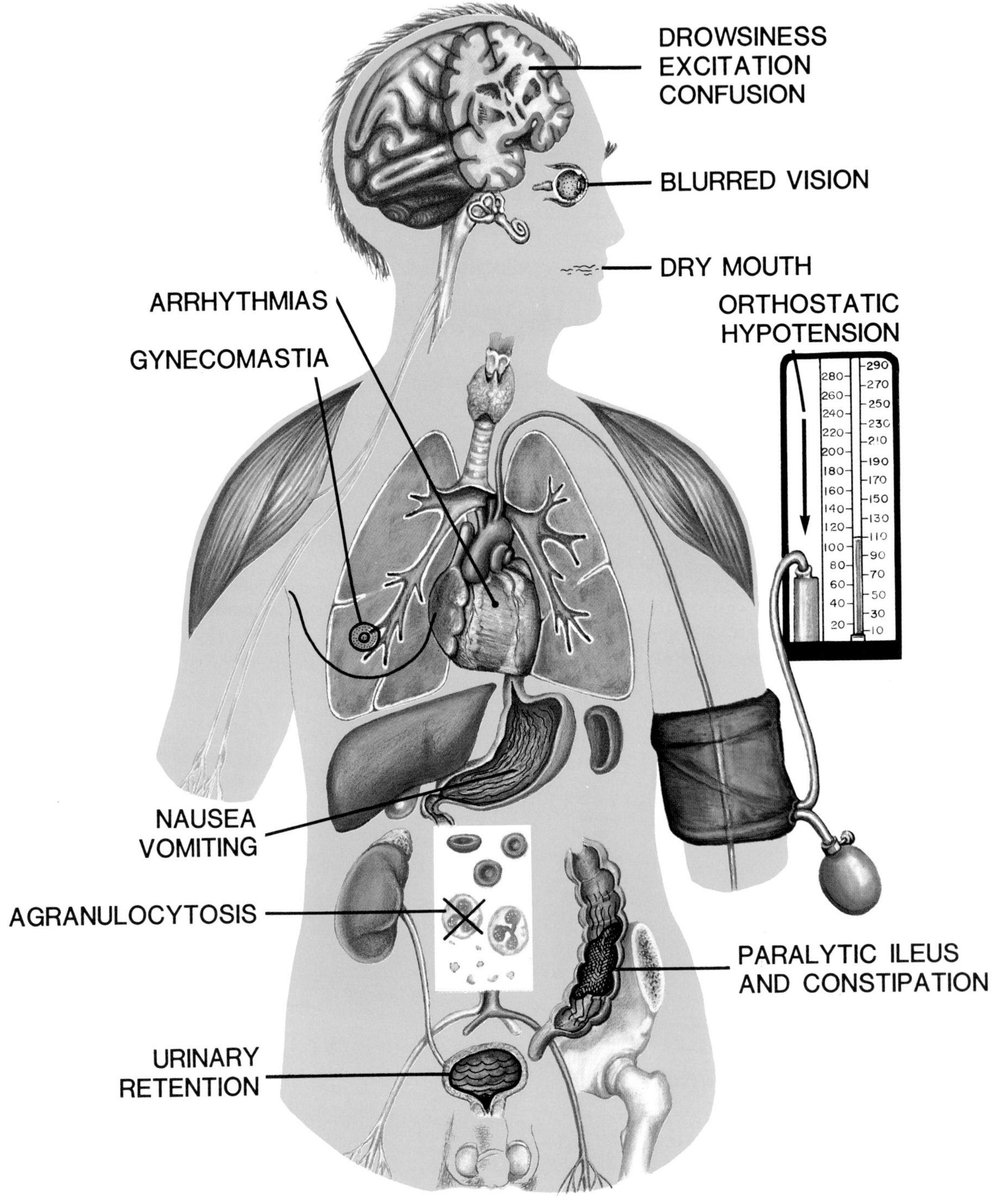

ANTIDEPRESSANTS

Tricyclic Antidepressants

Principal Drugs

Generic Name	Representative Trade Name
Doxepin hydrochloride	Sinequan
Amitriptyline hydrochloride	Elavil
Nortriptyline hydrochloride	Aventyl HCl
Protriptyline hydrochloride	Vivactil
Imipramine hydrochloride	Tofranil
Desipramine hydrochloride	Norpramin
Tricyclic antidepressants in combination with phenothiazines	Triavil

Toxicity Rating: Low because the incidence of severe toxicity (hypotension, arrhythmias, bone marrow depression, and hepatitis) is low, and the anticholinergic side effects seem to disappear with continued use.

Adverse Reactions

Cardiovascular Cardiovascular reactions include postural hypotension, arrhythmias, hypertension, and stroke.

Central Nervous System Tricyclic antidepressants often produce drowsiness shortly after administration; consequently these drugs are often given once daily at night. The opposite effect—agitation and restlessness, occasionally with tremor—may occur. Hallucinations, organic psychosis, neuropathy, cerebellar symptoms, and seizures occasionally occur. Any area of the nervous system may be involved.

Gastrointestinal Gastrointestinal reactions are secondary to the anticholinergic effects of tricyclics, and include dry mouth, constipation, and paralytic ileus.

Hepatobiliary Hepatitis occurs, but is fortunately rare.

Genitourinary Urinary retention may occur, but responds to the concomitant administration of bethanechol.

Hematologic Bone marrow depression has been reported.

Endocrine Tricyclic antidepressants, like phenothiazines, may cause gynecomastia, breast hypertrophy, and galactorrhea in women. Testicular swelling and decreased libido may also occur.

Other The anticholinergic effects of tricyclics may cause blurred vision and glaucoma. Allergic reactions occur but are rare. A withdrawal syndrome with nausea, headache, and malaise may occur upon abrupt cessation of the drugs.

Contraindications

Tricyclic antidepressants should not be given to patients with known hypersensitivity, nor to patients taking MAO inhibitors until 14 days after the MAO inhibitor has been discontinued. Tricyclic antidepressants should be given with caution in pregnancy until their safety has been more conclusively demonstrated.

MAO Inhibitors

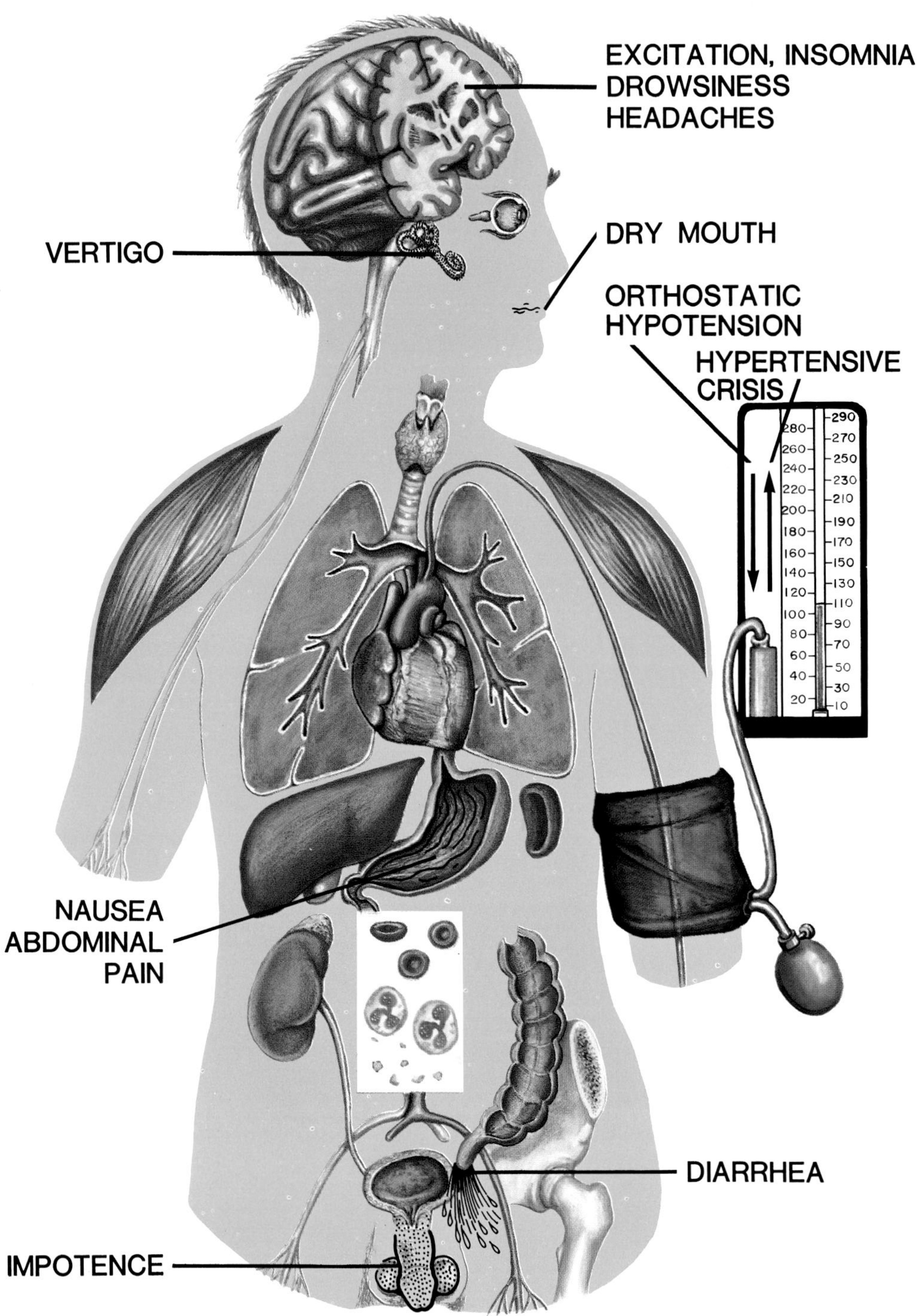
EXCITATION, INSOMNIA
DROWSINESS
HEADACHES
VERTIGO
DRY MOUTH
ORTHOSTATIC
HYPOTENSION
HYPERTENSIVE
CRISIS
NAUSEA
ABDOMINAL
PAIN
DIARRHEA
IMPOTENCE

Precautions

Tricyclic antidepressants may make schizophrenia worse. Careful observation for paralytic ileus, postural hypotension, hepatitis, and glaucoma should be done in patients who seem at risk.

Drug Interactions

The tricyclics may interfere with the action of guanethidine and clonidine, and should not be used concurrently with them. Tricyclics should be administered with caution to patients receiving ethchlorvynol or undergoing electroshock therapy. Since tricyclics act synergistically with other anticholinergics, they should be used with care in patients taking antiparkinsonian agents, phenothiazines, and antihistamines. Tricyclic antidepressants should be discontinued prior to elective surgery.

Treatment

Withdrawal of the drug and, when indicated, monitoring of hematologic and liver profiles is usually all that is necessary. As mentioned above, bethanechol will resolve urinary retention.

Monoamine Oxidase Inhibitors

Principal Drugs

Generic Name	Representative Trade Name
Tranylcypromine sulfate	Parnate
Phenelzine sulfate	Nardil
Isocarboxazid	Marplan

Toxicity Rating: The MAO inhibitors have a high toxicity rating because they may produce a hypertensive crisis with cerebral hemorrhage, are addictive, and are dangerous when taken with tyramine-containing foods.

Adverse Reactions

Central Nervous System Either overstimulation with agitation, anxiety, and manic symptoms may develop, or the opposite—weakness and drowsiness. Dizziness and headaches with or without blood pressure elevation may occur.

Cardiovascular Hypertensive crisis is the major cardiovascular reaction. Hypotension, postural or sustained, may also occur. Fatal syncope has been reported. Tachycardia and edema have also occurred.

Gastrointestinal Diarrhea, nausea, abdominal pain, and dry mouth are the principal gastrointestinal reactions. Hepatitis develops rarely.

Other Blurred vision, impotence, and inappropriate ADH secretion have occasionally been noted.

Contraindications

Because of their potential to induce a hypertensive crisis or hypotension, MAO inhibitors should not be used in patients with known or potential cardiovascular disease, hypertension, or a history of headache. Because MAO inhibitors inhibit the catabolism of catecholamines, they should not be given to patients with pheochromocytomas, or in combination with sympathomimetics (cold remedies, etc.). Patients taking MAO inhibitors must not eat foods high in tyramine (cheese, Chianti wine, liver, bananas, etc.), or take central nervous system depressants (alcohol,

Lithium Carbonate

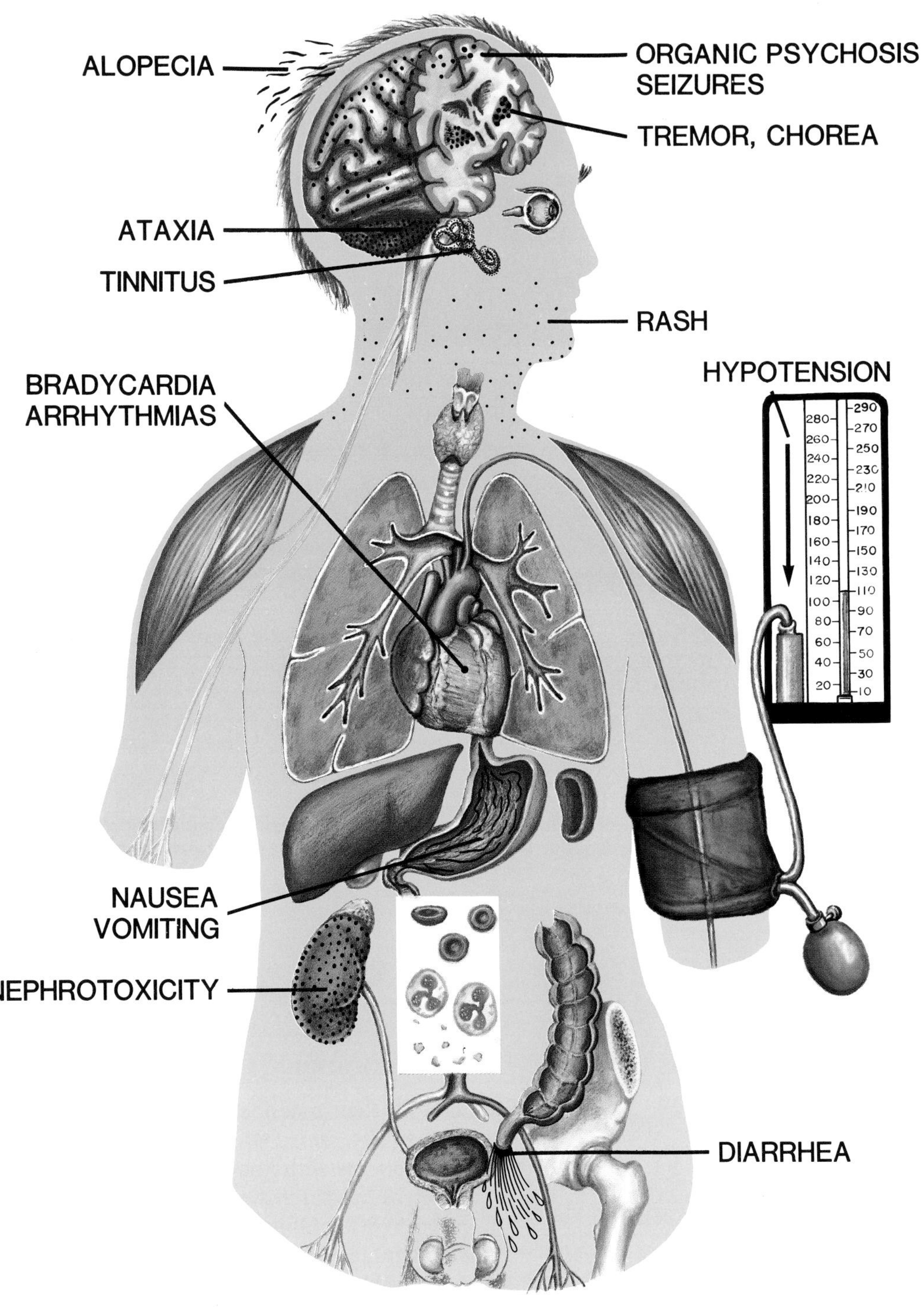

etc.). These drugs cannot be given concomitantly with the tricyclic antidepressants.

Precautions

In addition to the above dangers, caution should be observed in administering MAO inhibitors to outpatients and pregnant women. Patients must be given a list of the forbidden tyramine-containing foods and beverages, and should be warned to avoid caffeine and over-the-counter remedies. Patients on tricyclic antidepressants should be off these drugs for at least 14 days before beginning an MAO inhibitor.

Drug Interactions

Sympathomimetics, tricyclic antidepressants, caffeine, alcohol, and tyramine-containing foods increase MAO inhibitor toxicity.

Treatment

Most symptoms are treated by withdrawing the drug, but in a severe hypertensive crisis, phentolamine 5 mg IV slowly seems to be the drug of choice. Parenteral reserpine should not be used.

Lithium Carbonate

Representative Trade Name: Eskalith

Toxicity Rating: Lithium carbonate has a high toxicity rating because irreversible brain and kidney damage has occurred, and because therapeutic blood levels are very close to toxic levels.

Adverse Reactions

Central Nervous System Confusion, tremor, ataxia, chorea, seizures, and hyperirritability of the muscles and nervous system are among the many CNS symptoms that may occur. These symptoms are usually reversible, but may be irreversible when the patient is receiving haloperidol concomitantly.

Cardiovascular Hypotension, arrhythmias, bradycardia, and shock may occur.

Gastrointestinal Diarrhea, nausea, and vomiting are the most common symptoms, and indicate high lithium blood levels.

Genitourinary Atrophy of the nephron and interstitial fibrosis may result in albuminuria, polyuria, decreased creatinine clearance, and nephrogenic diabetis insipidus.

Dermatologic Almost any kind of skin change may be observed including alopecia, folliculitis, angioneurotic edema, and psoriasis.

Endocrinologic Euthyroid goiter and hypothyroidism may occur.

Other Lithium may produce numerous other symptoms, including fatigue, pruritus, impotence, polyarthalgias, and dental caries.

Contraindications

Lithium should not be given to patients with significant renal or cardiovascular diseases, dehydration, or debilitation, or to patients taking diuretics. The safety of lithium therapy in pregnant women and nursing mothers has not been established. Lithium cannot be recommended for children less than 12 years old.

Precautions

Precautions for lithium therapy are as above. Lithium blood levels should be determined frequently upon initiating therapy, and at regular intervals during therapy in patients at risk for toxicity.

Drug Interactions

Lithium may prolong neuromuscular blockade. Lithium should be used with caution in patients taking haloperidol, because irreversible brain damage is suspected to occur. Both diuretics and mazindol may enhance lithium toxicity.

Treatment

Lithium should be withdrawn. Intravenous administration of balanced electrolyte solutions will help to reduce lithium blood levels.

Benactyzine Hydrochloride

Representative Trade Name: Contained in Deprol

Toxicity Rating: Low

Adverse Reactions

Central Nervous System Dizziness, thought-blocking, a feeling of depersonalization, anxiety, insomnia, and a feeling of muscle flaccidity are seen occasionally.

Special Senses Blurred vision and dry mouth may occur secondary to anticholinergic effects.

Other Gastric distress, ataxia, and allergic reactions are occasionally seen.

Contraindications

Benactyzine should not be given to patients with glaucoma or hypersensitivity to the drug.

Treatment

Simple withdrawal of the drug is usually all that is necessary.

ANTIPSYCHOTIC DRUGS

Phenothiazines

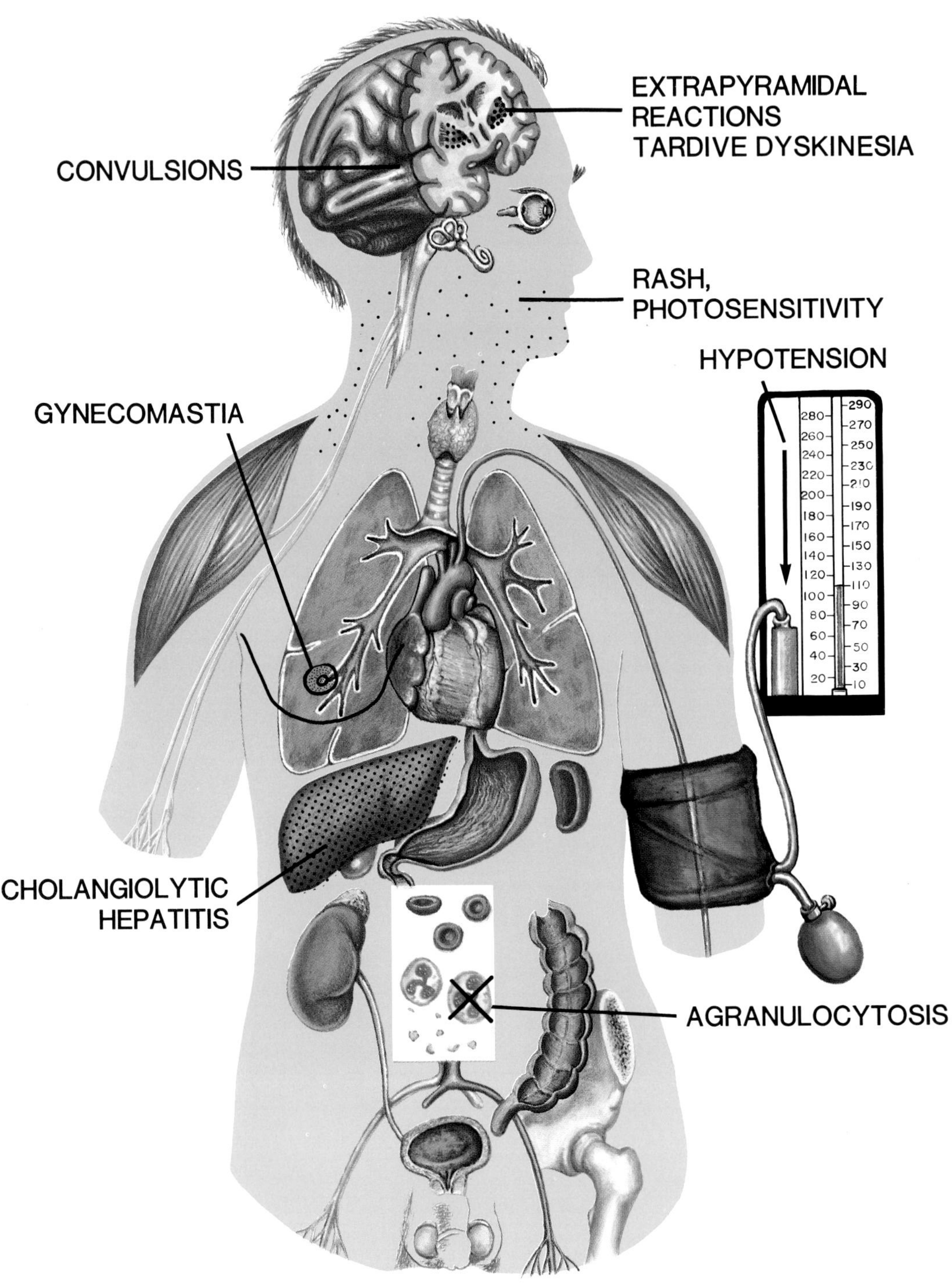

EXTRAPYRAMIDAL
REACTIONS
TARDIVE DYSKINESIA
CONVULSIONS
RASH,
PHOTOSENSITIVITY
HYPOTENSION
GYNECOMASTIA
CHOLANGIOLYTIC
HEPATITIS
AGRANULOCYTOSIS

ANTIPSYCHOTIC DRUGS

Phenothiazines

Principal Drugs

Generic Name	Representative Trade Name
Chlorpromazine	Thorazine
Prochlorperazine	Compazine
Perphenazine	in Etrafon and Triavil
Fluphenazine hydrochloride	Permitil, Prolixin
Thioridazine hydrochloride	Mellaril
Piperacetazine	Quide
Mesoridazine besylate	Serentil
Trifluoperazine hydrochloride	Stelazine
Triflupromazine hydrochloride	Vesprin
Thiothixene hydrochloride	Navane
Chlorprothixene	Taractan
Promazine hydrochloride	Sparine

Toxicity Rating: Moderate because of acute extrapyramidal reactions, cholestatic hepatitis, and persistent tardive dyskinesia.

Adverse Reactions

Central Nervous System The most significant CNS reactions to phenothiazines are extrapyramidal, and include dystonias such as opisthotonus, oculogyric crisis and torticollis, pseudoparkinsonism, hyperactivity, and tardive dyskinesia. Drowsiness occurs in initial stages of therapy. Cerebral edema is a rare complication. Convulsions may occur.

Hepatobiliary Cholangiolitic hepatitis is a dangerous reaction to these drugs.

Cardiovascular Cardiovascular reactions include hypotension and *sudden death* from cardiac arrest. EKG changes may occur. Severe hypotension occurs in patients with a pheochromocytoma or mitral insufficiency.

Hematologic Bone marrow depression manifested by leukopenia and thrombocytopenia has been reported. Anemia may also occur.

Endocrinologic Galactorrhea, gynecomastia, priapism, and menstrual irregularities have occurred.

Allergic Urticaria, photosensitivity, and exfoliative dermatitis occur. There may also be laryngeal edema and anaphylactoid reactions. Mild fever and a lupus-like syndrome have been noted rarely.

Other Miscellaneous side effects of phenothiazines include nausea, bloating, constipation, and dry mouth. Lenticular opacities are rare.

Contraindications

Phenothiazines should not be given to patients in coma or with bone marrow depression. It is also not wise to give them to children under two years of age or who weigh less than 20 pounds.

Precautions

Confusion and the extrapyramidal symptoms of Reye's syndrome and other encephalopathies may occur. Patients should be warned that phenothiazines may cause drowsiness and interfere with mental or physical abilities during the first few days of therapy. The safety of phenothiazines in pregnancy has not been established. They may mask the signs of overdosage from other drugs and make the diagnosis of other diseases, such as intestinal obstruction and brain tumors, difficult. Caution should be exercised in giving these drugs to patients with known cardiovascular disease because of their hypotensive effects. Because they may cause mydriasis, phenothiazines should be used with caution in glaucoma patients.

Drug Interactions

Phenothiazines decrease the effectiveness of oral anticoagulants and produce alpha-adrenergic blockade. When phenothiazines are administered with propranolol, the plasma levels of both drugs are increased. These drugs may also induce phenytoin toxicity.

Prophylaxis

An antiparkinsonian drug, such as trihexyphenidyl HCl or procyclidine HCl, may be given concomitantly with phenothiazines to prevent the extrapyramidal reactions. It is wise to monitor blood counts and liver function in patients with hematologic or hepatic disorders.

Treatment

Diphenhydramine HCl 50–100 mg IV or benztropine mesylate 1–2 mg IV may be given for acute extrapyramidal symptoms. Trihexyphenidyl HCl, benztropine mesylate, or other antiparkinsonian drugs may be given by mouth for the milder reactions. Diazepam or amobarbital sodium may be given for repeated convulsions, but usually all that is necessary is to discontinue the drug. Jaundice may resolve upon withdrawal of the drug, but if it persists, a 5 day course of prednisone 20 mg/day may be given ("steroid whitewash"), provided there is no contraindication. Hematologic and other types of reactions can usually be treated by simple withdrawal of the drug. Severe hypotension may necessitate administration of norepinephrine bitartrate or other pressor amines.

Side Effects of Specific Phenothiazines

Thioridazine and promazine seem to be less likely than other phenothiazines to cause exrapyramidal and convulsive reactions, while chlorpromazine is more likely to cause jaundice. Trifluoperazine and prochlorperazine seem to be more likely to cause hypotension. Cerebral edema, grand mal convulsions, and failure of ejaculation have not been reported with perphenazine.

Haloperidol

Haloperidol

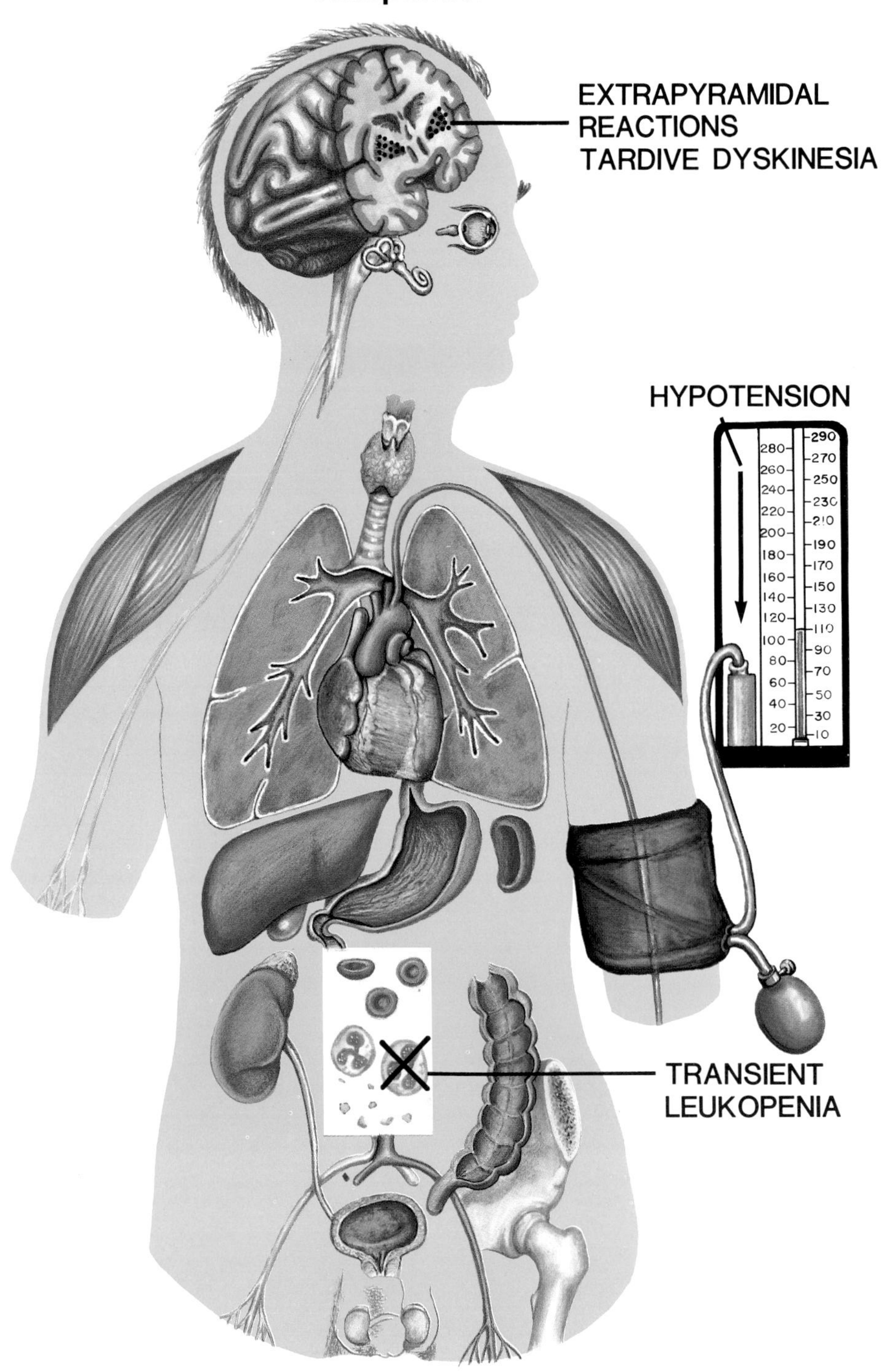
EXTRAPYRAMIDAL REACTIONS
TARDIVE DYSKINESIA
HYPOTENSION
280 260 240 220 200 180 160 140 120 100 80 60 40 20
290 270 250 230 210 190 170 150 130 110 90 70 50 30 10
TRANSIENT LEUKOPENIA

Haloperidol

Representative Trade Name: Haldol

Toxicity Rating: Moderate because of acute extrapyramidal reactions, laryngospasm, and persistent tardive dyskinesia.

Adverse Reactions

Central Nervous System As with the phenothiazines, the most common side effects of haloperidol are extrapyramidal reactions such as dystonias, opisthotonus, tremors, oculogyric crisis, psychomotor activity, and hyperreflexia. These may occur even with low doses. Tardive dyskinesia may persist after the drug is withdrawn. Insomnia, restlessness, and anxiety, and the opposite reactions—drowsiness and depression—are reported.

Hepatobiliary Jaundice and impaired liver function occur.

Cardiovascular Tachycardia, hypotension, and cardiac arrest have been reported.

Hematologic Agranulocytosis and anemia are rarely seen.

Endocrinologic Like the phenothiazines, haloperidol may cause gynecomastia, galactorrhea, decreased or increased libido, alopecia, and alterations in blood sugar.

Gastrointestinal Anorexia, nausea, vomiting, and diarrhea have been observed.

Other Almost any kind of allergic reaction may occur, including drug eruptions and hyperpyrexia. Dry mouth, blurred vision, and acute renal failure or urinary retention have been reported.

Contraindications

Parkinson's disease, known hypersensitivity, toxic encephalopathy, and coma are the major contraindications.

Precautions

The safety in pregnancy is not established. Care must be taken when giving haloperidol to patients with angina, epilepsy, hypomania, or hyperthyroidism, or who are taking CNS depressants.

Drug Interactions

Toxic encephalopathy sometimes resulting in irreversible brain damage may occur if haloperidol is given with lithium.

Treatment

Concomitant administration of an antiparkinson drug (trihexyphenidyl HCl, etc.) may be required to eliminate extrapyramidal side effects. Vasopressors may be necessary to control hypotension while the drug is being withdrawn. Other reactions usually subside after the drug is withdrawn. Acute extrapyramidal reactions may be treated with diphenhydramine HCl 50 – 100 mg IV or benztropine mesylate 1 – 2 mg IV.

Chapter 33

SKELETAL MUSCLE RELAXANTS

Skeletal Muscle Relaxants

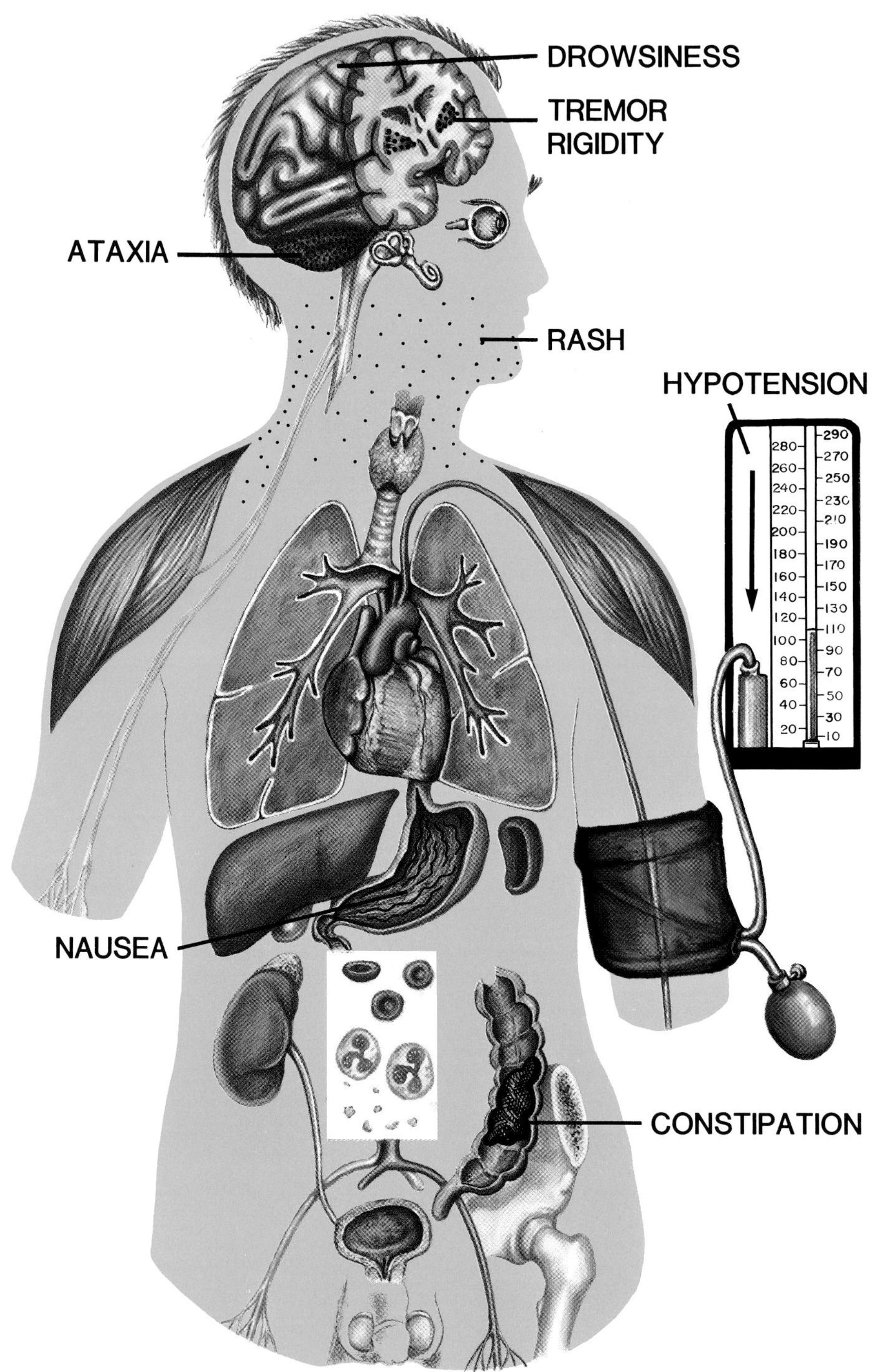

Skeletal Muscle Relaxants

Principal Drugs

Cyclobenzaprine hydrochloride
Dantrolene sodium
Carisoprodol
  Meprobamate (see page 261)
Chlorzoxazone
Methocarbamol
Orphenadrine citrate
Baclofen
Parenteral neuromuscular blockers
  Succinylcholine chloride
  Tubocurarine chloride
  Metocurine iodide
  Pancuronium bromide
Quinine sulfate
Diazepam (see page 259)
Chlordiazepoxide (see page 259)

Cyclobenzaprine Hydrochloride

Representative Trade Name: Flexeril

Toxicity Rating: The toxicity of this drug is low and rarely irreversible.

Adverse Reactions

This drug is closely related to the tricyclic antidepressants, and the reader is referred to page 263 for an illustration and more detailed discussion of its side effects. Drowsiness occurs in 20–40% of patients, and many anticholinergic effects, such as dry mouth, dizziness, tachycardia, constipation, urinary retention, and vasodilation may occur. Other central nervous system effects include ataxia, dysarthria, paresthesias, tremors, insomnia, and muscle twitching.

Contraindications

Cyclobenzaprine should not be given to patients taking MAO inhibitors until at least two weeks after the MAO inhibitors have been discontinued. Cyclobenzaprine should also not be administered to patients with hyperthyroidism, arrhythmias, or conduction disturbances, or during recovery from a myocardial infarction.

Precautions

Cyclobenzaprine should be given with care to patients with glaucoma or prostatic hypertrophy with urinary retention, as it can exacerbate these conditions. As with all CNS depressants, the patient should be warned to avoid driving or working around dangerous machinery while taking cyclobenzaprine.

Drug Interactions

Cyclobenzaprine interacts dangerously with MAO inhibitors, causing fever, convulsions, and death. Cyclobenzaprine may enhance the action of other CNS depressants. On the other hand, it may block the antihypertensive effects of guanethidine and compounds that act similarly.

Treatment

Withdrawal of the drug is usually sufficient; thus, diagnosis is the main step in treatment.

Dantrolene Sodium

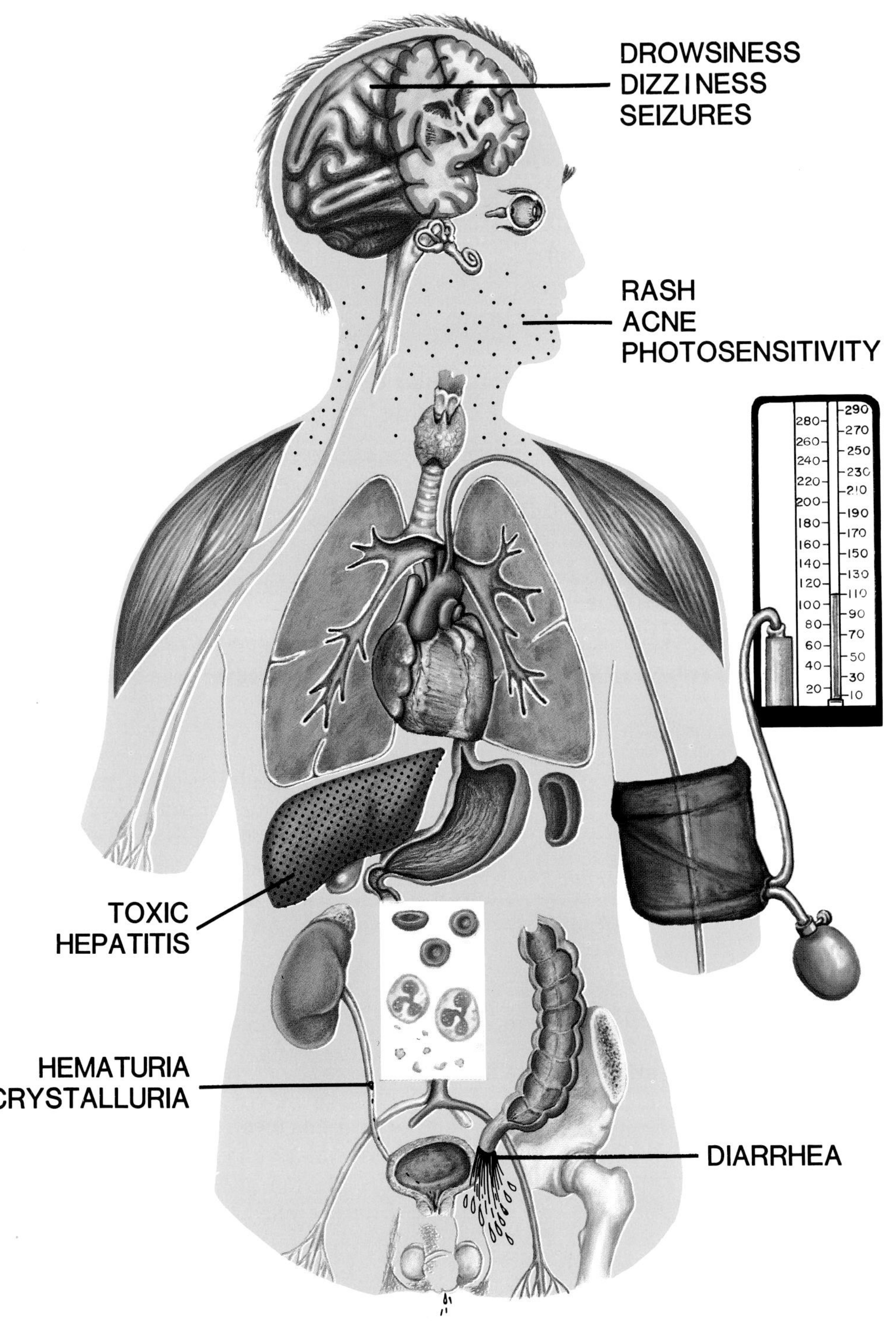

Dantrolene Sodium

Representative Trade Name: Dantrium

Toxicity Rating: This drug has a high toxicity rating by virtue of the high incidence of side effects and hepatitis.

Adverse Reactions

Central Nervous System Up to 75 percent of patients receiving this drug develop drowsiness, weakness, lightheadedness, and dizziness. The frequency of epileptic seizures may be increased.

Gastrointestinal Severe diarrhea may occur but constipation, abdominal cramps, and gastrointestinal bleeding are also possible.

Hepatobiliary Hepatitis, sometimes fatal, has been seen with this drug.

Cardiovascular Tachycardia, blood pressure variations, and phlebitis may occur.

Genitourinary Genitourinary reactions to dantrolene include hematuria, urinary frequency, crystalluria, and impotence. Both urinary incontinence and retention have been noted.

Dermatologic Of course, allergic skin reactions occur. However, photosensitivity, abnormal hair growth, sweating, and acne are peculiar to this muscle relaxant.

Other Headache, myalgia, fever, and an allergic pleural effusion with pericarditis may occur.

Contraindications

Liver disease and hypersensitivity to the drug are absolute contraindications. If spasticity is necessary for upright posturing or other functions, the drug should not be given. The safety in pregnancy is not established.

Precautions

It is wise to monitor liver function during the early stages of therapy. The safety of dantrolene in children under 5 years old has not been established. Patients with emphysema and cardiac disease must be observed for decompensation.

Drug Interactions

Estrogen may enhance the hepatotoxicity of dantrolene.

Treatment

Withdrawal of the drug and measures to prevent hepatic coma (low-protein diet, etc.) and crystalluria (IV fluids), are recommended. Endotracheal intubation may be necessary in cases of severe muscle flaccidity.

Carisoprodol

Principal Drugs

Generic Name	Representative Trade Names
Carisoprodol	Soma
Related drug:	
Meprobamate (see page 261)	Equanil, Miltown

Toxicity Rating: This drug deserves a low toxicity rating, but rare cases of idiosyncratic reactions (see below) and anaphylactoid shock have been reported.

Adverse Reactions

Central Nervous System Drowsiness is the main CNS effect of carisoprodol, but, like baclofen, this drug may affect any area of the nervous system. Consequently, tremor, ataxia, vertigo, agitation, and depression have been observed. A rare idiosyncratic reaction may occur with the first dose of carisoprodol—temporary extreme weakness, quadriplegia, ataxia, loss of vision, dysarthria, and disorientation. Hospitalization may be necessary.

Allergic Like penicillin, carisoprodol can cause acute and immediate (first to fourth dose) drug eruptions, drug fever, and anaphylactoid shock.

Cardiovascular Like baclofen, carisoprodol can cause hypotension (usually postural) and tachycardia. Facial flushing has also been noted.

Gastrointestinal Carisoprodol may cause nausea, vomiting, hiccups, and epigastric distress.

Other Transient bone marrow depression may occur.

Contraindications

Carisoprodol, like the barbiturates, is contraindicated in patients with intermittent porphyria. It is also contraindicated in patients with known hypersensitivity to it, and in pregnancy.

Precautions

As with all central nervous system depressants, patients should be warned about driving or working near hazardous machinery while taking carisoprodol. Caution should be observed when using this drug in patients with known liver or kidney disease.

Drug Interactions

Carisoprodol can enhance the effect of other central nervous system depressants.

Treatment

Most reactions subside upon withdrawal of the drug. If an idiosyncratic reaction develops, hospitalization may be indicated. Anaphylactic shock and other allergic reactions may require epinephrine, corticosteroids, and antihistamines.

Chlorzoxazone

Representative Trade Names: Parafon Forte, Paraflex

Toxicity Rating: This drug has earned a low toxicity rating over many years of clinical usage.

Adverse Reactions

Central Nervous System Drowsiness is not uncommon. Less common side effects include dizziness, malaise, and overstimulation.

Gastrointestinal Nausea and rarely vomiting or hepatitis may occur. Rare instances of gastrointestinal bleeding have been reported.

Other Obviously, allergic reactions are possible, but they are exceedingly rare. Discoloration of the urine may occur but is of no clinical consequence.

Contraindications

Aside from known hypersensitivity, there are no contraindications. Chlorzoxazone may be used in pregnancy if the benefits outweigh the possible risks to the fetus.

Drug Interactions

Chlorzoxazone may enhance the effects of other CNS depressants.

Treatment

Withdrawal of the drug is sufficient.

Methocarbamol

Representative Trade Name: Robaxin

Toxicity Rating: This is another muscle relaxant with a low toxicity rating.

Adverse Reactions

Central Nervous System As might be expected, drowsiness, lightheadedness, and dizziness are the most frequent side effects.

Gastrointestinal Like chlorzoxazone, methocarbamol sometimes causes nausea.

Other Allergic reactions, such as conjunctivitis, rash, and fever occasionally occur.

Contraindications

Known hypersensitivity to the drug is the only contraindication. The benefits of methocarbamol in pregnancy must be weighed against the possibility of risk to the fetus, as with so many other drugs.

Drug Interactions

Methocarbamol may enhance the effects of alcohol and other central nervous system depressants.

Treatment

Simple withdrawal of the drug is all that is necessary unless there is a serious overdose, in which case more vigorous measures are needed.

Orphenadrine Citrate

Representative Trade Names: Norflex, Norgesic

Toxicity Rating: Low

Adverse Reactions

The adverse reactions to orphenadrine are largely due to its mild anticholinergic effects (see Chapter 4). Dry mouth, mydriasis, mental confusion, and urinary retention may occur, although they are not common. Glaucoma may be precipitated.

Contraindications

Known hypersensitivity to the drug is the only significant contraindication.

Precautions

Patients with tachycardia and cardiac arrhythmias may not tolerate orphenadrine.

Drug Interactions

The effects of orphenadrine and other anticholinergics are additive. Concurrent use of orphenadrine and tolbutamide may induce hypoglycemia. Severe hypoglycemia has been observed when orphenadrine has been given with chlorpromazine.

Treatment

Simple withdrawal of the drug is usually effective.

Baclofen

Representative Trade Name: Lioresal

Toxicity Rating: This drug is low to moderate in toxicity. The toxicity would be low if it were not for the seizures and hallucinations that result from abrupt withdrawal—the other side effects are generally reversible.

Adverse Reactions

Central Nervous System Transient drowsiness occurs in almost two-thirds of patients using this drug. Other neurologic reactions include dizziness, fatigue, confusion, hallucinations, ataxia, tremor, and rigidity. Almost any area of the nervous system may be affected.

Cardiovascular Hypotension is not uncommon. Syncope, palpitations, chest pain, and dyspnea are rare and are usually secondary to the hypotension.

Gastrointestinal Nausea and constipation are common but other gastrointestinal symptoms are rare. There may be blood in the stool.

Genitourinary Urinary frequency, urinary retention, and impotence may occur.

Other Allergic skin reactions, edema, excessive perspiration, and weight gain may occur. Abnormal liver function and hyperglycemia have been observed.

Contraindications

The only contraindications are known hypersensitivity to the drug, and pregnancy.

Precautions

Caution should be observed in patients with known renal disease, stroke, and other diseases with preexisting central nervous system depression. Patients with known epilepsy should be warned that abrupt withdrawal may induce hallucinations and seizures.

Drug Interactions

The effects of any central nervous system depressant (alcohol, etc.) may be increased by baclofen.

Treatment

Most side effects are treated by gradual withdrawal of the drug. In cases of severe nervous system depression, intubation and large doses of balanced electrolyte solution intravenously (with appropriate monitoring) will be necessary to promote maximal renal excretion of the drug.

Parenteral Neuromuscular Blockers

Parenteral Neuromuscular Blockers

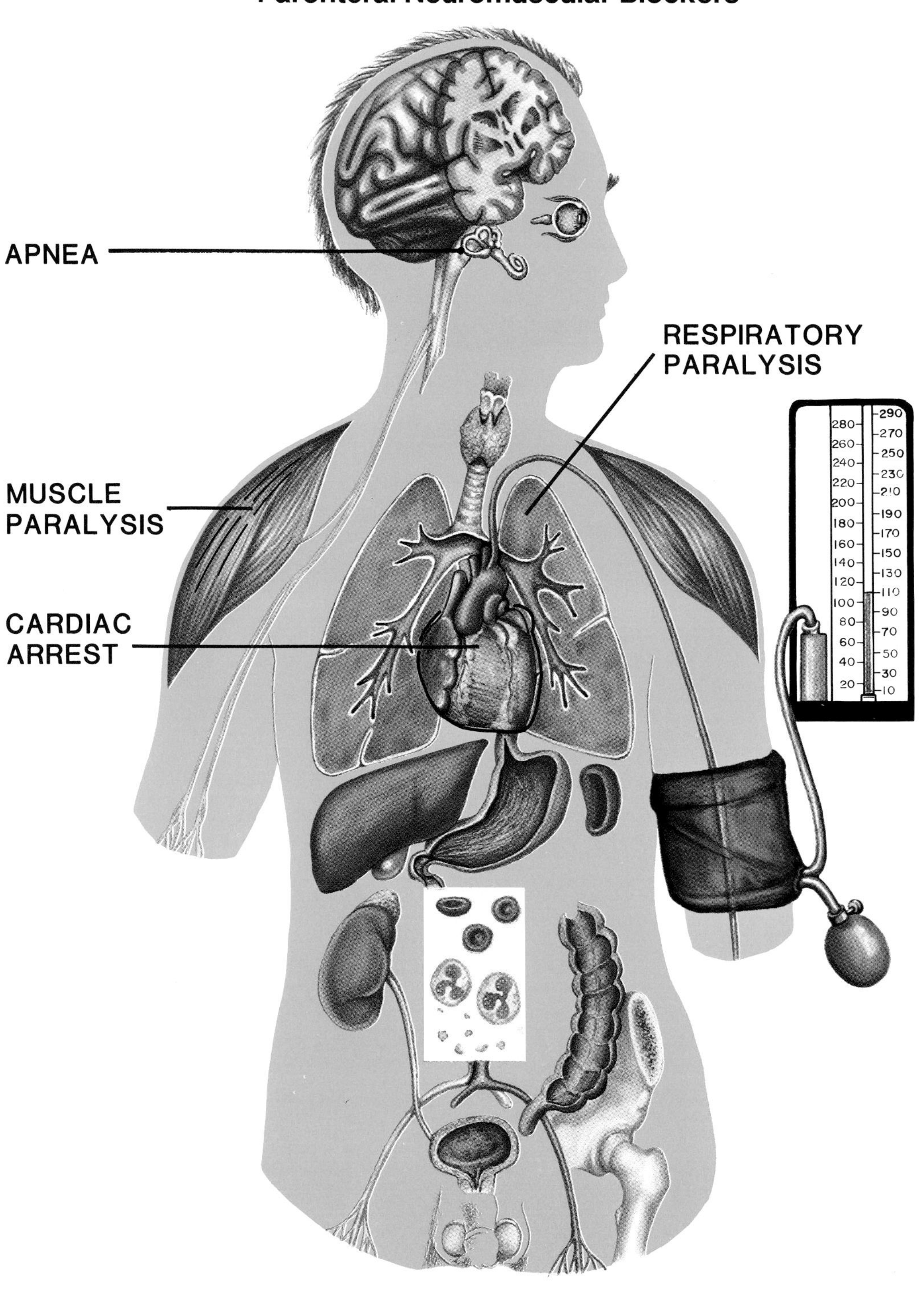

Parenteral Neuromuscular Blockers

Principal Drugs

Generic Name	Representative Trade Name
Succinylcholine chloride	Anectine
Tubocurarine chloride	Tubocurarine Chloride
Metocurine iodide	Metubine Iodide
Pancuronium bromide	Pavulon

Toxicity Rating: These drugs can be highly toxic in some patients. Only physicians specially trained in their use should administer them.

Adverse Reactions

Central Nervous System Muscular relaxation may be so profound as to cause severe respiratory depression or apnea. This effect is of course therapeutic if anesthesia and assisted ventilation is planned.

Allergic Hypersensitivity reactions occur rarely.

Other Succinylcholine may cause cardiac arrest, malignant hyperthermia, hypertension, arrhythmias, glaucoma, and hemoglobinemia, and muscle cramps may occur rarely.

Adverse Reactions to Tubocurarine Like succinylcholine, tubocurarine may cause circulatory depression and release of histamine.

Contraindications

Known hypersensitivity to the drug is the most significant contraindication.

Precautions

Physicians using these drugs should be skilled in the management of artificial respiration, and all necessary equipment should be immediately available. Equipment to treat hypotension and shock must also be available. Caution must be used in giving parenteral neuromuscular blockers to patients in shock or with renal disease.

Drug Interactions

These drugs can potentiate the action of any other drug that causes even minimal neuromuscular blockade. Some nonpenicillin antibiotics, such as streptomycin, kanamycin, and gentamicin, may potentiate the effects of the parenteral neuromuscular blockers. Certain general anesthetics have neuromuscular blocking effects, which may be *either* synergistic with or antagonistic to the effects of parenteral neuromuscular blockers. Quinidine may cause a recurrence of neuromuscular blockade if given shortly after recovery from parenteral neuromuscular blockers. Magnesium sulfate may potentiate the neuromuscular blockade. Beta blockers, procainamide, lithium, promazine, and oxytocin may also enhance neuromuscular blockade. Pancuronium bromide should not be given until the side effects of previously administered succinylcholine have worn off.

Quinine Sulfate

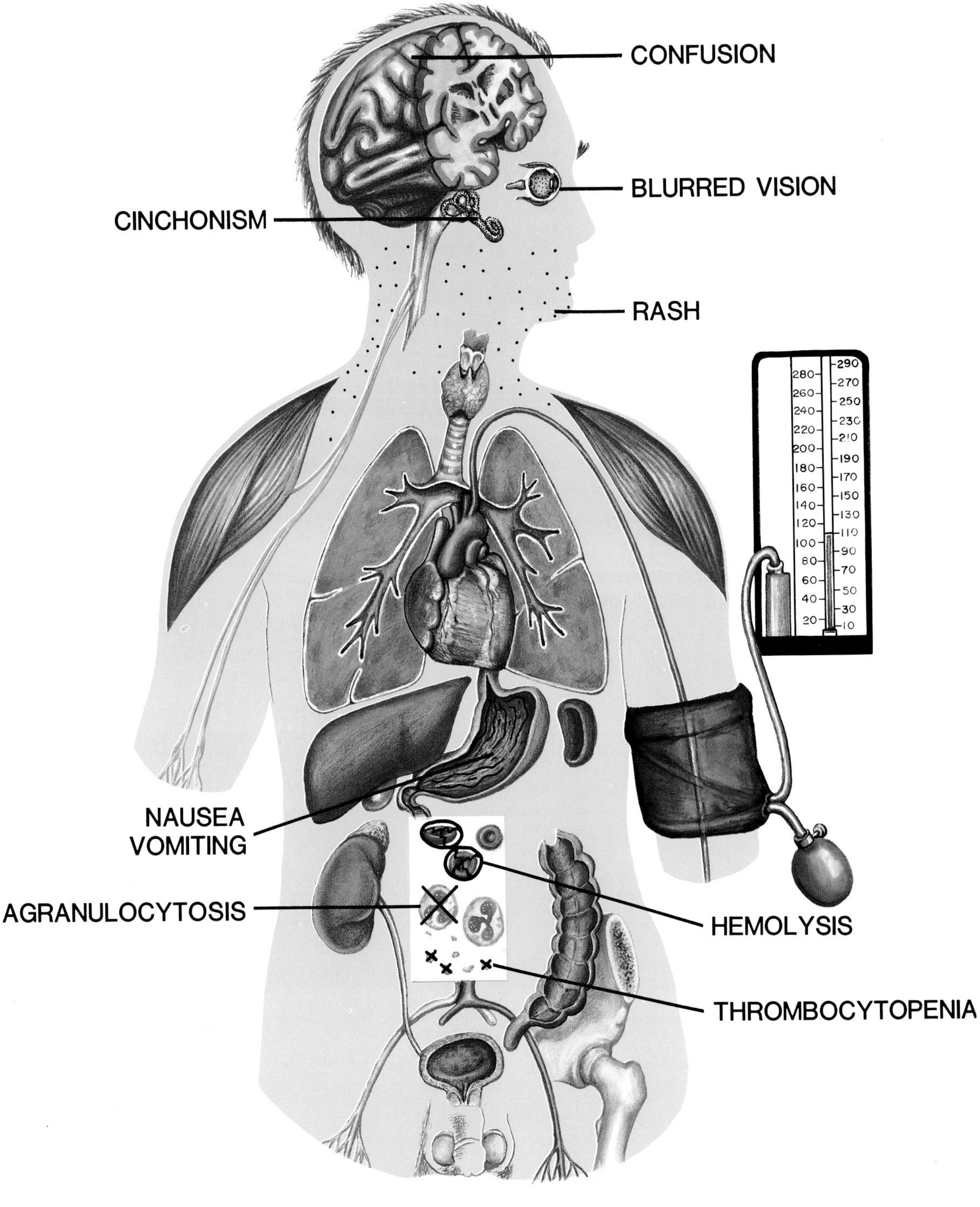

CONFUSION

BLURRED VISION

CINCHONISM

RASH

NAUSEA
VOMITING

AGRANULOCYTOSIS

HEMOLYSIS

THROMBOCYTOPENIA

Quinine Sulfate

Representative Trade Names: Quinamm, Quinite

Toxicity Rating: Moderate

Adverse Reactions

Central Nervous System Most of the CNS reactions are related to cinchonism—scotomata, tinnitus, deafness, vertigo, blurred vision, and confusion. Other visual disturbances, headache, and apprehension occur.

Gastrointestinal Nausea and vomiting are common.

Hematologic Quinine sulfate may cause acute hemolysis, agranulocytosis, and thrombocytopenic purpura. Hypoprothrombinemia may also occur.

Dermatologic Numerous types of skin rashes, flushing, sweating, and edema of the face may occur.

Other Asthmatic symptoms, angina, fever, and epigastric pain may occur.

Contraindications

Pregnancy, known quinine hypersensitivity, and glucose-6-phosphate dehydrogenase deficiency are the most important contraindications.

Drug Interactions

Quinine may increase plasma levels of digoxin. The absorption of quinine may be delayed or decreased by aluminum-containing antacids. Quinine may enhance the effect of oral anticoagulants. Quinine drugs potentiate the neuromuscular blockade produced by succinylcholine and analgesic compounds. Drugs that cause alkaline urine (antacids, acetazolamide, etc.) may precipitate quinine toxicity.

Treatment

Withdrawal of the drug, gastric lavage, and vasopressors to maintain blood pressure may be necessary. Fluid and electrolyte solutions should be given according to blood electrolyte determinations. Acidification of the urine may promote quinine excretion.

Chapter 34

SYMPATHOMIMETIC DRUGS

Sympathomimetic Drugs

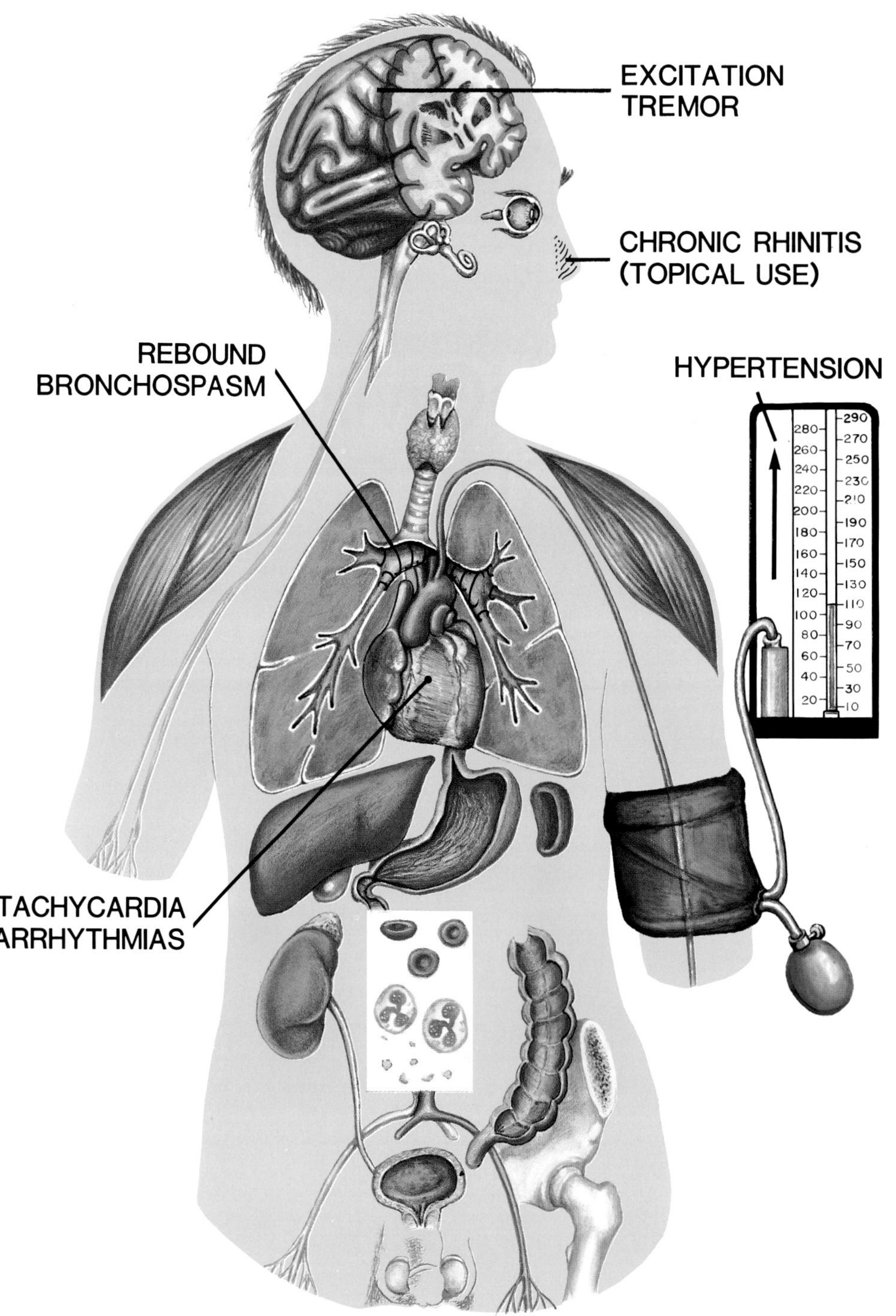

Sympathomimetic Drugs

Principal Drugs

Generic Name	Representative Trade Name
Epinephrine	Adrenalin Chloride
Pseudoephedrine hydrochloride	Sudafed; in Actifed, Novafed
Terbutaline sulfate	Brethine, Bricanyl
Ethylnorepinephrine hydrochloride	Bronkephrine Hydrochloride
Isoetharine	Bronkometer, Bronkosol
Phenylephrine hydrochloride	Neo-Synephrine Hydrochloride; in Comhist, Dimetapp, and numerous other drug combinations
Phenylpropanolamine hydrochloride	in Nolamine, CoTylenol, Dimetapp, and numerous other drug combinations
Methamphetamine hydrochloride	Desoxyn
Dextroamphetamine sulfate	Dexedrine
Benzphetamine hydrochloride	Didrex
Isoproterenol hydrochloride	in Isuprel
Norepinephrine bitartrate	Levophed Bitartrate
Methoxamine hydrochloride	Vasoxyl
Ephedrine sulfate	Bronkotabs
Ephedrine	Quibron Plus
Ephedrine hydrochloride	Tedral, Quadrinal
Metaraminol bitartrate	Aramine
Mephentermine sulfate	Wyamine Sulfate
Dopamine hydrochloride	Intropin
Tetrahydrozoline hydrochloride	Tyzine
Naphazoline hydrochloride	Privine Hydrochloride
Phentermine hydrochloride	Fastin
Phentermine resin	Ionamin
Diethylpropion hydrochloride	Tenuate, Tepanil
Fenfluramine hydrochloride	Pondimin
Mazindol	Sanorex

Toxicity Rating: Low if used topically or orally. Moderate if used intravenously.

Adverse Reactions

Adverse reactions to sympathomimetics are mostly secondary to the vasoconstrictive effects of these drugs.

Cardiovascular Hypertension, tachycardia, and arrhythmias occur.

Central Nervous System Anxiety, tremor, headache, dizziness, and restlessness occur.

Respiratory Rebound bronchospasm may occur.

Table 34-1. Side Effects of Sympathomimetics

Drug	Hyper-tension	Tachycardia	Arrhythmias	CNS Symptoms	Headache	Gastro-intestinal Effects	Seizures	Urinary Retention	Tremor
Epinephrine	+	++	+	++	+	+	+	+	+
Norepinephrine	+++	+ (sometimes bradycardia)	−	+	+	−	−	−	+
Isoproterenol	−	++	−	+	+	+	+	−	+
Ephedrine	+	+	−	+	+	+	−	+	+
Terbutaline	−	+	−	+	+	+	−	+	++
Dextroamphetamine	+	+	−	++	+	+	+	+	+
Ethylnorepinephrine	+ (rare)	+	−	+	+	+	−	−	+
Dopamine HCl	+ (sometimes hypotension)	+ (sometimes bradycardia)	−	+	+	+	−	−	+

Genitourinary Urinary retention in patients with benign prostatic hypertrophy has been noted.

Other Sweating is common. Local necrosis at the site of injection has been observed. When sympathomimetics are applied topically to the nasal mucosa, chronic rhinitis may occur.

Contraindications

Patients with hypertension, hyperthyroidism, ischemic heart disease, or cerebrovascular disease do not tolerate these drugs well. Sympathomimetics should not be given to patients known to be hypersensitive to them.

Precautions

Sympathomimetics should be used in pregnancy only if the benefits outweigh the risk to the fetus. These drugs should be used with caution in the presence of diabetes, hyperthyroidism, cardiac diseases, hypertension, and epilepsy.

Drug Interactions

Dangerous reactions may occur when these drugs are used with MAO inhibitors.

Treatment

Withdrawal of the drug is usually all that is necessary. If blood pressure rises to extreme levels, phentolamine or phenoxybenzamine HCl and beta blockers (propranolol HCl, etc.) may be given. Tachycardia can be treated by beta blockers. Arrhythmias should be treated according to the type of arrhythmia. Rapid digitalization may be necessary.

Reactions to Specific Sympathomimetics

Epinephrine

Epinephrine is contraindicated in narrow angle glaucoma and should not be given with local anesthetics in the fingers and toes because tissue sloughing may occur. Epinephrine will deteriorate if exposed to light. Epinephrine tachyphylaxis may occur.

Norepinephrine bitartrate

This drug has four times the hypertensive effects of epinephrine; therefore, it must be given with careful blood pressure monitoring. It should not be given when hypotension is due to a blood volume deficit.

Mazindol

While this drug is really a tricyclic compound (see page 263), it prevents the re-uptake of norepinephrine by afferent sympathetic neurons and thus has indirect sympathomimetic effects. Constipation and CNS stimulation are common.

Isoproterenol

Hypertension is rare but tachycardia may be more frequent. Otherwise the side effects are similar to those of epinephrine.

Terbutaline

In general, the side effects of terbutaline are those typical of sympathomimetics. Hypertension, arrhythmia, and seizures are uncommon.

Dopamine

In contrast to epinephrine, this drug may induce hypotension and bradycardia, although tachycardia is more common. Widening of the QRS complex, dyspnea, and angina are infrequently observed, but nausea and vomiting are more frequent than with other sympathomimetics.

Chapter 35

VASODILATORS

Vasodilators

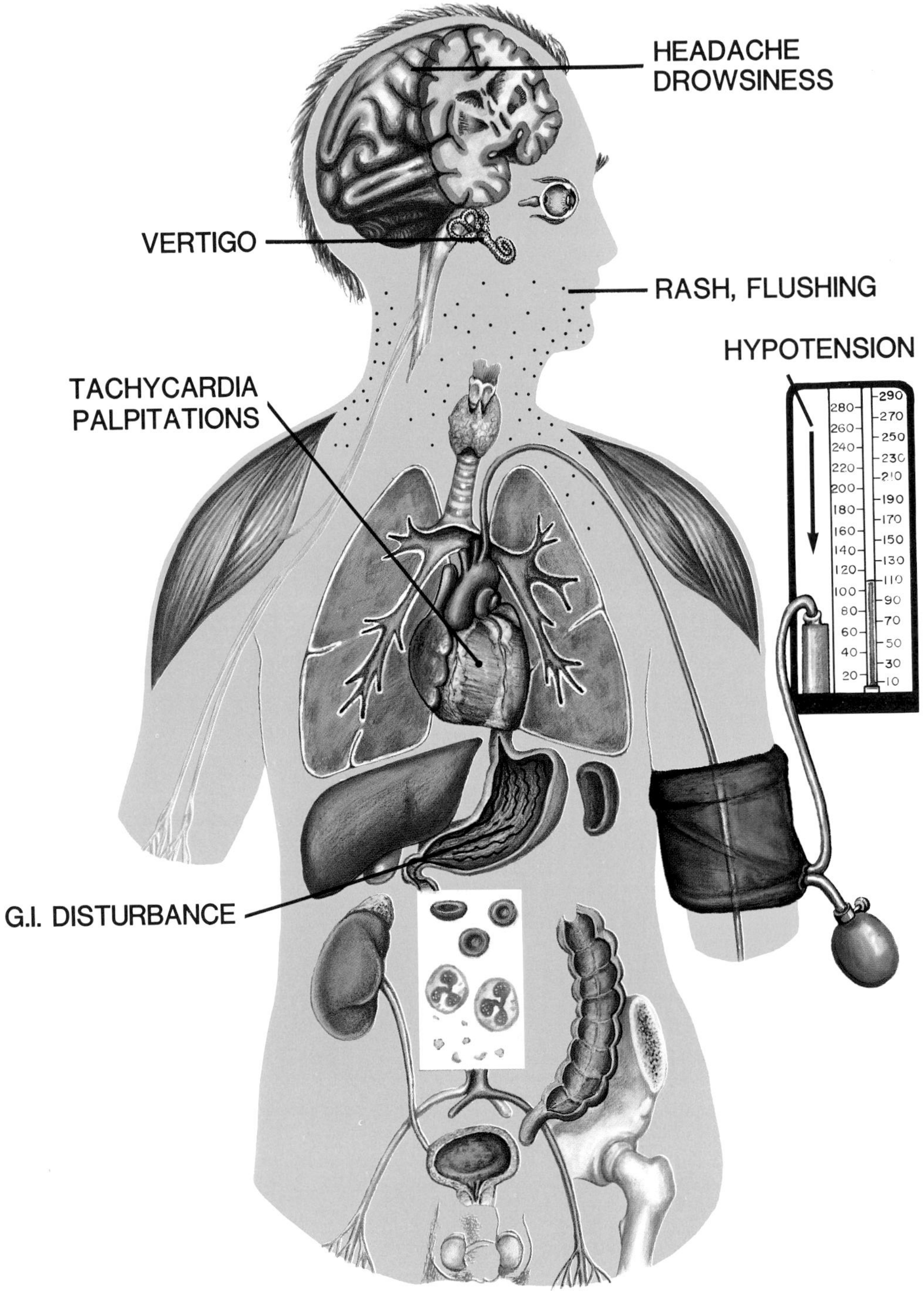

HEADACHE
DROWSINESS

VERTIGO

RASH, FLUSHING

HYPOTENSION

TACHYCARDIA
PALPITATIONS

G.I. DISTURBANCE

Introduction

Principal Vasodilators

Papaverine hydrochloride
  Related drug:
    Ethaverine hydrochloride
Isoxsuprine hydrochloride
Cyclandelate
Nylidrin
Niacin
  Related drug:
    Nicotinyl alcohol
Tolazoline hydrochloride
Phenoxybenzamine hydrochloride
Phentolamine
Ergoloid mesylates
Reserpine (see page 81)
Guanethidine sulfate (see page 83)
Methyldopa (see page 75)
Nitroglycerine compounds (see page 9)

The side effects of all vasodilators are very similar. All are capable of causing hypotension — postural or general — which may be severe when the drugs are administered parenterally. Most of the CNS and cardiovascular side effects (tachycardia, etc.) are secondary to hypotension. Vasodilators can also produce gastrointestinal irritation, flushing, tingling, sweating, and allergic skin reactions.

Vasodilators are of low toxicity except when administered parenterally. They should be used with caution in patients with cardiovascular diseases that may be aggravated by hypotension. The only other common precaution for vasodilator use is peptic ulcer disease; tolazoline HCl in particular should be avoided in these patients. Simple withdrawal of the drug is usually sufficient therapy for reactions to vasodilators. Severe hypotension may need to be treated with a vasopressor.

Papaverine Hydrochloride

Principal Drugs

Generic Name	Representative Trade Names
Papaverine hydrochloride	Pavabid, Vasospan
Related drug:	
Ethaverine hydrochloride	Ethaquin

Toxicity Rating: Low

Adverse Reactions

Central Nervous System Headache, drowsiness, vertigo, and malaise are reported infrequently.

Cardiovascular Hypotension and postural hypotension rarely occur.

Gastrointestinal Nausea, anorexia, abdominal distress, diarrhea, and constipation are infrequently reported.

Other Skin rashes, hepatic hypersensitivity with jaundice and eosinophilia, and sweating may occur.

Contraindications

Known hypersensitivity to papaverine is the only contraindication.

Precautions

The drug must be used with caution in patients with glaucoma.

Treatment

Simple withdrawal of the drug is usually sufficient.

Isoxsuprine Hydrochloride

Representative Trade Name: Vasodilan

Toxicity Rating: Low

Adverse Reactions

Cardiovascular System Hypotension, postural hypotension, tachycardia, dizziness, and chest pain are the main reactions to isoxsuprine, but are infrequent.

Gastrointestinal Nausea, vomiting, and abdominal distress occur.

Other Skin rashes, sometimes severe, are rare.

Contraindications and Precautions

There are no absolute contraindications other than known hypersensitivity. Hypocalcemia, hypoglycemia, and hypotension have occurred in newborns whose mothers received this drug during labor.

Treatment

Simple withdrawal of the drug is sufficient.

Cyclandelate

Representative Trade Name: Cyclospasmol

Toxicity Rating: Low

Adverse Reactions

Adverse reactions to cyclandelate are infrequent. However, gastrointestinal distress (especially on an empty stomach), flushing, headache, weakness, tachycardia, and occasional hypotension occur.

Contraindications

Known hypersensitivity is the major contraindication.

Precautions

Glaucoma may be worsened by the drug.

Treatment

Simple withdrawal of the drug is usually sufficient.

Nylidrin

Representative Trade Name: Arlidin

Toxicity Rating: Low

Adverse Reactions

Central Nervous System Trembling, nervousness, lack of energy, and dizziness occur.

Cardiovascular Palpitations and postural hypotension may occur but are infrequent.

Contraindications

Nylidrin is contraindicated in patients with acute myocardial infarction, paroxysmal tachycardia, severe coronary insufficiency, and thyrotoxicosis.

Precautions

Patients with arrhythmias, coronary disease, or congestive heart failure should be given this drug only with caution.

Treatment

Simple withdrawal of the drug is usually sufficient.

Niacin

Principal Drugs

Generic Name	Representative Trade Names
Niacin	Nicobid, Nicolar
Related drug:	
Nicotinyl alcohol	Roniacol

Toxicity Rating: Low

Adverse Reactions

Most reactions are mild and temporary. They include temporary flushing, headache, itching, tingling, and gastric distress. Skin rashes and allergies may occur. Postural hypotension may develop with large doses.

Contraindications

The major contraindications for niacin therapy are known hypersensitivity, hepatic disease, and peptic ulcer. Administration of large doses during pregnancy is not advisable.

Precautions

Niacin may cause decreased glucose tolerance, elevated uric acid, and sensitivity to beta blockers. Monitoring of liver function may be wise in patients predisposed to hepatic disorders.

Treatment

Simple withdrawal of the drug is usually adequate.

Tolazoline Hydrochloride

Representative Trade Name: Priscoline Hydrochloride

Toxicity Rating: Low to moderate because tolazoline is given intravenously and intraarterially.

Adverse Reactions

Central Nervous System Confusion, hallucinations, dizziness, and vertigo occur rarely.

Cardiovascular Like all the vasodilators, tolazoline may cause flushing, tachycardia, hypotension, palpitations, and edema. Cardiac arrhythmias, angina, and hypertension can develop in susceptible individuals.

Gastrointestinal Nausea, vomiting, diarrhea, hepatitis, and aggravation of peptic ulcer disease may occur.

Other Allergic reactions, paradoxical vasospasm of the peripheral blood vessels, hematuria, bone marrow depression, and a burning sensation have been reported.

Contraindications

Tolazoline must not be used following a stroke or in patients with known hypersensitivity or preexisting coronary disease.

Precautions

Caution must be exercised when tolazoline is used in the presence of known peptic ulcer and mitral stenosis.

Treatment

All but the most severe effects may be treated by withdrawing the drug. Severe hypotension should be treated with ephedrine, as epinephrine and norepinephrine may cause an ''epinephrine reversal'' (paradoxical drop in blood pressure).

Phenoxybenzamine Hydrochloride

Representative Trade Name: Dibenzyline

Toxicity Rating: Low

Adverse Reactions

Adverse reactions to phenoxybenzamine HCl are primarily due to adrenergic blockade and include hypotension, tachycardia, miosis, nasal congestion, and inhibition of ejaculation. Nausea, gastric distress, drowsiness, and fatigue are reported.

Contraindications

Phenoxybenzamine is contraindicated in patients with any vascular disorder (stroke, coronary insufficiency, etc.) in which a drop in blood pressure may have serious consequences. Known hypersensitivity is also a contraindication but is rare.

Precautions

Phenoxybenzamine should not be given with compounds that stimulate both alpha and beta receptors, because an exaggerated hypotensive response may occur.

Treatment

Simple withdrawal of the drug should be sufficient. Where severe hypotension and shock develop, intravenous solutions of norepinephrine will reverse the alpha blockade.

Phentolamine

Representative Trade Name: Regitine

Toxicity Rating: Low to moderate because the drug is administered intravenously.

Adverse Reactions

Adverse reactions to phentolamine, as to phenoxybenzamine, are primarily due to adrenergic blockade. They include hypotension, tachycardia, arrhythmias, nasal congestion, flushing, dizziness, and weakness. Nausea, vomiting, and diarrhea may occur.

Contraindications

In addition to known hypersensitivity, contraindications for phentolamine include present or past myocardial infarction, other coronary disease, and other conditions that may be aggravated by hypotension.

Precautions

Phentolamine has been known to produce cerebrovascular and myocardial occlusions. Urine catecholamine determination and other laboratory tests, and roentgenography, have replaced phentolamine as a method for ruling out the presence of a pheochromocytoma.

Treatment

Mild hypotension and adrenergic blockade can be treated by withdrawal of the drug and supportive measures. Severe hypotension may necessitate norepinephrine therapy.

Ergoloid Mesylates

Representative Trade Name: Hydergine

Toxicity Rating: Low

Adverse Reactions

These drugs do not have the vasoconstrictive effects of other ergot alkaloids. However, they may cause transient nausea and gastric disturbances.

Contraindications

Known hypersensitivity and acute or chronic psychosis are the important contraindications.

Precautions

A careful diagnosis of the cause of decreased mental alertness and ability should be made before these drugs are prescribed.

Treatment

Withdrawal of the drug is usually adequate treatment.

Chapter 36

VITAMINS

Vitamins (Overdose)

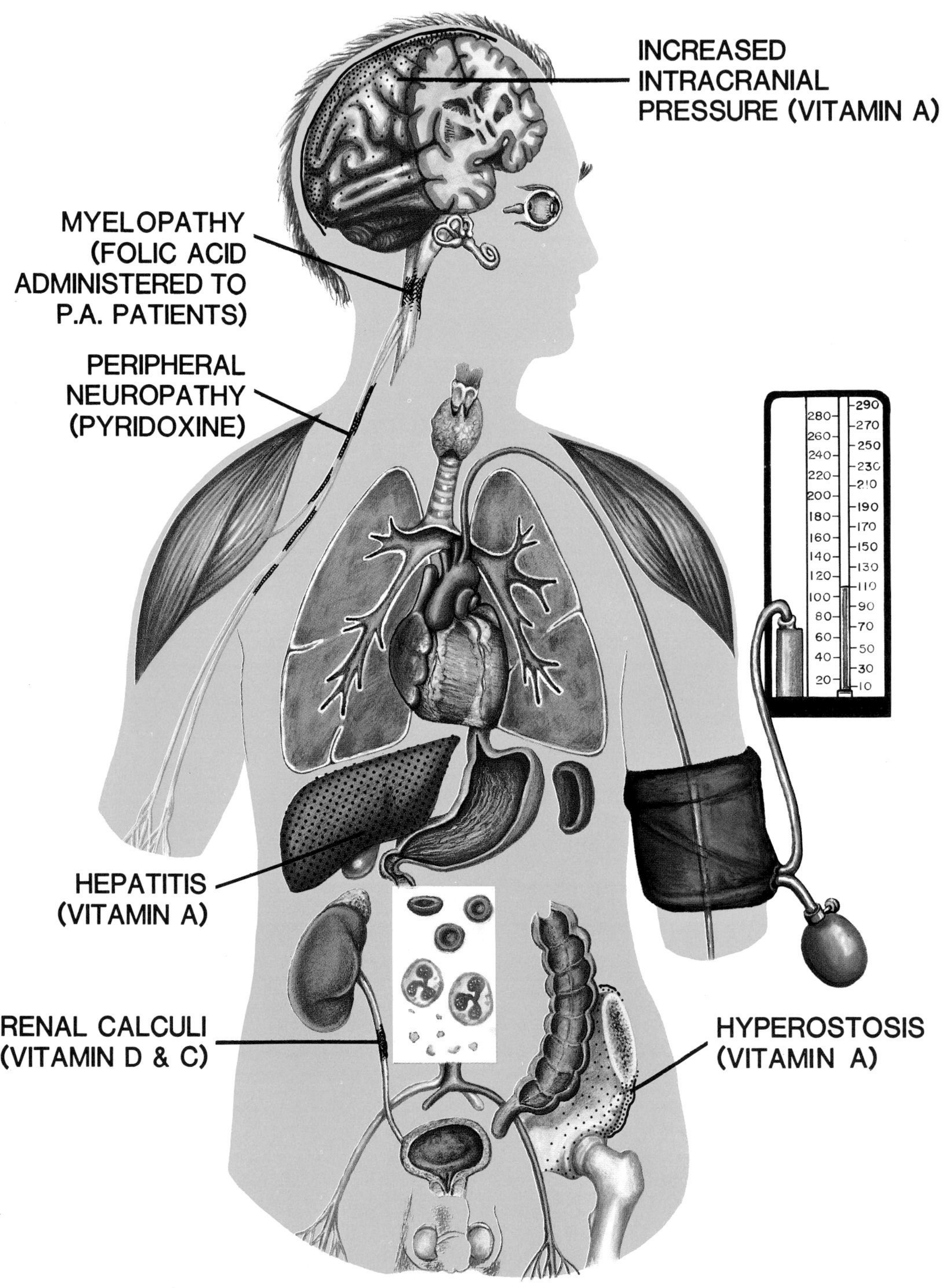
INCREASED INTRACRANIAL PRESSURE (VITAMIN A)
MYELOPATHY (FOLIC ACID ADMINISTERED TO P.A. PATIENTS)
PERIPHERAL NEUROPATHY (PYRIDOXINE)
HEPATITIS (VITAMIN A)
RENAL CALCULI (VITAMIN D & C)
HYPEROSTOSIS (VITAMIN A)
280 260 240 220 200 180 160 140 120 100 80 60 40 20
290 270 250 230 210 190 170 150 130 110 90 70 50 30 10

Vitamins

With one exception, vitamins given in therapeutic doses have no significant side effects except rare allergic reactions. The exception is folic acid, which can precipitate or aggravate neurological deficits in patients with pernicious anemia unless cyanocobalamin (vitamin B_{12}) is given concomitantly. Overdosage of certain vitamins will precipitate toxic reactions.

Vitamin A

Acute overdosage of this vitamin is associated with nausea, vomiting, headache, vertigo, and, in infants, increased intracranial pressure with bulging fontanelles. Chronic overdosage of vitamin A is associated with hepatitis, marked hypercalcemia, and neurological changes including headache, nystagmus, diplopia, and depression. In children there may be hyperostosis, periosteal swelling, and premature closure of the epiphyses. Large doses of vitamin A may increase the prothrombin time in patients on coumarin drugs. Almost all patients taking excessive doses of vitamin A develop skin changes. These include pruritus, alopecia, dry and desquamating skin, and angular stomatitis.

Vitamin D

Chronic overdosage of vitamin D causes hypercalcemia, renal stones, and calcification in the soft tissues of almost any organ of the body. Pancreatitis, hypertension, and renal failure may develop. There are reports of increased susceptibility to myocardial infarctions during long-term overdosage. Mental retardation and growth retardation may occur in children.

Vitamin E

Overdosage of vitamin E is not definitely known to produce any side effects. It may decrease the action of iron in anemic children. Overdosage may deplete vitamin A stores, but this is controversial. Overdosage may also increase prothrombin time in patients taking coumarin drugs.

Vitamin K

Excessive oral intake of vitamin K is probably harmless except when patients are taking coumarin drugs, in which case vitamin K may neutralize the anticoagulant effect of the drugs. Intravenous vitamin K (phytonadione) can cause flushing, diaphoresis, cyanosis, and anaphylactoid shock; fatalities have occurred. Parenteral administration of vitamin K to infants may cause hyperbilirubinemia and hemolytic anemia.

Thiamine Hydrochloride (Vitamin B_1)

Aside from hypersensitivity reactions to parenteral use, there are no known reactions to thiamine.

Riboflavin (Vitamin B_2)

No toxic effects of this vitamin have been reported.

Pyridoxine (Vitamin B_6)

Toxic effects are unusual in healthy individuals taking this vitamin, but Parkinson's disease patients will require more levodopa because pyridoxine enhances the peripheral catabolism of levodopa. Pyridoxine may also decrease the action of phenobarbital and phenytoin. Pyridoxine overdosage may produce a sensory neuropathy.

Niacin and Niacinamide

Most patients taking large doses of these drugs report harmless flushing, pruritus, headache, and paresthesias at some time or another. Unusually large doses may activate a peptic ulcer, decrease glucose tolerance, or produce jaundice. Rare cases of anaphylaxis have been reported upon intravenous administration.

Pantothenic Acid

Even large doses of this drug are not known to produce adverse reactions in man.

Ascorbic Acid (Vitamin C)

Excessive doses of vitamin C may cause diarrhea, nonspecific urethritis, and renal calculi (hyperoxaluria). Plasma levels of ethenyl estradiol may increase. Iron absorption may increase and constitute a potential hazard in patients with hemochromatosis, sideroblastic anemia, or various hemolytic anemias. Diabetics need to be careful with overdoses of vitamin C because it may produce false positive or false negative urine tests for sugar with the various home-test kits available.

Cyanocobalamin (Vitamin B_{12})

There are no known adverse effects from overdosage.

Treatment of Hypervitaminosis

Simple withdrawal of the vitamin is usually sufficient.

Chapter 37

MINERALS

Minerals

Principal Mineral Drugs

- Ferrous sulfate
  - Related drugs:
    - Ferrous gluconate
    - Iron dextran
- Gold sodium thiomalate
  - Related drug:
    - Aurothioglucose
- Fluoride
- Other miscellaneous minerals

Ferrous Sulfate

Principal Drugs

Generic Name	Representative Trade Names
Ferrous sulfate	Ferrous Sulfate, Feosol
Related drugs:	
Ferrous gluconate	Fergon
Iron dextran	Imferon

Toxicity Rating: Low

Adverse Reactions

Gastrointestinal Nausea, vomiting, constipation, diarrhea, or abdominal cramps may be noted with various preparations. These reactions can often be obviated by IM injection, but this has its own disadvantages.

Allergic Allergic reactions occur with parenteral iron (iron dextran) and include anaphylactic shock, urticaria, bronchial asthma, and drug fever.

Other Local reactions to parenteral iron include sterile abscesses, phlebitis, lymphadenopathy, and brownish skin discoloration. Local sarcomas have occurred in laboratory animals.

Contraindications

Known hypersensitivity and pregnancy are the major contraindications to parenteral iron. There are no contraindications to oral iron therapy.

Precautions

Excessive iron administration may produce hemosiderosis, especially if the iron is given parenterally for hemolytic anemias. Parenteral iron administration may also exacerbate joint symptoms in rheumatoid arthritis.

Treatment

Simple withdrawal of the drug is usually all that is necessary. Deferoxamine mesylate may be given in cases of acute or chronic iron overload.

Gold Sodium Thiomalate

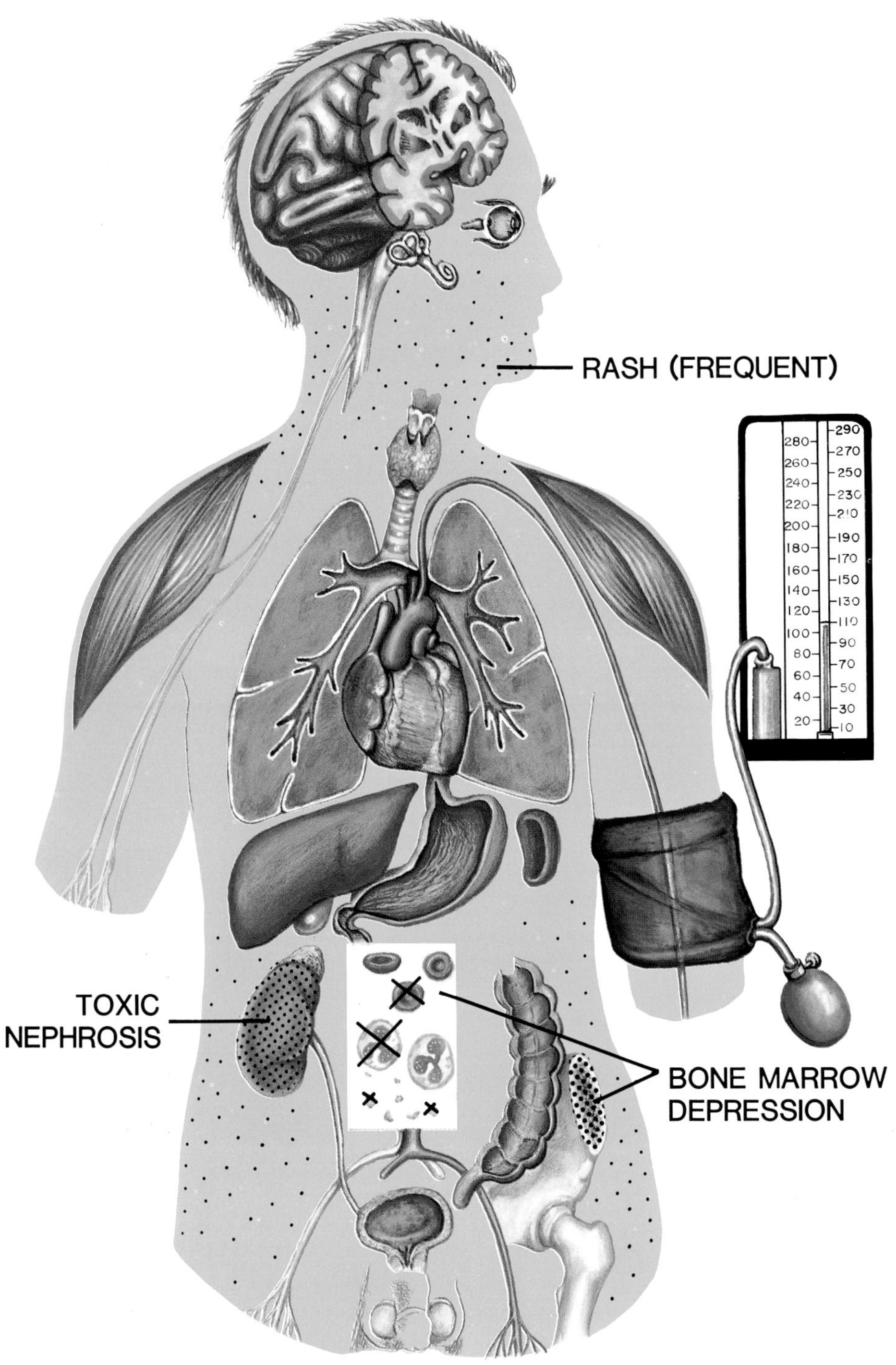

Gold Sodium Thiomalate

Principal Drugs

Generic Name	Representative Trade Name
Gold sodium thiomalate	Myochrysine
Related drug:	
Aurothioglucose	Solganal

Toxicity Rating: High because of severe dermatitis, nephrosis, and bone marrow depression.

Adverse Reactions

Dermatologic Dermatitis is the most common reaction to gold therapy and may vary from erythema to severe exfoliative dermatitis. Gold dermatitis is aggravated by sunlight. There may be stomatitis, gingivitis, and glossitis as well.

Renal Nephrosis is not uncommon and may be severe.

Hematologic Bone marrow depression is infrequent but may lead to aplastic anemia, severe agranulocytosis, or thrombocytopenia.

Allergic Anaphylactoid reactions and drug fever may occur in addition to the many dermatologic reactions.

Other Nausea, vomiting, gastritis, or colitis may occur. Any mucous membrane may be affected—vaginal, pharyngeal, tracheal, and conjunctival. Iritis and corneal ulcers may also occur. Encephalitis and toxic hepatitis have been reported.

Contraindications

Contraindications are known hypersensitivity, uncontrolled diabetes, preexisting renal disease, collagen disease, severe hypertension or blood dyscrasias, and previous irradiation or infectious hepatitis.

Precautions

Repeated evaluations of hepatic and renal function and blood counts should be done during therapy. Patients should be warned to notify the physician promptly of dermatitis or other symptoms.

Drug Interactions

No serious drug interactions have been reported.

Treatment

Mild reactions are treated by simple withdrawal of the drug. Dermatitis may respond to soothing lotions and topical corticosteroids. For severe dermatitis, nephrosis, and hematologic reactions systemic corticosteroids should be given. A chelating agent such as dimercaprol may be used if these reactions continue despite adequate systemic steroid therapy. Anabolic steroids and penicillamine may be useful in selected cases, especially when there is significant bone marrow depression.

Fluoride

Representative Trade Names: Adeflor, Luride

Toxicity Rating: Low

Adverse Reactions

Allergic rash and other idiosyncrasies have rarely been reported with therapeutic doses. Mottled enamel, osteomalacia, and osteosclerosis may occur.

Contraindications

This drug should not be used when adequate fluoride has been added to the drinking water. Children under the age of 3 should not be given this drug.

Treatment

Simple withdrawal of the drug is usually all that is necessary. Unfortunately, no other treatment is available for chronic fluorosis.

Miscellaneous Minerals

Adverse Reactions

Calcium preparations administered orally may cause renal stones and nephrocalcinosis. Parenteral calcium (calcium chloride) may cause local tissue necrosis and sloughing. Transient hypercalcemia may cause weakness, cardiac arrhythmias, and cardiac arrest. Intravenous magnesium may cause neuromuscular blockade, cardiac arrest, or respiratory depression. Intravenous potassium may also cause cardiac arrhythmias and arrest; oral potassium chloride may cause jejunal ulcers with perforation. Excessive ingestion of zinc may cause copper and iron deficiency and nausea, vomiting, and abdominal pain. Headache, chills, fever, and weakness occur. Overdose of selenium is unusual.

Treatment

Intravenous calcium gluconate may reverse the effects of hyperkalemia and hypermagnesemia. Steroids may lower serum calcium levels.

Chapter 38

MISCELLANEOUS DRUGS

Aminocaproic Acid

Representative Trade Name: Amicar

Toxicity Rating: Moderate if used intravenously because of the potential for thrombophlebitis and intravascular clotting.

Adverse Reactions

Central Nervous System Headache, dizziness, tinnitus, and weakness may occur.

Cardiovascular Hypotension and bradycardia may occur. Thrombophlebitis has been reported with intravenous use.

Gastrointestinal As with most drugs, nausea, cramps, and diarrhea can occur.

Other Skin rashes and nasal and conjuctival congestion have been noted.

Contraindications

Active intravascular clotting is the major contraindication.

Precautions

Caution must be exercised in administering this drug to patients with cardiac, hepatic, or renal disorders. The safety in pregnancy has not been established.

Drug Interactions

Oral contraceptives may increase the chances of intravascular clotting when used with this drug.

Treatment

Simple withdrawal of the drug is usually all that is necessary.

Apomorphine Hydrochloride

Toxicity Rating: Moderate since acute circulatory failure may occur, especially in the elderly.

Adverse Reactions

Central Nervous System CNS reactions include drowsiness, confusion, and depression, but the opposite (restlessness, tremor, or euphoria) may occur.

Respiratory Like most narcotics, apomorphine may cause respiratory depression, a potentially dangerous side effect.

Cardiovascular Acute circulatory failure and death may occur, especially with overdosage.

Other Apomorphine is used to induce vomiting, and as expected it can sometimes cause excessive vomiting.

Contraindications

Known hypersensitivity to narcotics is the major contraindication. Emetics such as apomorphine are often used to induce vomiting in cases of poisoning; it must be remembered that emesis is dangerous with poisons (gasoline, oil, etc.) that can damage the esophagus or respiratory tree on the way back up. Endotracheal intubation prior to administering the emetic may be useful to prevent aspiration of the poison into the respiratory tree.

Treatment

Naloxone 0.1 mg/kg may be given to stop excessive vomiting. Otherwise, simple withdrawal of the drug will usually be sufficient. Supportive measures and vasopressors may be indicated in acute circulatory collapse.

Benzquinamide Hydrochloride

Representative Trade Name: Emete-con

Toxicity Rating: Low

Adverse Reactions

Central Nervous System Drowsiness is common. Paradoxical excitation may occur, with insomnia, tremors, restlessness, and anxiety. Headache has also been reported.

Cardiovascular Hypertension, hypotension, and arrhythmias (mostly harmless) occur.

Dermatologic Allergic reactions include fever and chills, urticaria, and various other skin rashes.

Gastrointestinal Anorexia and nausea are infrequent. Hiccoughs, dry mouth, or excessive salivation have occasionally been reported.

Contraindications

Known hypersensitivity and pregnancy are the significant contraindications.

Precautions

Intravenous use is associated with more frequent cardiovascular side effects than oral, so careful monitoring is necessary. Patients with hypertension or hypotension need careful monitoring, especially if they are using other drugs that affect blood pressure. Benzquinamide may mask the signs of intoxication by other drugs. Other causes of vomiting should be ruled out before initiating benzquinamide therapy.

Treatment

Simple withdrawal of the drug is effective therapy for most reactions. Blood pressure support or antiarrhythmic therapy may occasionally be necessary.

Calcitonin

Representative Trade Name: Calcimar Solution

Toxicity Rating: Moderate because the drug is given parenterally and allergic reactions may be severe.

Adverse Reactions

Central Nervous System Headache, tingling, and unusual taste sensations may occur.

Gastrointestinal Nausea, vomiting, and diarrhea are noted occasionally.

Allergic Rashes and anaphylaxis can occur.

Other Local inflammation at the injection site occurs in 10 percent of patients.

Contraindications

Known hypersensitivity to the drug or its vehicle are the major contraindications. The safety in pregnant women, nursing mothers, and children has not been established.

Precautions

Patients should be skin tested for sensitivity before calcitonin is administered. Epinephrine should be on hand. Parenteral calcium solutions should also be available in case hypocalcemia develops. Patients on chronic therapy need periodic urinalysis.

Treatment

Allergic reactions are treated with epinephrine, oxygen, IV solutions, and steroids. Hypocalcemia may necessitate IV calcium gluconate. Other reactions are treated by simple withdrawal of the drug.

Chenodiol (Chenodeoxycholic Acid)

Representative Trade Name: Chenix

Toxicity Rating: Low

Adverse Reactions

Dyspepsia and diarrhea are the most common side effects. Mild hepatitis occurs but is usually transient.

Contraindications

Acute cholecystitis, cholangitis, obstructive jaundice, inflammatory bowel disease, and pregnancy are the major contraindications.

Drug Interactions

Aluminum-containing antacids may bind this drug and prevent absorption.

Treatment

Halving the dose of chenodeoxycholic acid will usually resolve diarrhea. The dose is then gradually increased to therapeutic levels again. Rarely, diarrhea and other symptoms necessitate that the drug be stopped.

Cholestyramine Resin

Representative Trade Names: Questran, Cuemid

Toxicity Rating: Low

Adverse Reactions

Constipation is the main side effect; it can be reduced or reversed by decreasing the dosage. Nausea, vomiting, diarrhea, steatorrhea, and hypoprothrombinemia occur rarely. Cholestyramine binds bile salts and as a result inhibits absorption of all fat-soluble vitamins. This may lead to osteoporosis. There are reports of calcification in the biliary tree, but this may not be drug related. Since cholestyramine preparations contain FD & C Yellow No. 5 (tartrazine), hypersensitivity reactions to this substance may be observed.

Contraindications

Complete biliary obstruction is the major contraindication.

Precautions

When cholestyramine is given for prolonged periods, concomitant administration of fat-soluble vitamin supplements may be wise. Sometimes folic acid is also given. Younger patients should be observed for hyperchloremic alkalosis. Patients should be watched for the complications of chronic constipation such as fecal impaction.

Drug Interactions

Cholestyramine may delay the absorption of phenylbutazone, warfarin, chlorothiazide, tetracycline, penicillin, phenobarbital, thyroid hormones, and digitalis. It is therefore wise to administer these drugs no closer than 1 hour before or 4 hours after giving cholestyramine.

Treatment

Simple withdrawal of the drug is usually all that is necessary.

Cimetidine

Cimetidine

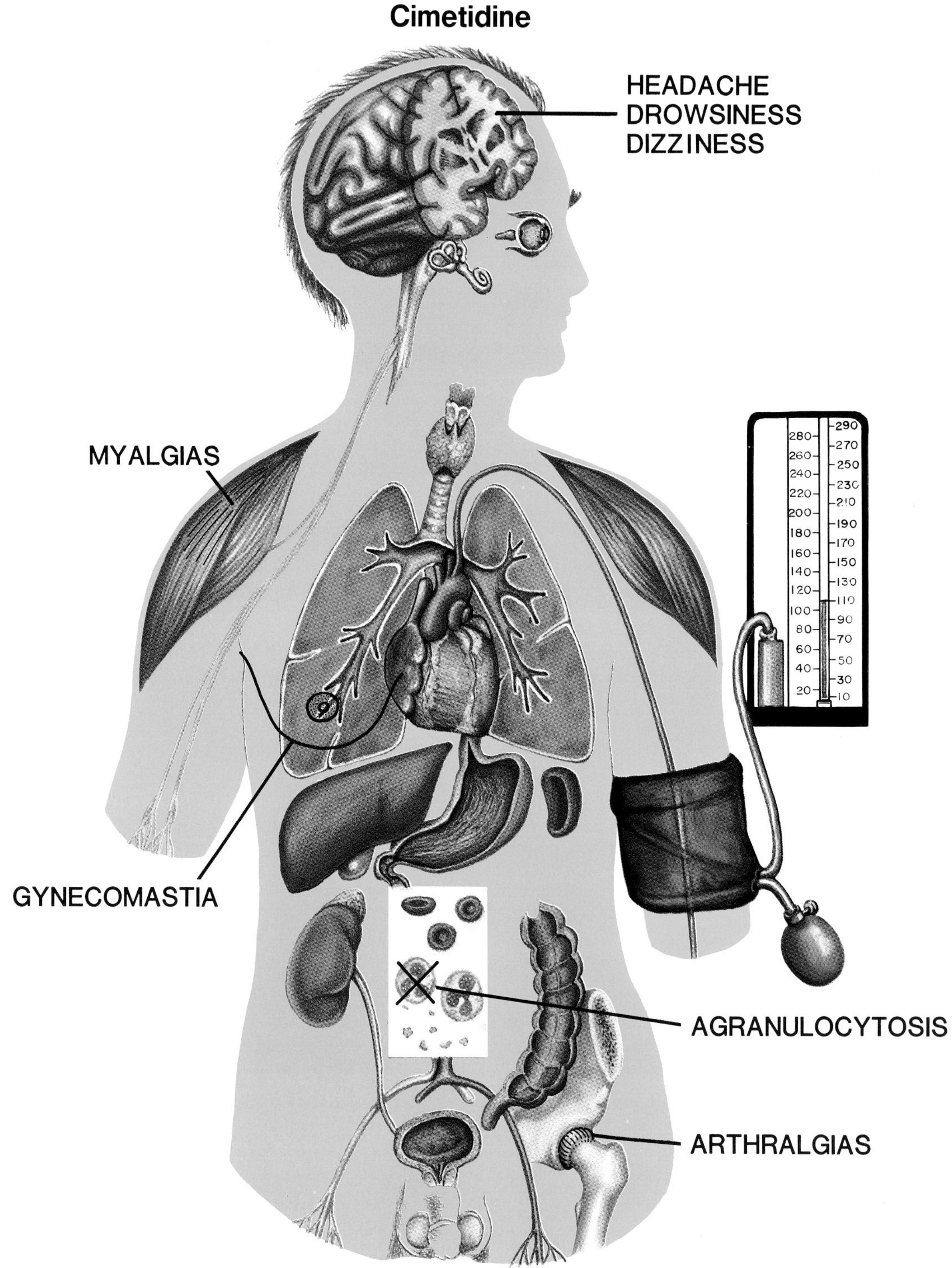
HEADACHE
DROWSINESS
DIZZINESS
MYALGIAS
GYNECOMASTIA
AGRANULOCYTOSIS
ARTHRALGIAS
280 260 240 220 200 180 160 140 120 100 80 60 40 20
290 270 250 230 210 190 170 150 130 110 90 70 50 30 10

Cimetidine

Principal Drugs

Generic Name	Representative Trade Name
Cimetidine	Tagamet
Related drug:	
Ranitidine hydrochloride	Zantac

Toxicity Rating: Low

Adverse Reactions

Central Nervous System Mild drowsiness, dizziness, and moderate to severe headache have been reported.

Gastrointestinal Transient diarrhea may occur.

Musculoskeletal Mild arthralgias, myalgias, and exacerbation of preexisting arthritis have been observed.

Hematologic Rare cases of agranulocytosis, thrombocytopenia, and aplastic anemia have been reported.

Endocrinologic Gynecomastia, reversible impotence, and loss of libido may occur. The causal relationship between impotence and cimetidine is questionable.

Other Rare cases of hepatic and renal toxicity have been reported.

Contraindications

There are none.

Precautions

Elderly and severely ill patients may develop confusional states. The drug is not recommended in children and pregnant women unless the benefits outweigh the potential risk. Close monitoring of the prothrombin time is indicated.

Drug Interactions

Cimetidine reduces the hepatic metabolism of coumarin drugs, phenytoin, propranolol, chlordiazepoxide, diazepam, lidocaine, and theophylline, with associated increased blood levels of these drugs. There is an additive effect when cimetidine is administered with other drugs that depress the white blood cell count.

Treatment

Almost invariably, withdrawal of the drug alleviates the side effects.

Clofibrate

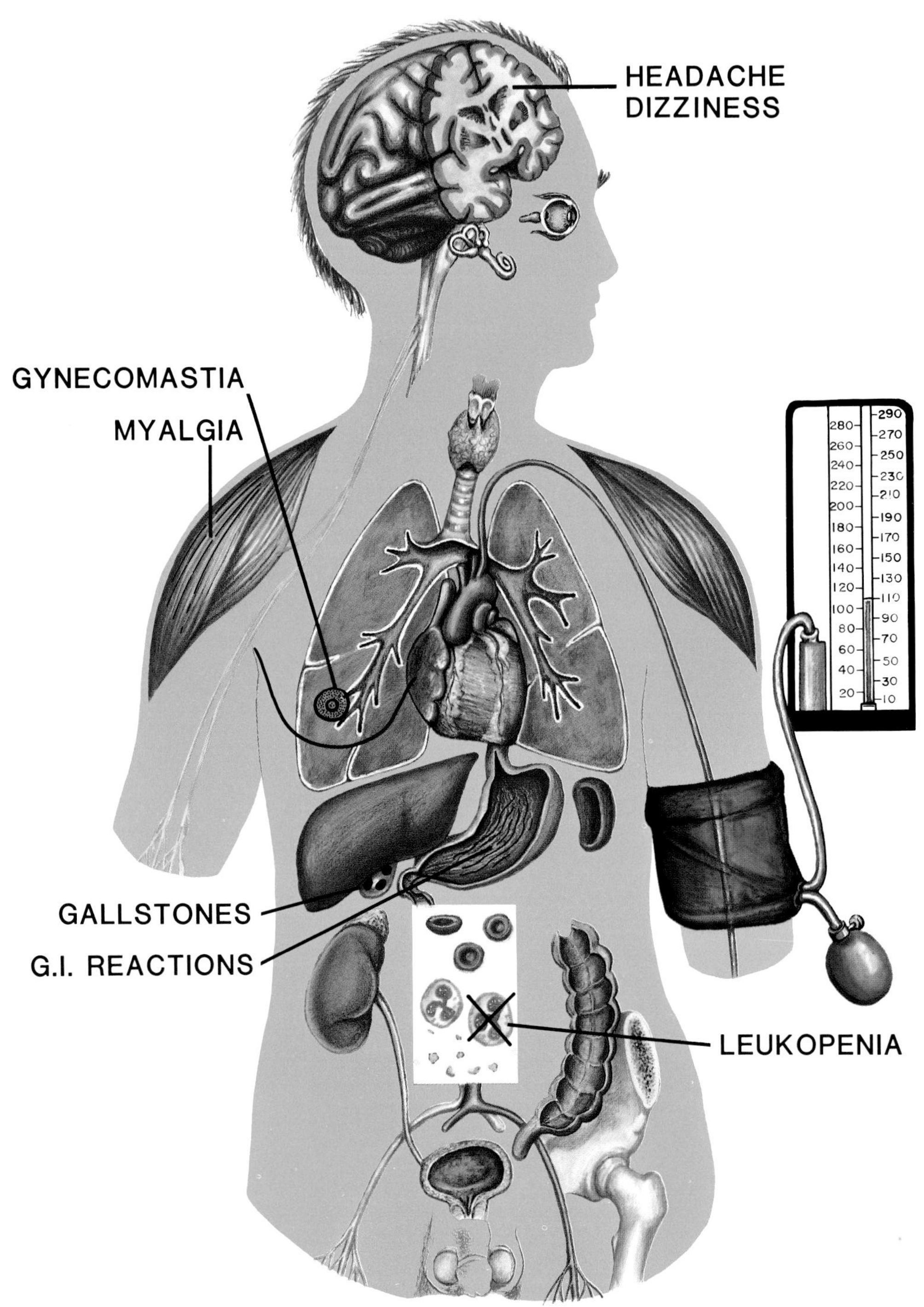
HEADACHE
DIZZINESS
GYNECOMASTIA
MYALGIA
GALLSTONES
G.I. REACTIONS
LEUKOPENIA

Clofibrate

Principal Drugs

Generic Name	Representative Trade Name
Clofibrate	Atromid-S
Related drug:	
Gemfibrozil	Lopid

Toxicity Rating: Low

Adverse Reactions

Gastrointestinal Nausea, vomiting, diarrhea, dyspepsia, and abdominal cramps may occur. Gallstones and hepatomegaly occur.

Nervous System Myalgia is more common than previously realized. In addition, patients may experience headache, dizziness, and fatigue.

Hematologic Although rare, leukopenia, anemia, and eosinophilia may occur. Clofibrate may potentiate the action of anticoagulants.

Endocrinologic Gynecomastia, alopecia, and decreased libido are reported.

Other Myocardial ischemia, arrhythmias, skin rashes, urticaria, pruritus, renal dysfunction, abnormal liver function, weight gain, and polyphagia occur.

Contraindications

Pregnant women, nursing mothers, and patients with significant liver and renal disease should not receive clofibrate.

Precautions

Frequent serum lipid determinations should be done during therapy to be certain the drug is effective. Liver function studies and blood counts should be done occasionally in the early stages of therapy because of the possibility of elevated transaminases and anemia. Dosages of anticoagulants should be halved when clofibrate therapy is begun, and then adjusted according to prothrombin times.

Drug Interactions

Clofibrate potentiates the action of phenytoin, coumarin drugs, and tolbutamide.

Treatment

Simple withdrawal of the drug is usually all that is necessary.

Clomiphene Citrate

Representative Trade Name: Clomid

Toxicity Rating: Moderate because of increased incidence of ovarian cysts.

Adverse Reactions

In addition to ovarian cysts there may be abdominal pain, nausea, hot flashes, and breast discomfort. Multiple pregnancies have occurred.

Drug Interactions

Clomiphene may antagonize the action of estrogen.

Treatment

Withdrawal of the drug is effective therapy for most side effects.

Cromolyn Sodium

Representative Trade Name: Intal

Toxicity Rating: Low

Adverse Reactions

Respiratory Cough, wheezing, nasal congestion, sneezing, and nasal itching or burning can occur. Eosinophilic pneumonia occurs rarely.

Gastrointestinal Nausea, epigastric discomfort, and esophagitis have been reported.

Central Nervous System Headache and dizziness occur.

Allergic Urticaria, serum sickness, dermatitis, and anaphylaxis occur infrequently.

Contraindications

Cromolyn sodium is contraindicated in acute asthmatic attacks and in patients with known hypersensitivity to the drug.

Precautions

Patients with hepatic or renal insufficiency may require reduced dosage; patients should be warned that asthmatic symptoms may recur when the dosage is reduced.

Treatment

Simple withdrawal of the drug is usually all that is necessary.

Deferoxamine Mesylate

Representative Trade Name: Desferal Mesylate

Toxicity Rating: Moderate because severe allergic reactions and hypotension may occur on IV administration.

Adverse Reactions

Allergic reactions, including urticaria, drug fever, and anaphylaxis, are the most common side effects of deferoxamine. There may be pain and induration at the site of injection. Long-term use may be associated with diarrhea, tachycardia, leg cramps, dysuria, and blurred vision.

Contraindications

Deferoxamine is contraindicated in patients with severe renal insufficiency and with known hypersensitivity.

Precautions

Since rare cataracts are reported with chronic administration of deferoxamine, periodic slit-lamp examinations are advised. Because of the possibility of anaphylaxis, this drug should not be given rapidly intravenously.

Drug Interactions

None are known.

Treatment

Simple withdrawal of the drug is usually sufficient, but anaphylaxis should be treated aggressively.

Dexpanthenol

Representative Trade Name: Ilopan

Toxicity Rating: Low

Adverse Reactions

Gastrointestinal Since dexpanthenol is used to stimulate the bowels, excessive flatus, diarrhea, and hyperperistalsis are side effects.

Hematologic Oddly enough, prolonged bleeding time occurs in a few patients.

Other Allergic reactions are rarely reported.

Contraindications

There are no absolute contraindications, but if allergic reactions to this drug are suspected to have occurred in the past, it should not be used. Pregnancy is a relative contraindication.

Precautions

Mechanical intestinal obstruction should be ruled out before using dexpanthenol.

Drug Interactions

Dexpanthenol may enhance the duration of succinylcholine neuromuscular blockade.

Treatment

Simple withdrawal of the drug is all that is necessary.

Dextrothyroxine Sodium

Representative Trade Name: Choloxin

Toxicity Rating: Low

Adverse Reactions

The major reaction to this drug is hyperthyroidism. Weight loss, tremor, insomnia, tachycardia, menstrual irregularities, and diarrhea may occur. Patients sensitive to iodine may develop rashes.

Contraindications

Dextrothyroxine should not be given to patients with preexisting myocardial ischemia or arrhythmias.

Precautions

Care should be taken when administering dextrothyroxine to pregnant women and patients with preexisting hypertension, or hepatic or renal disease. Since this drug may decrease glucose tolerance, diabetics taking it may need higher dosages of insulin or oral antidiabetic drugs.

Drug Interactions

Dextrothyroxine, like clofibrate, may potentiate the effects of oral anticoagulants.

Treatment

Simple withdrawal of the drug is usually all that is necessary.

Dimercaprol

Representative Trade Name: BAL in Oil

Toxicity Rating: Moderate because tachycardia and rise in blood pressure are consistently associated with the drug.

Adverse Reactions

Cardiovascular The most frequent side effect of this drug is hypertension and tachycardia.

Central Nervous System CNS reactions include headache, paresthesias, anxiety, and weakness.

Disulfiram

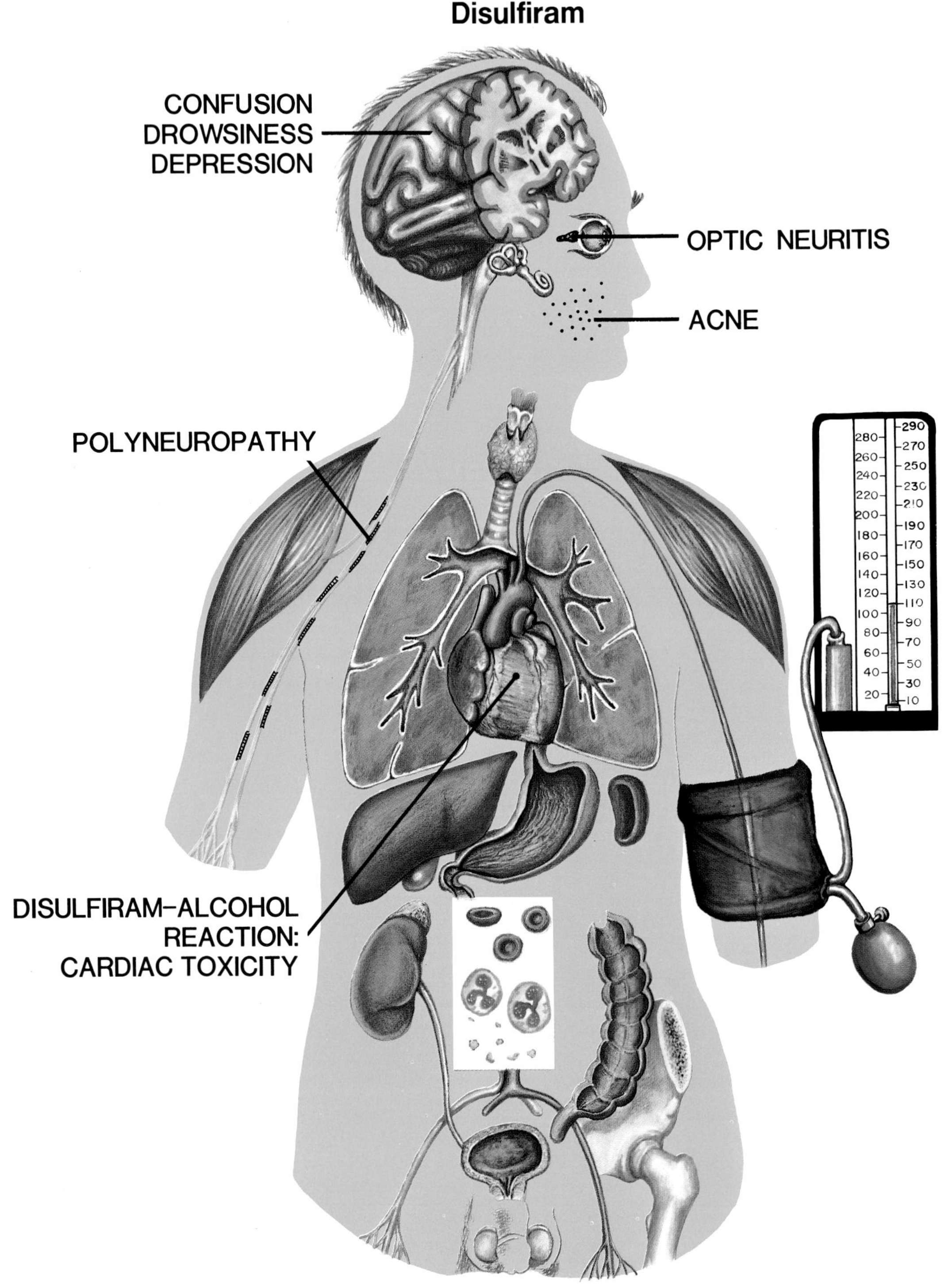
CONFUSION
DROWSINESS
DEPRESSION
OPTIC NEURITIS
ACNE
POLYNEUROPATHY
DISULFIRAM–ALCOHOL
REACTION:
CARDIAC TOXICITY

Gastrointestinal Nausea, vomiting, abdominal pain, and burning of the lips, mouth, and throat occur.

Special Senses Blepharospasm, conjunctivitis, and a peculiar taste or odor of the breath may occur.

Genitourinary Toxic nephrosis with renal failure has occurred but is rare if the urine is kept alkaline.

Other Metabolic acidosis, penile pain, and excessive lacrimation, salivation, and sweating occur. Sterile abscesses may occur at the injection site.

Contraindications

Dimercaprol is contraindicated in severe hepatic and renal insufficiency.

Precautions

The urine should be kept alkaline to prevent toxic nephrosis. Fever occurs in 30 percent of children receiving dimercaprol. The safety in pregnancy has not been established.

Drug Interactions

Iron should not be given to patients on dimercaprol therapy. Uptake of iodine I 131 is decreased during dimercaprol therapy.

Treatment

An antihistamine will relieve most of the side effects. Toxic nephrosis can be managed by discontinuing therapy and alkalinizing the urine. Most symptoms disappear on discontinuing the drug.

Disulfiram

Representative Trade Name: Antabuse

Toxicity Rating: Moderate to high because of cardiac reactions that may occur when disulfiram is used with alcohol.

Adverse Reactions

The most serious reaction from this drug is the disulfiram–alcohol reaction manifested by dyspnea, nausea, sweating, and even cardiac arrhythmias, myocardial infarction, congestive heart failure, shock, and death.

Central Nervous System Optic neuritis, polyneuritis, drowsiness, headache, confusion, and depression may occur.

Dermatologic In addition to allergic reactions, acneform eruptions may develop with chronic administration.

Other Impotence and a metallic or garlic-like aftertaste may occur.

Contraindication

Obviously, the major contraindication is alcoholic intoxication. This drug should not be given to patients who have recently ingested alcohol-containing preparations such as cough syrups or any other "elixirs." Patients with myocardial disease, coronary insufficiency, psychoses, or hypersensitivity to the drug should not receive disulfiram.

Precautions

This drug should be given with care in patients with diabetes, epilepsy, hyperthyroidism, nephritis, hepatitis, cirrhosis, or encephalopathy. Patients need to wear disulfiram-use identifying tags.

Drug Interactions

Disulfiram may cause ataxia or behavior changes when given with isoniazid and metronidazole. Disulfiram may also increase serum phenytoin to toxic levels. Concomitant administration of disulfiram and paraldehyde may lead to toxic levels of acetaldehyde. Use with coumarin drugs may further prolong the prothrombin time.

Treatment

The disulfiram–alcohol reaction is treated with vasopressors, a mixture of 95 percent oxygen and 5 percent carbon dioxide, massive doses of intravenous vitamin C (1 g), and ephedrine sulfate. Potassium levels should be monitored as hypokalemia may occur. Other reactions may be treated with simple withdrawal of the drug.

Ergotamine Tartrate

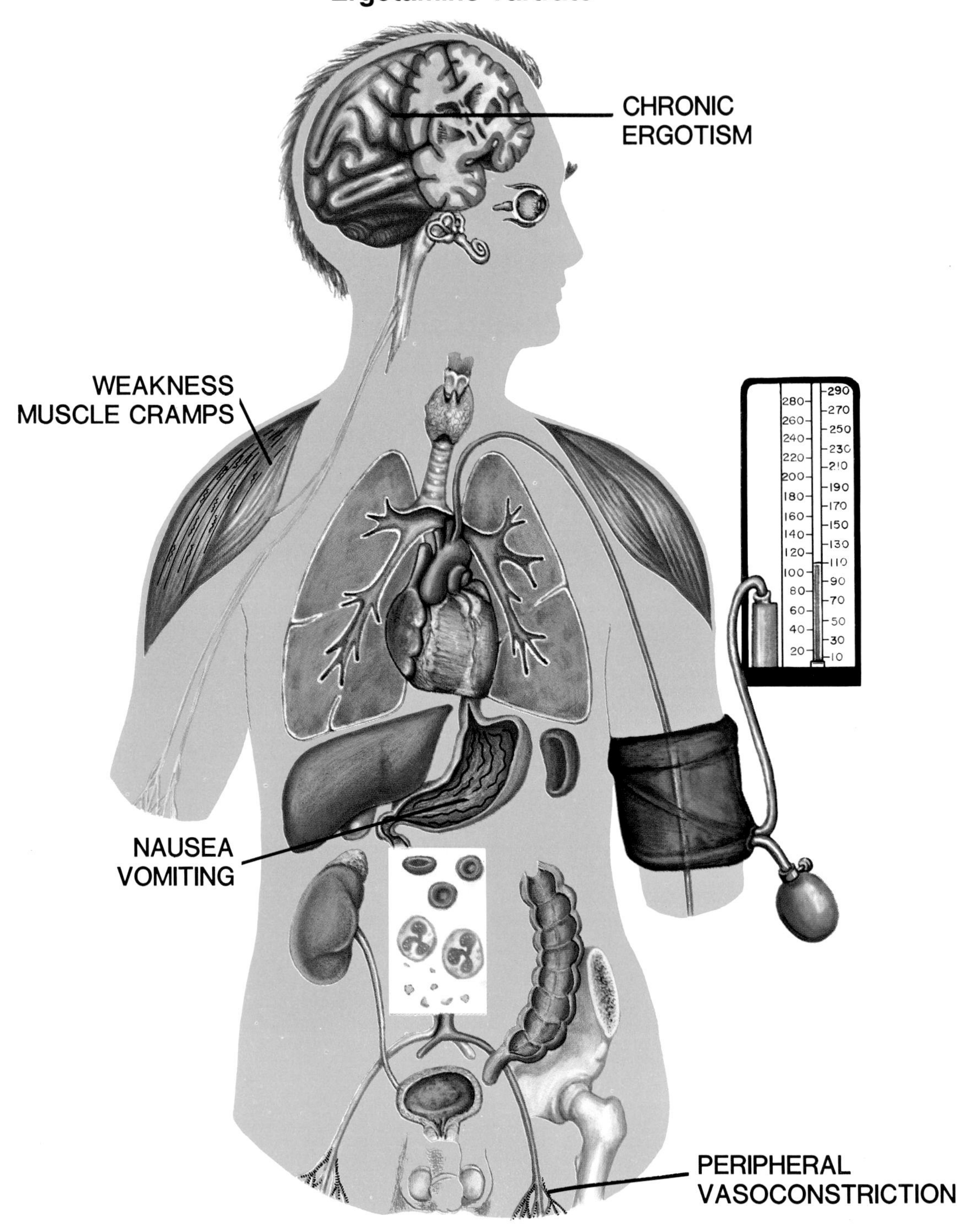

Edetate Disodium

Representative Trade Name: E.D.T.A.

Toxicity Rating: Moderate to high because of renal tubular necrosis and occasional fatal nephrosis.

Adverse Reactions

Reactions to edetate disodium are similar to those to dimercaprol.

Central Nervous System Frequent CNS reactions are paresthesias of the mouth and extremities, headache, fatigue, and myalgia.

Gastrointestinal Nausea, vomiting, diarrhea, and abdominal cramps occur.

Cardiovascular Both hypertension and hypotension may occur. Thrombophlebitis has been reported.

Genitourinary Renal tubular necrosis can occasionally be a fatal reaction to edetate disodium.

Other Marked hypocalcemia and pain at the site of injection occur.

Contraindications

Edetate disodium should not be used in patients with severe renal insufficiency or known hypersensitivity to the drug.

Precautions

Edetate disodium should not be used in hypercalcemia unless there is a real threat to life. Calcium disodium edetate should not be used to treat hypercalcemia because it is already chelated to calcium. Edetate disodium should not be used to treat lead poisoning.

Treatment

An IV solution of calcium should be kept on hand in case severe hypocalcemia occurs. EKG and serum calcium levels should be monitored frequently during therapy. Other reactions are usually treated by withdrawing the drug.

Ergotamine Tartrate

Principal Drugs

Generic Name	Representative Trade Names
Ergotamine tartrate	Ergomar, Gynergen
Ergotamine combinations:	
With caffeine	Cafergot
With belladonna and phenobarbital	Bellergal
Related drug:	
Dihydroergotamine mesylate	D.H.E. 45

Toxicity Rating: Low

Adverse Reactions

Central Nervous System Weakness, pains, and cramps of the legs occur. Paresthesias of the fingers and toes are not uncommon.

Gastrointestinal Nausea, vomiting, and abdominal cramps are perhaps the commonest side effects of ergotamine.

Cardiovascular Peripheral vasospasm, gangrene, angina, and myocardial infarction have been reported rarely.

Methysergide Maleate

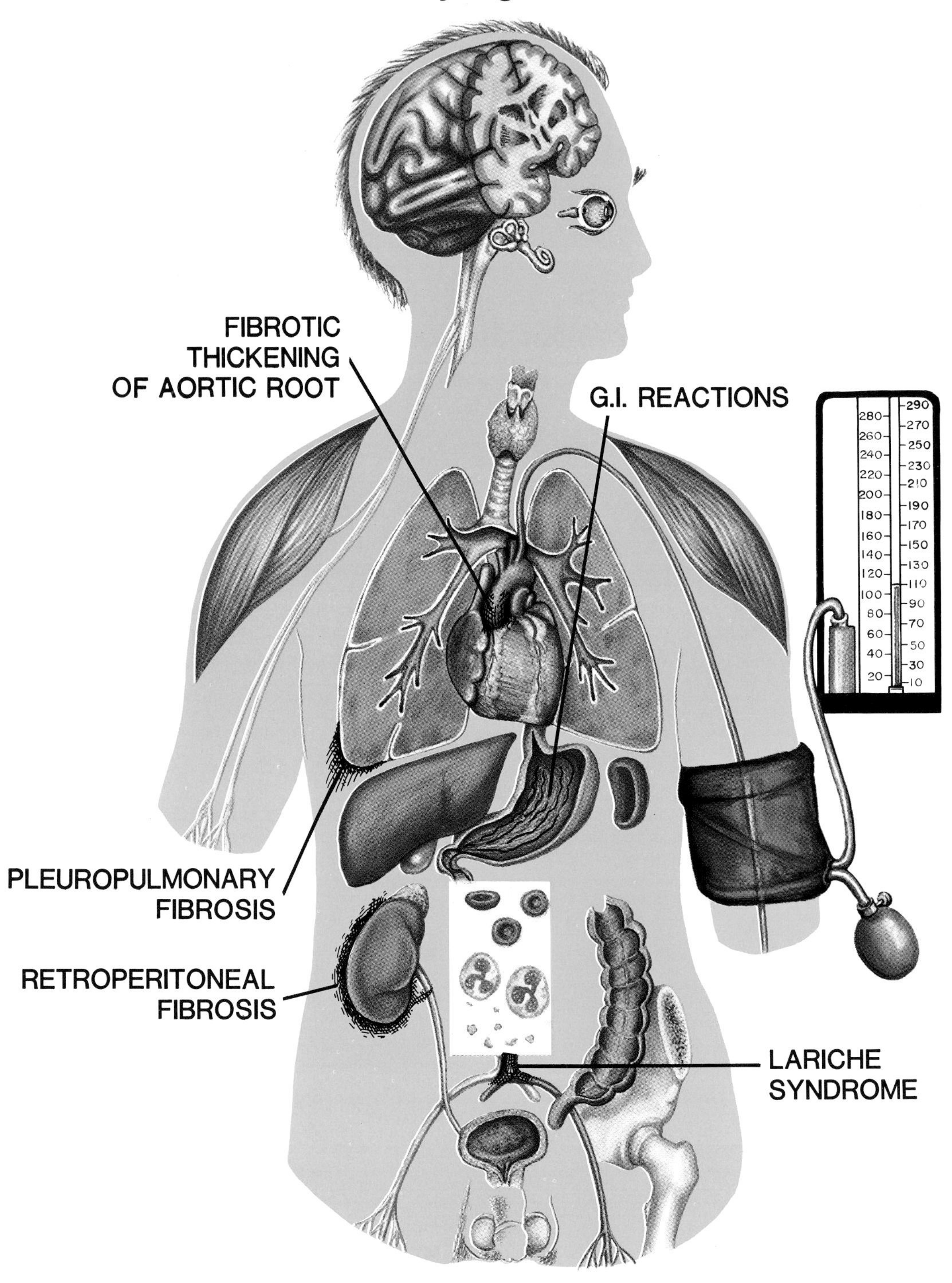

Other Chronic ergotism characterized by drowsiness, depression, loss of appetite, coldness of the extremities, and rebound headache may be more common than is realized. Consequently, patients should be warned not to take more than 10 mg a week.

Contraindications

Ergotamine should not be given to patients with a history of any type of serious vascular disease (severe hypertension, coronary insufficiency, or peripheral arteriosclerosis). It is also unwise to give this drug to patients with hepatic or renal insufficiency or to pregnant women. Known hypersensitivity is a contraindication.

Precautions

Patients should be cautioned not to use more than 6 mg for any attack or more than 10 mg a week.

Treatment

Simple withdrawal of the drug will be sufficient therapy for most reactions. Severe peripheral ischemia may be reversed by an infusion of sodium nitroprusside or oral prazosin.

Ipecac Alkaloids

Representative Trade Name: Ipecac syrup

Toxicity Rating: Low

Adverse Reactions

Reactions to ipecac include persistent vomiting and aspiration, and many of the reactions that occur with apomorphine, although with ipecac they are much milder.

Precautions

Ipecac should not be given to infants under 6 months old.

Methysergide Maleate

Representative Trade Name: Sansert

Toxicity Rating: Moderate because of potential retroperitoneal and pleuropulmonary fibrosis.

Adverse Reactions

Connective Tissue Retroperitoneal and pleuropulmonary fibrosis are the most serious complications of this drug. Fortunately they are infrequent, and can usually be prevented by interrupting methysergide therapy for 1 month every 6 months.

Cardiovascular Fibrotic thickening of the aortic root and the aortic and mitral valves may occur. The retroperitoneal fibrosis may encroach upon the abdominal aorta, producing a Lariche syndrome, or upon the inferior vena cava causing thrombophlebitis and venous obstruction. Intrinsic obstruction of large and small arteries may also occur.

Gastrointestinal Nausea, vomiting, diarrhea, heartburn, or constipation may occur early in the course of therapy but can be prevented by administering the drug with meals.

Central Nervous System Drowsiness, insomnia, ataxia, dizziness, delusions, and hallucinations may occur. These symptoms may be due to an associated migraine attack.

Dermatologic Flushing, telangiectasia, various rashes, and transient hair loss have been reported.

Other Edema, weight gain, neutropenia, eosinophilia, myalgias, and arthralgias have occurred. Hypersensitivity to FD & C Yellow No. 5, contained in Sansert, has occurred.

Contraindications

Patients with known vascular disease of any kind, severe hypertension collagen disease, valvular heart disease, pregnancy, and significant liver or renal disease should not take this drug.

Precautions

Patients should be warned of the risk of fibrosis, and an intravenous pyelogram and other studies should be ordered at the first sign of one of these conditions. Therapy should be interrupted for 1 month every 6 months to prevent these conditions. Dosage should be reduced gradually to prevent a rebound headache.

Treatment

Most symptoms including fibrosis and cardiac valvular disease regress once therapy is terminated. Surgical intervention may still be necessary in obstructive uropathy or arterial or venous insufficiency.

Metoclopramide Hydrochloride

Representative Trade Name: Reglan

Toxicity Rating: Low

Adverse Reactions

Gastrointestinal Nausea, vomiting, diarrhea, or other bowel disturbances may occur.

Central Nervous System There may be drowsiness, fatigue, or lassitude. On the other hand, insomnia and extrapyramidal reactions such as torticollis, oculogyric crisis, and dystonias may occur.

Contraindications

Gastrointestinal hemorrhage, obstruction, or perforation are contraindications. The drug may precipitate a hypertensive crisis in patients with a pheochromocytoma. The drug is also contraindicated in patients with known hypersensitivity to it.

Precautions

Patients should not engage in activities requiring agility and alertness (driving, etc.) for a few hours after taking the drug.

Drug Interactions

This drug may enhance the extrapyramidal and convulsive effects of other drugs. Anticholinergics and narcotics will antagonize the action of this drug on the gastrointestinal tract. The drug may enhance the action of CNS depressants such as sedatives, alcohol, and tranquilizers. This drug influences the rate of absorption of certain drugs from the GI tract.

Treatment

Simple withdrawal of the drug is usually all that is necessary. However, if extrapyramidal reactions are severe, diphenhydramine 50 mg IV may be given to counteract them.

Pancreatin

Principal Drugs

Generic Name	Representative Trade Names
Pancreatin	Panteric, Viokase
Related drug:	
Pancrelipase	Cotazym

Toxicity Rating: Low

Adverse Reactions

Adverse reactions consist of rare allergic reactions and precipitation of gouty arthritis due to the high content of purine in these agents.

Contraindications

Known hypersensitivity to the drug and to pork protein are the major contraindications. The drug should be used in pregnancy only if the benefits outweigh the possible risk.

Treatment

Simple withdrawal of the drug is all that is necessary.

Penicillamine

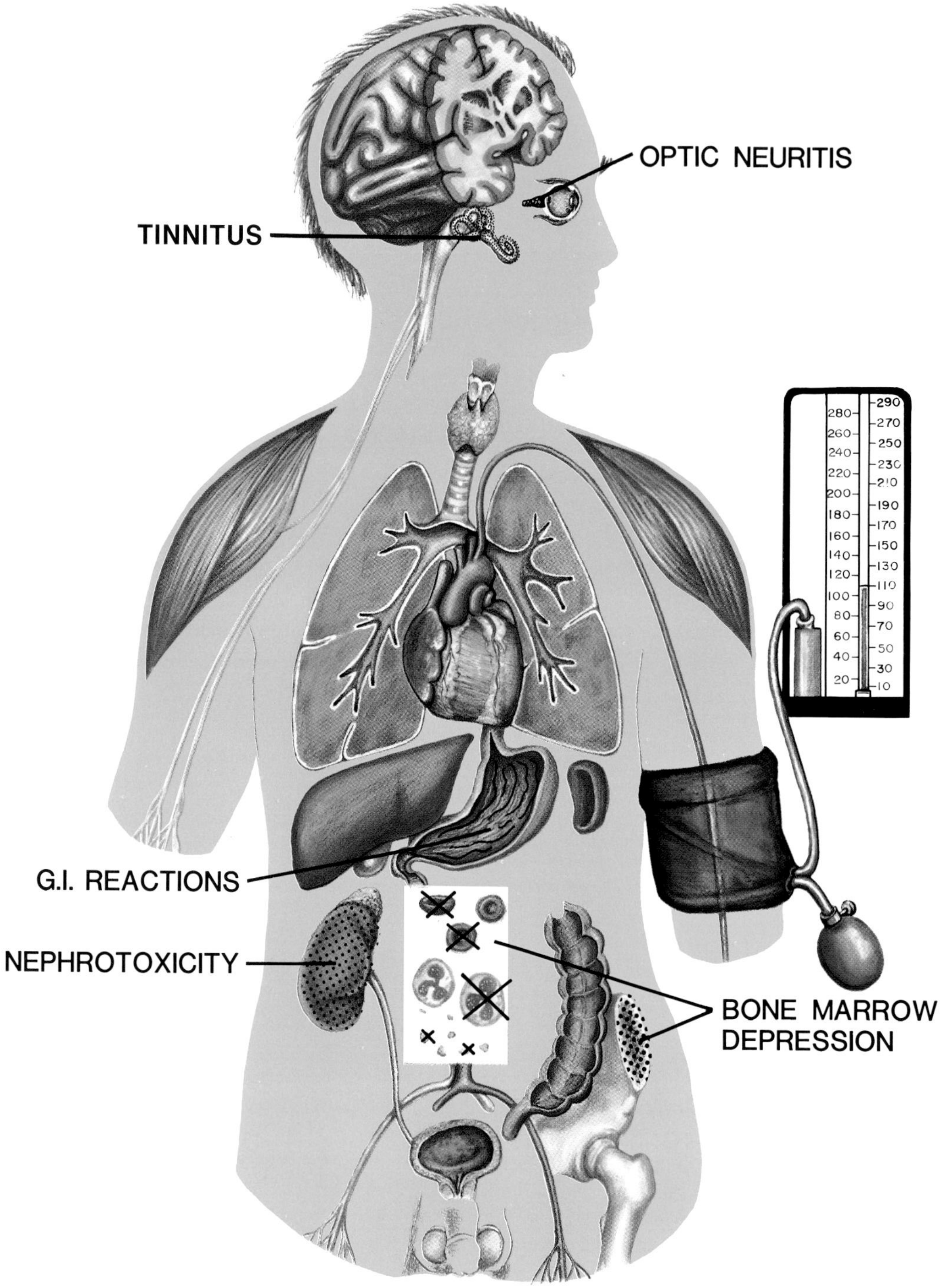

OPTIC NEURITIS
TINNITUS
G.I. REACTIONS
NEPHROTOXICITY
BONE MARROW DEPRESSION

Penicillamine

Representative Trade Name: Cuprimine

Toxicity Rating: High because of reports of fatal bone marrow depression and nephrotic syndrome.

Adverse Reactions

Hematologic The major side effect of penicillamine is bone marrow depression which may manifest as agranulocytosis, thrombocytopenia, or aplastic anemia. Hemolytic anemia and thrombotic thrombocytopenic purpura may also occur.

Renal Approximately 6 percent of patients taking this drug develop proteinuria or hematuria, and occasionally a nephrotic syndrome develops.

Gastrointestinal Nausea, vomiting, abdominal pain, and anorexia develop frequently. Diarrhea may also occur. Cases of reactivation of peptic ulcer, hepatitis, and pancreatitis have occurred.

Central Nervous System Tinnitus and optic neuritis have occurred.

Other Allergic reactions including urticaria, maculopapular eruptions, alopecia, and a lupus-like syndrome have occurred. Pyridoxine and iron deficiencies may also occur.

Contraindications

Penicillamine is contraindicated in pregnant women with rheumatoid arthritis and in patients who have suffered severe bone marrow depression while on the drug. Rheumatoid arthritis patients with known renal disease should not be given this drug.

Precautions

Patients should be carefully observed for skin reactions, and appropriate tests to detect nephrosis and bone marrow depression should be done frequently. Penicillamine should be given with caution to pregnant women and patients with rheumatoid arthritis.

Treatment

Allergic reactions can usually be managed by reducing the dosage and administering an antihistamine. If this is unsuccessful, the drug is discontinued for two weeks and restarted at a low dosage with a corticosteroid. Other more severe reactions (nephrotic syndrome, etc.) are treated by discontinuing the drug. Once recovery from the reaction is complete, the drug may be started again at decreased dosages with or without a corticosteroid. Pyridoxine (50 mg weekly) can be given to prevent pyridoxine deficiency.

Phenazopyridine Hydrochloride

Representative Trade Name: Pyridium

Toxicity Rating: Low

Adverse Reactions

The only significant reactions are headache, and nausea or vomiting, methemoglobinemia, and hemolytic anemia. Hepatic or renal insufficiency may occur, usually with excessive doses.

Contraindications

This drug should not be given to patients with significant renal or hepatic insufficiency.

Precautions

Patients should be warned that their urine may turn red or orange. Phenazopyridine should be stopped if the skin or sclera develops a yellow tinge.

Treatment

Simple withdrawal of the drug is usually all that is necessary. Methemoglobinemia is treated with methylene blue intravenously 1–2 mg/kg body weight or ascorbic acid 100–200 mg orally.

Probucol

Representative Trade Name: Lorelco

Toxicity Rating: Low

Adverse Reactions

Gastrointestinal Diarrhea, nausea, vomiting, and cramps are the most common side effects of this drug.

Cardiovascular The QT interval may be prolonged; the significance of this reaction is not certain.

Central Nervous System Occasionally an idiosyncratic reaction involving dizziness, nausea, vomiting, chest pain, and syncope occurs. Headaches and paresthesias may occur also.

Other Rash, pruritus, thrombocytopenia, peripheral neuropathy, and dulling of taste and smell occur rarely. Transient elevations of liver and renal function have occurred.

Contraindications

Patients with known hypersensitivity and recent myocardial damage should not take this drug.

Precautions

Baseline serum lipids and EKG should be done and repeated at intervals during therapy.

Treatment

Simple withdrawal of the drug is all that is necessary.

Sucralfate

Representative Trade Name: Carafate

Toxicity Rating: Low

Adverse Reactions

Adverse reactions to sucralfate are few because the drug is only minimally absorbed.

Gastrointestinal Nausea, gastric discomfort, constipation, and diarrhea may occur.

Central Nervous System Dizziness and drowsiness are the most common CNS symptoms.

Contraindications

There are no contraindications.

Precautions

While there is no evidence of serious toxic side effects to the fetus or mother, this drug should only be used in pregnancy if clearly needed. Peptic ulceration may recur once treatment is discontinued.

Drug Interactions

None are known.

Treatment

The reactions will usually respond to withdrawal of the drug.

Chapter 39

BIOLOGICAL PREPARATIONS

Biological Preparations

Principal Drugs

Generic Name	Representative Trade Name
Antigens	
Poison ivy extract	Rhus Tox
Staphylococcus bacterial antigen	Staphage Lysate
Antisera	
Rabies antiserum	
Black widow spider antivenin	Antivenin *(Micrurus fulvius)*
Rattlesnake antivenin	Antivenin (Crotalidae)
Hepatitis B immune globulin	HyperHep
Tetanus immune globulin	Homo-Tet
Gamma globulin	
Antirabies serum	
Pertussis immune globulin	
Antitoxins	
Diphtheria antitoxin	
Tetanus antitoxin	
Botulism antitoxin	
Rh_0 (D) immune globulins	
Serum extracts	
Human serum albumin	Albuminar-5
Antihemophilic factor	Factorate
Anti-inhibitor coagulant complex	Autoplex
Factor IX complex	
Immune serum globulin	
Toxoids	
Diphtheria toxoid	
Tetanus toxoid	
Vaccines	
BCG vaccine	
Cholera vaccine	
Influenza virus vaccine	
Measles virus vaccine (live or live attenuated)	
Rubella vaccine	
Smallpox vaccine	
Typhoid vaccine	
Yellow fever vaccine	
Rabies vaccine	
Pertussis vaccine	
Poliovirus vaccine	
Pneumococcal vaccine	
Plague vaccine	
Meningitis vaccines	
Mumps vaccine	

Toxicity Rating: Moderate because fatal anaphylaxis may occur.

Adverse Reactions

These are almost always allergic and may be divided into systemic and local reactions.

Systemic Anaphylactic shock is the major reaction to biological preparations. Serum sickness may manifest itself as rash, fever, chills, malaise, arthralgias, and lymphadenopathy. Influenza vaccine (swine-flu type) has been associated with a Guillain-Barré syndrome. Measles vaccine may cause febrile convulsions in susceptible children. Smallpox and rabies vaccine may cause neuropathy, encephalopathy, or transverse myelitis. Thrombocytopenic purpura and leukopenia have been infrequently noted with rubella. Black widow spider antivenin may cause neurotoxicity.

Local Local reactions include pain, erythema, and even ulceration at the injection site. There may be regional lymphangitis and lymphadenopathy.

Contraindications

Known hypersensitivity to the serum or vaccine is the only absolute contraindication.

Precautions

If hypersensitivity to sera or other vaccines has occurred in the past, administration must be initiated with the smallest dose and gradual desensitization accomplished over several hours. Any antiserum (especially equine) should be skin tested first before the full dose is given.

Treatment

Anaphylactoid reactions are treated with epinephrine, intravenous fluids, oxygen, steroids, and CPR procedures when necessary. Equipment for these procedures should be immediately available whenever biological preparations, especially antisera, are being administered parenterally.

Chapter 40

TOPICAL PREPARATIONS

Dermatologic Preparations

Principal Types of Drugs

Steroid creams, ointments, lotions
Antibiotic creams, ointments, lotions
Antifungal creams, ointments, lotions
Antipruritic creams, ointments, lotions
Emolient creams, lotions, oils
Antiviral ointment (e.g., acyclovir)
Combination steroid, antibiotic, and/or antifungal creams, ointments, and lotions
Antiacne preparations
Keratolytic preparations
Pediculicides
Shampoos
Depigmenting agents
Coal tar preparations
Soaps
Sulfur preparations
Selenium sulfide preparations (e.g., Selsun)
Enzyme creams and ointments
Topical anesthetics
Miscellaneous dermatologic preparations

Toxicity Rating: Low

Adverse Reactions

All dermatologic preparations may produce a local *chemical* reaction manifested by irritation, burning, desquamation, and perhaps lichenification, or a local *allergic* reaction mainfested by erythema, rash, and pruritus. There may also be *systemic* urticaria, angioneurotic edema, or other generalized reactions, but this is unusual. The important point to remember is that the allergic reaction may be to ingredients in the preparation other than the active ingredient. This is especially true of corticosteroid preparations.

Reactions Peculiar to Specific Drugs In addition to the above chemical and allergic reactions, *steroid* preparations may produce atrophy of the skin, depigmentation, and hypertrichosis, and may predispose to secondary infections in addition to the above complications. Furthermore, they may be absorbed systemically, especially after long-term use, and cause various manifestations of Cushing's syndrome. Systemic absorption of *boric acid* may cause convulsions, delirium, tachycardia, and circulatory collapse. Systemic absorption of *hexachlorophene* may cause neurotoxic effects, including convulsions and opisthotonus, especially if used on premature infants or on burns. Systemic absorption of *podophyllin* may cause blood dyscrasias and peripheral neuropathy. Systemic absorption of *anthralin* is suspected to cause nephrotoxicity. Surprisingly, *methoxsalen* is occasionally associated with nervousness or insomnia, hepatic toxicity, and nausea or diarrhea. Argyria may result from long-term local use of *silver nitrate.*

Contraindications

Hexachlorophene should not be used in infants. Known hypersensitivity to any ingredient in a preparation is the major contraindication.

Precautions

Long-term use of topical steroids should be avoided. This precaution also applies to silver nitrate and many other topical skin preparations. The safety of these topical agents in pregnancy has not been established. Prolonged use of any of these preparations, especially the steroids, is often associated with overgrowth of resistant bacteria and fungi.

Treatment

Simple withdrawal of the drug is usually all that is necessary.

Topical Ophthalmic Preparations

Principal Types of Drugs

- Antibiotics
- Corticosteroids
- Antiviral agents (e.g., idoxuridine)
- Silver nitrate preparations
- Vidarabine preparations
- Boric acid preparations
- Mydriatics and cycloplegics
- Ophthalmic vasoconstrictors (sympathomimetics)
- Local anesthetics
- Miotics

Toxicity Rating: Low

Adverse Reactions

Local Local reactions to ophthalmic preparations include chemical conjunctivitis, allergic conjunctivitis, burning, and itching. Contact dermatitis may develop on the eyelids. The antibiotics may predispose to conjunctivitis from nonsusceptible organisms. The corticosteroids predispose to glaucoma, cataracts, and superinfections. Corneal ulceration is a possible complication. Mydriatics may precipitate glaucoma and blurred vision, while topical anesthetics predispose to corneal ulcers.

Systemic Systemic effects include Cushing's syndrome and adrenal insufficiency from long-term steroid use, bone marrow depression with chloramphenicol, headache, nausea, vomiting, bradycardia, hypotension, eye cysts, and lens opacities with the miotics while the sympathomimetics may cause tachycardia, urinary retention, somnolence, and convulsions.

Contraindications

Known hypersensitivity is the major contraindication. The sympathomimetics and mydriatics are contraindicated in corneal ulcers, especially ulcers due to herpes simplex.

Precautions

Mydriatics and local anesthetics should be used cautiously in patients with corneal ulcers, cardiac disease, and hyperthyroidism.

Drug Interactions

The sympathomimetics should not be given concomitantly with MAO inhibitors. Guanethidine may increase the mydriasis of the sympathomimetics, whereas levodopa reduces mydriasis. Miotics may precipitate a cholinergic crisis in myasthenia patients. Also, when miotics are used with organophosphorus insecticides, an additive effect may be noted. Pilocarpine should not be used with phenylephrine or carbachol.

Treatment

Simple withdrawal of the drug is usually all that is necessary.

Topical Oral and Nasal Preparations

Principal Drugs

Generic Name	Representative Trade Name
Beclomethasone dipropionate	Vancenase Nasal Inhaler
Benzocaine	Orabase, Trocaine
Carbamide peroxide	Gly-Oxide
Cocaine HCl	Cocaine HCl
Dexamethasone	Decadron Phosphate Turbinaire, Decadron Phosphate Respihaler
Ephedrine sulfate	Isofedrol
Flunisolide	Nasalide Nasal Solution
Lidocaine hydrochloride	Xylocaine
Naphazoline hydrochloride	Privine Hydrochloride
Phenylephrine hydrochloride	Neo-Synephrine
Piperocaine hydrochloride	Metycaine Hydrochloride
Tetrahydrozoline hydrochloride	Tyzine
Triamcinolone acetonide	Kenalog

Toxicity Rating: Low

Adverse Reactions

Local reactions include burning, irritation, sneezing, rebound congestion, rhinitis, dermatitis medicamentosa, gingivitis, and allergic reactions. Systemic reactions to sympathomimetics (phenylephrine HCl, etc.) include nervousness, tachycardia, hypertension, nausea, and occasional arrhythmias. Prolonged use of topical steroids may result in Cushing's syndrome, adrenal insufficiency, and predisposition to local infections.

Contraindications

Known hypersensitivity is the major contraindication. Tetrahydrozoline HCl is contraindicated in glaucoma.

Precautions

Careful observation is advised when giving sympathomimetics to patients with hyperthyroidism, coronary artery disease, hypertension, glaucoma, and diabetes.

Drug Interactions

Hypertensive crisis may occur when sympathomimetics are administered concomitantly with MAO inhibitors.

Treatment

Simple withdrawal of the drug is usually all that is necessary.

Topical Otologic Preparations

Principal Types of Drugs

Antibiotics
Corticosteroids
Local anesthetics
Boric acid preparations
Carbamide peroxide preparations
Triethanolamine polypeptide oleate-condensate (e.g. Cerumenex)

Toxicity Rating: Low

Adverse Reactions

Local Local reactions include chemical irritation, burning, and rash as well as allergic reactions (erythema, pruritus, urticaria, and maculopapular rashes). There may be overgrowth by nonsusceptible organisms with topical antibiotics and various bacterial superinfections with the topical corticosteroids. Neomycin and colistin may cause ototoxicity in patients with a perforated eardrum.

Systemic Systemic reactions include Cushing's syndrome and adrenal insufficiency with long-term use of corticosteroids, and sore throat or angioneurotic edema with topical chloramphenicol.

Contraindications

The major contraindication is known hypersensitivity to any of these drugs. Corticosteroids are contraindicated in local herpes simplex, vaccinia, or varicella infections. Known perforation is a relative contraindication.

Precautions

Patients should be warned that their otitis externa may get worse if superinfection develops. Also, patients with perforation or chronic otitis media should be warned about ototoxicity with neomycin and colistin. Triethanolamine polypeptide should be administered under the supervision of a physician.

Treatment

Simple withdrawal of the drug is usually all that is necessary.

Topical Parasiticidal Agents, Scabicides, and Pediculicides

Principal Drugs

Generic Name	Representative Trade Name
Benzyl benzoate lotion	Scobanca
Copper oleate solution	Cuprex
Crotamiton	Eurax
Lindane	Kwell

Toxicity Rating: Low

Adverse Reactions

These are almost always local and consist of chemical and allergic dermatitis.

Contraindications

Known hypersensitivity to these drugs is the major contraindication. If the skin is already raw and inflamed, these preparations may be contraindicated.

Precautions

Other members of the family may also require treatment. To prevent reinfections, all recently used clothes and bed linens should be sterilized. Care should be taken not to apply these drugs to the face and eyes.

Drug Interactions

None reported.

Treatment

Simple withdrawal of the drug is usually all that is necessary.

Appendix A

GENERIC INDEX

A

Acetaminophen (nonnarcotic analgesic)
Acetazolamide (diuretic)
Acetohexamide (oral antidiabetic agent)
Acetylcysteine (expectorant)
ACTH (corticosteroid)
Acyclovir (antiviral agent)
Albuterol (sympathomimetic)
Allopurinol (antigout agent)
Alphaprodine HCl (narcotic analgesic)
Alprazolam (nonsteroidal antiinflammatory agent)
Alseroxylon (antihypertensive)
Aluminum hydroxide (antacid)
Amantadine HCl (antiparkinson agent)
Ambenonium chloride (cholinergic)
Amcinonide (topical corticosteroid)
Amikacin sulfate (antibiotic)
Amiloride HCl (diuretic)
Aminacrine (topical antimicrobial agent)
Aminobenzoic acid (nonnarcotic analgesic)
Aminocaproic acid (enzyme)
Aminoglutethamide (corticosteroid inhibitor)
Aminophylline (bronchodilator)
Aminosalicylic acid (antimycobacterial)
Amitriptyline HCl (antidepressant)
Ammonium chloride (expectorant)
Amobarbital sodium (hypnotic)
Amodiaquine HCl (parasiticidal agent)
Amoxapine (antidepressant)
Amoxicillin trihydrate (antibiotic)
Amphetamine sulfate (sympathomimetic)
Amphotericin B (antifungal agent)
Ampicillin sodium (antibiotic)
Amylolytic enzyme (digestive enzyme)
Anisotropine methylbromide (anticholinergic)
Anthralin preparations (dermatologic preparations)
Anthraquinone (laxative)
Antihemophilic factor (biological preparation)
Anti-inhibitor coagulant complex (biological preparation)
Antipyrine (topical and analgesic)
Antirabies serum (biological preparation)
Apomorphine hydrochloride (emetic)
Antivenin (Crotalidae) (biological preparation)
Antivenin *(Micrurus fulvius)* (biological preparation)
Aprobarbital (hypnotic)
Ara-A (antiviral agent)
Ascorbic acid (vitamin C)
Asparaginase (antineoplastic agent)
Aspirin (nonsteroidal antiinflammatory agent)
Atenolol (antihypertensive)
Atropine sulfate (anticholinergic)
Aurothioglucose (antiarthritic mineral)
Azatadine maleate (antihistamine)
Azathioprine (immunosuppressant, antineoplastic agent)
Azlocillin sodium (antibiotic)
Azosulfisoxazole (antimicrobial agent)

B

BCG vaccine (biological preparation)
Bacampicillin hydrochloride (antibiotic)
Bacitracin (topical antibiotic)
Baclofen (skeletal muscle relaxant)
BAL (heavy metal antagonist)
Barbiturate preparations (hypnotics)
Beclomethasone (corticosteroid)
Belladonna Preparations (anticholinergics)
Benactyzine HCl (antidepressant)
Bendroflumethiazide (diuretic)
Benzethonium chloride (antimicrobial, antifungal agent)
Benzocaine (topical anesthetic)
Benzoic acid (used in urinary antiseptic preparations)
Benzonatate (antitussive agent)
Benzoyl peroxide (dermatologic antimicrobial preparation)
Benzphetamine HCl (sympathomimetic anorexant)
Benzquinamide HCl (antiemetic)
Benzthiazide (diuretic)
Benztropine mesylate (antiparkinson agent)
Benzylpenicilloyl-polylysine (penicillin allergy test)
Bephenium hydroxynaphthoate (anthelmintic)
Betaine HCl (hydrochloric acid agent)
Betamethazone (corticosteroid)
Bethanechol chloride (cholinergic)
Bioflavonoids (vitamin analogs)
Biperiden (antiparkinson agent)
Bisacodyl (laxative)
Bismuth preparations (antacid)
Bithionol (anthelmintic)
Bleomycin sulfate (antineoplastic agent)
Boric acid (soothing topical agent)
Bornyl acetate (nasal decongestant)
Botulism antitoxin (biological preparation)
Bretylium tosylate (antiarrhythmic agent)
Bromelains (proteolytic enzyme)
Bromocriptine mesylate (antiparkinson agent)
Bromodiphenhydramine HCl (antihistamine)
Brompheniramine maleate (antihistamine)
Buclizine HCl (antihistamine)
Bupivacaine HCl (local anesthetic)
Buprenorphine (narcotic analgesic)
Busulfan (antineoplastic agent)
Butabarbital (hypnotic)
Butalbital (hypnotic)
Butamben picrate (topical anesthetic)
Butorphanol tartrate (narcotic analgesic)

C

Caffeine (CNS stimulant)
Calamine (topical antipruretic)
Calcifediol (vitamin D analogue)
Calciferol (vitamin D analogue)
Calcitonin (calcium lowering hormone)
Calcitriol (vitamin D analogue)
Calcium carbonate (antacid)
Calcium chloride (mineral)
Calcium disodium edetate (chelating agent)
Calcium gluconate (mineral)
Calcium glycerophosphate (injectible mineral)
Calcium iodide (expectorant)
Calcium lactate (mineral)
Calcium phosphate (mineral)
Calcium polycarbophil (laxative)
Candicidin (antifungal agent)
Cantharidin (topical keratolytic agent)
Capreomycin sulfate (antimycobacterial agent)
Captopril (antihypertensive)
Caramiphen edisylate (antitussive agent)
Carbamazepine (anticonvulsant)
Carbamide peroxide (dermatologic preparation)
Carbarsone (amebicidal agent)
Carbenicillin disodium (antibiotic)
Carbetapentane tannate (antitussive agent)
Carbidopa (antiparkinsonian agent)
Carbinoxamine maleate (antihistamine)
Carisoprodol (muscle relaxant)
Carmustine (antineoplastic agent)
Casanthranol (laxative)
Cascara sagrada (laxative)
Castor oil (laxative)
Cefaclor (antibiotic)
Cefadroxil monohydrate (antibiotic)
Cefamandole nafate (antibiotic)
Cefazolin sodium (antibiotic)
Cefoxitin sodium (antibiotic)
Cellulase (digestive enzyme)
Cephalexin (antibiotic)
Cephalothin sodium (antibiotic)
Cephapirin sodium (antibiotic)
Cephotaxime sodium (antibiotic)
Cephradine (antibiotic)
Cetylpyridinium chloride (topical antimicrobial and fungicidal agent)
Chenodeoxycholic acid (gallstone solvent)
Chlophedianol HCl (antitussive agent)
Chloral hydrate (hypnotic)
Chlorambucil (antineoplastic agent)
Chloramphenicol (antibiotic)
Chlorazepate dipotassium (antianxiety agent)
Chlorcyclizine HCl (antihistamine)
Chlordiazepoxide (antianxiety agent)
Chlorhexidine gluconate (topical antimicrobial agent)
Chlormezanone (antianxiety agent)
Chloroprocaine HCl (local anesthetic)
Chloroquine HCl (antimalarial agent)
Chloroquine phosphate (antimalarial agent)
Chlorothiazide (diuretic)
Chlorotrianisene (hormone)
Chloroxine (topical antimicrobial agent)
Chloroxylenol (topical antifungal agent)
Chlorphenesin carbamate (antiinflammatory agent)
Chlorpheniramine (antihistamine)
Chlorpromazine HCl (antipsychotic agent)
Chlorpropamide (oral antidiabetic agent)
Chlorprothixene (antianxiety agent)
Chlortetracycline HCl (antibiotic)
Chlorthalidone (diuretic)
Chlorzoxazone (skeletal muscle relaxant)
Cholestyramine (antilipemic agent)
Choline bitartrate (vitamin)
Choline magnesium trisalicylate (nonsteroidal antiinflammatory agent)
Choline salicylate (nonsteroidal antiinflammatory agent)
Chorionic, gonadotropin (hormone)
Chromic chloride (mineral)
Chromium (mineral)
Chymotrypsin (digestive enzyme)
Cimetidine (histamine H_2 receptor antagonist)
Cinnamedrine HCl (antispasmodic)
Cinoxacin (antibiotic)
Cisplatin (antineoplastic agent)
Citric acid (alkalizing agent)
Clemastine fumarate (antihistamine)
Clidinium bromide (anticholinergic)
Clindamycin (antibiotic)
Clocortolone pivalate (topical corticosteroid)
Clofibrate (antilipemic agent)
Clomiphene citrate (infertility agent)
Clonazepam (anticonvulsant)
Clonidine HCl (antihypertensive)
Clorazepate dipotassium (antianxiety agent)
Clotrimazole (antifungal agent)
Cloxacillin (antibiotic)
Coal tar (dermatologic preparation)
Cocaine HCl (local anesthetic)
Codeine (narcotic analgesic)
Colchicine (antigout agent)
Colestipol HCl (antilipemic agent)
Colistimethate sodium (antibiotic)
Colistin sulfate (antibiotic)
Collangenase (topical enzyme)
Copper (mineral)
Cortisone acetate (topical corticosteroid)

Coumarin drugs (anticoagulants)
Cromolyn sodium (antiasthmatic agent)
Cryptenamine (antihypertensive)
Cyanocobalamin (vitamin)
Cyclandelate (vasodilator)
Cyclizine (antihistamine)
Cyclobenzaprine HCl (skeletal muscle relaxant)
Cyclopentamine HCl (antihistamine)
Cyclophosphamide (antineoplastic agent)
Cycloserine (antibiotic)
Cyclothiazide (diuretic)
Cycrimine HCl (antiparkinson agent)
Cyproheptadine HCl (antihistamine)
Cytarabine (antineoplastic agent)

D

Dacarbazine (antineoplastic agent)
Dactinomycin (antineoplastic agent)
Danazol (hormone inhibitor)
Danthron (laxative)
Dantrolene sodium (skeletal muscle relaxant)
Dapsone (antileprosy agent)
Daunorubicin HCl (antineoplastic agent)
Deanol (CNS stimulant)
Deferoxamine mesylate (heavy metal antagonist)
Dehydrocholic acid (laxative)
Demeclocycline (antibiotic)
Deserpidine (antihypertensive)
Desipramine HCl (antidepressant)
Deslanoside (antiarrhythmic agent)
Desmopressin acetate (hormone)
Desonide (topical corticosteroid)
Desoximetasone (topical corticosteroid)
Desoxycorticosterone (corticosteroid)
Desoxyribonuclease (proteolytic enzyme)
Dexamethasone (corticosteroid)
Dexbrompheniramine maleate (antihistamine)
Dexclorpheniramine maleate (antihistamine)
Dexpanthenol (anticholinergic)
Dextran (biological preparation)
Dextroamphetamine preparations (sympathomimetic, anorexant)
Dextromethorphan hydrobromide (antitussive agent)
Dextrothyroxine (thyroid hormone)
Diazepam (antianxiety agent)
Diazoxide (antihypertensive)
Dibucaine (topical anesthetic)
Dichloralphenazone (sympathomimetic)
Dichlorophen (anthelmintic)
Dicloxacillin (antibiotic)
Dicoumarol (anticoagulant)
Dicyclomine HCl (anticholinergic)
Dienestrol (estrogen)
Diethylcarbamazine citrate (anthelmintic)
Diethylpropion HCl (sympathomimetic anorexant)
Diethylstilbestrol (estrogen)
Diflorazone diacetate (topical corticosteroid)
Diflunisal (nonsteroidal antiinflammatory agent)
Digitalis preparations (antiarrhythmic agents)
Digitoxin (antiarrhythmic agent)
Digoxin (antiarrhythmic agent)
Dihydrocodeinone bitartrate (narcotic analgesic)
Dihydroergotamine mesylate (antimigraine agent)
Dihydromorphinone HCl (narcotic analgesic)
Dihydrotachysterol (vitamin D derivative)
Diisopropyl sebacate (dermatologic preparation)
Diltiazem HCl (antianginal agent)
Dimenhydrinate (antihistamine)
Dimercaprol (heavy metal antagonist)
Dimethindene maleate (antihistamine)
Dimethyl sulfoxide (topical bladder preparation)
Dioctyl sodium succinate (*see* Docusate sodium)
Dioxybenzone (dermatologic preparation)
Diperodon (dermatological preparation)
Diphenhydramine (antihistamine)
Diphenidol (anitemetic, antivertigo agent)
Diphenoxylate (antidiarrheal agent)
Diphenylhydantoin sodium (anticonvulsant)
Diphenylpyraline HCl (antihistamine)
Diphtheria toxoid (biological preparation)
Diphylline (bronchodilator)
Dipyridamole (antianginal agent)
Disopyramide phosphate (antiarrhythmic agent)
Disulfiram (alcohol antagonist)
Dobutamine HCl (sympathomimetic)
Docusate calcium (laxative)
Docusate potassium (laxative)
Docusate sodium (laxative)
Dopamine HCl (sympathomimetic)
Doxapram HCl (respiratory stimulant)
Doxepin HCl (antidepressant)
Doxorubicin HCl (antineoplastic agent)
Doxycycline monohydrate (antibiotic)
Doxylamine succinate (antihistamine)
Dromostanolone (antineoplastic agent)
Droperidol (preanesthetic agent)
Dyphylline (bronchodilator)

E

Echothiophate iodide (topical ophthalmic preparation)
Edetate disodium (calcium antagonist)
Edrophonium chloride (cholinergic)
Emetidine HCl (amebicidal)
Entsufon sodium (dermatologic preparation)
Ephedrine preparations (sympathomimetics)
Epinephrine preparations (sympathomimetics)

Hydroxyurea (antineoplastic agent)
Hydroxyzine HCl (antihistamine)
Hyoscyamine preparations (anticholinergics)
Hyoscyamus preparations (anticholinergics)

I

Ibuprofen (nonsteroidal antiinflammatory agent)
Imipramine (antidepressant)
Indomethacin (nonsteroidal antiinflammatory agent)
Inositol (vitamin)
Insulin preparations (hormones)
Iodine preparations (expectorants)
Iodochlorhydroxyquin (topical antimicrobial agent)
Iodoquinol (amebicidal)
Ipecac preparations (emetic)
Iron dextran (mineral)
Iron preparations (mineral)
Isocarboxazid (MAO inhibitor antidepressant)
Isoetharine (sympathomimetic)
Isometheptene mucate (sympathomimetic, antimigraine drug)
Isoniazid (antimycobacterial agent)
Isopropamide iodide (anticholinergic)
Isopropyl alcohol (dermatologic preparation)
Isoproterenol preparations (sympathiomimetics)
Isosorbide dinitrate (antianginal agent)
Isotretinoin (antiacne preparation)
Isoxsuprine HCl (vasodilator)

K

Kanamycin sulfate (antibiotic)
Kaolin (antidiarrheal agent)
Ketamine HCl (general anesthetic)
Ketoconazole (antifungal agent)

L

Lactase (digestive enzyme)
Lactic acid (dermatologic preparation)
Lactobacillus acidophilus (miscellaneous gastrointestinal agent)
Lactulose (miscellaneous gantrointestinal agent)
Leucovorin calcium (folinic acid vitamin)
Levallorphan tartrate (narcotic antagonist)
Levodopa (antiparkinsonian agent)
Levonordefrin (local anesthetic)
Levopropoxyphene (antitussive)
Levorphanol tartrate (narcotic analgesic)
Levothyroxine sodium (thyroid hormone)
Lidocaine (local anesthetic)
Lincomycin HCl monohydrate (antibiotic)
Lindane (scabicide)
Liothyronine sodium (thyroid hormone)
Liotrix (thyroid hormone)
Lipolytic enzyme (pancreatic enzyme)
Lithium carbonate (antidepressant)
Lithium citrate (antidepressant)
Liver preparations (vitamin preparations)
Lomustine (antineoplastic agent)
Loperamide HCl (antidiarrheal agent)
Lorazepam (antianxiety agent)
Loxapine HCl (antipsychotic agent)
Lypressin (antidiuretic hormone)
Lysine (amino acid)

M

Mafenide acetate (topical antimicrobial agent)
Magaldrate (antacid)
Magnesium compounds (antacids)
Magnesium sulfate (electrolyte replacement solution)
Malathion (pediculicide)
Maprotiline HCl (antidepressant)
Mazindol (sympathomimetic anorexant)
Mebendazole (anthelmintic)
Mechlorethamine HCl (antineoplastic agent)
Meclizine HCl (antihistamine)
Meclocycline sulfosalicylate (antiacne agent)
Meclofenamate sodium (nonsteroidal antiinflammatory agent)
Medroxyprogesterone acetate (progestin)
Mefenamic acid (analgesic)
Megestrol acetate (estrogen hormone)
Melphalan (antineoplastic agent)
Menadiol sodium diphosphate (vitamin K preparation)
Menotropins (gonadotropin hormones)
Mepenzolate bromide (anticholinergic)
Meperidine HCl (narcotic analgesic)
Mephentermine sulfate (sympathomimetic)
Mephenytoin (anticonvulsant)
Mephobarbital (anticonvulsant)
Mepivacaine HCl (local anesthetic)
Meprobamate (hypnotic)
Mercaptopurine (antineoplastic agent)
Mesoridazine (antipsychotic agent)
Mestranol preparations (estrogen)
Metaproterenol sulfate (sympathomimetic)
Metaraminol bitartrate (sympathomimetic)
Methacycline HCl (antibiotic)
Methadone HCl (narcotic analgesic)
Methamphetamine HCl (sympathomimetic anorexant)
Methaqualone (hypnotic)
Metharbital (anticonvulsant)
Methazolamide (*see* Acetazolamide)
Methdilazine (antipruritic phenothiazine)
Methenamine preparations (urinary antiseptics)
Methicillin sodium (antibiotic)

Paraldehyde (hypnotic)
Paramethadione (anticonvulsant)
Paramethasone acetate (corticosteroid)
Paregoric (narcotic antidiarrheal agent)
Pargyline HCl (antihypertensive)
Paromomycin sulfate (amebicide)
Pectin (antidiarrheal agent)
Pemoline (CNS stimulant)
Penicillamine (heavy metal antagonist)
Penicillin preparations (antibiotics)
Pentaerythritol tetranitrate (antianginal agent)
Pentagastrin (digestive hormone)
Pentazocine HCl (narcotic analgesic)
Pentylenetetrazol (CNS stimulant)
Pepsin (digestive enzyme)
Peroxide preparations (dermatologic preparations)
Perphenazine (antipsychotic agent)
Pertussis immune globulin (biological preparation)
Pertussis vaccine (biological preparation)
Phenacemide (anticonvulsant)
Phenacetin (nonnarcotic analgesic)
Phenazopyridine (urinary analgesic)
Phendimetrazine (sympathomimetic)
Phendimetrazine tartrate (sympathomimetic)
Phenelzine sulfate (antidepressant)
Phenindamine tartrate (sympathomimetic)
Pheniramine maleate (antihistamine)
Phenmetrazine HCl (sympathomimetic-anorexant)
Phenobarbital (hypnotic-anticonvulsant)
Phenobarbital sodium (hypnotic-anticonvulsant)
Phenol (topical antifungal agent)
Phenolphthalein (laxative)
Phenothiazines (antipsychotic agents)
Phenoxybenzamine HCl (vasodilator)
Phenprocoumon (anticoagulant)
Phensuximide (anticonvulsant)
Phentermine HCl (sympathomimetic anorexant)
Phentermine resin (sympathomimetic anorexant)
Phentolamine (vasodilator)
Phenylbutazone (nonsteriodal antiinflammatory agent)
Phenylephrine compounds (sympathomimetics)
Phenylpropanolamine compounds (sympathomimetics)
Phenyltoloxamine compounds (sympathomimetics)
Phenytoin (anticonvulsant)
Phosphorated carbohydrate solution (antiemetic)
Phosphorus preparations (urinary acidifiers)
Physostigmine salicylate (cholinergic)
Physostigmine sulfate (cholinergic)
Phytonadione (vitamin K preparation)
Pilocarpine (cholinergic)
Pindolol (antihypertensive)
Piperacetazine (antipsychotic agent)
Piperacillin sodium (antibiotic)
Piperazine preparations (anthelmintic)
Piperonyl butoxide (pediculicide)
Piroxicam (nonsteroidal antiinflammatory agent)
Pitressin tannate (antidiuretic hormone)
Plague vaccine (biological preparation)
Plasma fractions, human (biological preparations)
Plicamycin (antineoplastic agent)
Pneumococcal vaccine (biological preparation)
Podophyllin (dermatological preparation)
Poison ivy extract (biological preparation)
Poliomyelitis vaccine (biological preparation)
Poliovirus vaccine (biological preparation)
Polyestradiol phosphate (estrogen)
Polymyxin B sulfate (antibiotic)
Polyoxyethylene dodecanol (expectorant)
Polythiazide (diuretic)
Potassium acetate (potassium replacement solution)
Potassium acid phosphate (potassium replacement solution)
Potassium bicarbonate (potassium replacement solution)
Potassium bitartrate (potassium replacement solution)
Potassium chloride (potassium replacement solution)
Potassium citrate (potassium replacement solution)
Potassium gluconate (potassium replacement solution)
Potassium guaiacolsulfonate (expectorant)
Potassium hetacillin (antibiotic)
Potassium iodide (expectorant)
Potassium phosphate (phosphorus replacement solution)
Potassium salicylate (analgesic)
Potassium sorbate (topical vaginal solution)
Povidone-iodine (topical antimicrobial agent)
Pralidoxime chloride (cholinesterace reactivator)
Pramoxine HCl (dermatologic preparation)
Prazepam (antianxiety agent)
Prazosin HCl (antihypertensive)
Prednisolone (corticosteroid)
Prednisolone acetate (corticosteroid)
Prednisolone sodium phosphate (corticosteroid)
Prednisolone tebutate (corticosteroid)
Prednisone (corticosteroid)
Prilocaine HCl (local anesthetic)
Primaquine phosphate (antimalarial drug)
Primidone (anticonvulsant)
Probenecid (uricosuric agent)
Probucol (antilipemic agent)
Procainamide HCl (antiarrhythmic drug)
Procaine HCl (local anesthetic)
Procarbazine HCl (antineoplastic agent)
Prochlorperazine, (antipsychotic drug)
Procyclidine HCl (anticholinergic)
Progesterone (progestin hormone)
Promazine HCl (antipsychotic agent)
Promethazine (antihistamine, antipsychotic agent)

Propantheline bromide (anticholinergic)
Propoxyphene HCl (narcotic analgesic)
Propoxyphene napsylate (narcotic analgesic)
Propranolol HCl (antihypertensive, antiarrhythmic)
Propylene glycol (topical otic preparation)
Propylthiouracil (antithyroid drug)
Protamine sulfate (heparin antagonist)
Proteolytic preparations (enzymes)
Protriptyline HCl (antidepressant)
Pseudoephedrine HCl (sympathomimetic)
Psyllium preparations (laxatives)
Pyrantel pamoate (anthelmintic)
Pyrethrins (pediculicide)
Pyrethroids (pediculicide)
Pyridostigmine bromide (cholinergic)
Pyridoxine (vitamin)
Pyrilamine maleate (antihistamine)
Pyrilamine tannate (antihistamine)
Pyrimethamine (antimalarial)
Pyrrobutamine phosphate (antihistamine)
Pyrvinium pamoate (anthelmintic)

Q

Quinestrol (estrogen)
Quinethazone (diuretic)
Quinidine gluconate (antiarrhythmic agent)
Quinidine preparations (antiarrhythmic agents)
Quinine sulfate (neuromuscular blocker)

R

Rabies antiserum and vaccines (biological preparations)
Racemethionine (dermatologic preparation)
Ranitidine HCl (histamine H_2 receptor antagonist)
Rauwolfia preparations (antihypertensives)
Rescinnamine (antihypertensive)
Reserpine (antihypertensive)
Resorcinol (dermatologic preparation)
Rh_0 (D) immune globulin (biological preparation)
Riboflavin (vitamin)
Ricinoleic acid (topical vaginal preparation)
Rifampin (antimycobacterial agent)
Ritodrine HCl (uterine stimulant)

S

Salicylamide (nonsteroidal, antiinflammatory agent)
Salicylic acid (dermatologic preparation)
Salicylsalicylic acid (nonsteroidal antiinflammatory agent)
Salsalate (*see* Salicylsalicylic acid)
Scopolamine hydrobromide (anticholinergic)
Scopolamine preparations (anticholinergics)
Secobarbital sodium (hypnotic)
Selenium (mineral)
Selenium sulfide (dermatologic preparation)
Senna (laxative)
Silver nitrate (ophthalmic preparation)
Silver sulfadiazine (topical antimicrobial agent)
Simethicone (antacid, antifoaming agent)
Smallpox vaccine (biological preparation)
Sodium ampicillin (antibiotic)
Sodium bicarbonate (antacid)
Sodium borate (topical vaginal preparation)
Sodium butabarbital (hypnotic)
Sodium dextrothyroxine (antilipemic agent)
Sodium diethyl barbiturate (hypnotic)
Sodium fluoride (mineral)
Sodium hyaluronate (local ophthalmic preparation)
Sodium iodide (antithyroid drug)
Sodium iodide I 131 (antithyroid drug)
Sodium lauryl sulfate (dermatologic preparation)
Sodium levothyroxine (thyroid hormone)
Sodium liothyronine (thyroid hormone)
Sodium nitroprusside (antihypertensive)
Sodium oxychlorosene (topical antimicrobial solution)
Sodium pentobarbital (hypnotic)
Sodium phosphate (topical enema)
Sodium polystyrene sulfonate (ion exchange resin)
Sodium salicylate (nonsteroidal antiinflammatory agent)
Sodium sulfacetamide (topical ophthalmic preparation)
Sodium sulfate (dermatologic preparation)
Sodium tetradecyl sulfate (local sclerosing solution)
Sodium thiopentol (hypnotic)
Sodium thiosulfate (dermatologic preparation)
Somatropin (growth hormone)
Spectinomycin HCl (antibiotic)
Spironolactone (diuretic)
Stanozolol (anabolic-androgen steroid)
Staphylococcus vaccine (biological preparation)
Stibocaptate (anthelmintic)
Streptodornase (enzyme)
Streptokinase (enzyme)
Streptomycin sulfate (antimicrobial agent)
Succinylcholine chloride (neuromuscular blocker)
Sucralfate (miscellaneous gastrointestinal agent)
Sulfabenzamide (topical antimicrobial preparation)
Sulfacetamide (topical antimicrobial preparation)
Sulfacetamide sodium (topical ophthalmic preparation)
Sulfadiazine (antimicrobial agent)
Sulfamethizole (antimicrobial agent)
Sulfamethoxazole (antimicrobial agent)
Sulfanilamide (topical vaginal preparation)
Sulfapyridine (antimicrobial agent)
Sulfasalazine (antimicrobial antiinflammatory agent)
Sulfathiazole (topical vaginal preparation)

Sulfinpyrazone (uricosuric agent)
Sulfisoxazole (antimicrobial agent)
Sulfur (dermatologic preparation)
Sulindac (nonsteroidal antiinflammatory agent)
Sutilains (topical enzyme preparation)

T

Tamoxifen citrate (antiestrogen, antineoplastic agent)
Tar preparations (dermatologic preparations)
Temazepam (hypnotic)
Terbutaline sulfate (sympathomimetic)
Testolactone (antineoplastic agent)
Testosterone preparations (androgens)
Tetanus immune globulin (biological preparation)
Tetanus toxoids and antitoxins (biological preparations)
Tetracaine HCl (topical anesthetic)
Tetracycline compounds (antibiotics)
Tetrahydrozoline HCl (sympathomimetic)
Theophylline preparations (bronchodilators)
Thiabendazole (anthelmintic)
Thiamine HCl (vitamin)
Thiamylal sodium (general anesthetic)
Thiethylperazine (antiemetic, antipsychotic)
Thioguanine (antineoplastic agent)
Thioridazine (antipsychotic agent)
Thiotepa (antineoplastic agent)
Thiothixene (antipsychotic agent)
Thiphenamil HCl (gastrointestinal antispasmotic)
Thymol (nasal inhalant)
Thyroglobulin (thyroid hormone)
Thyroid, dessicated (thyroid hormone)
Thyrotropic hormone (pituitary hormone)
Thyroxine (thyroid hormone)
Ticarcillin disodium (antibiotic)
Timolol maleate (calcium channel blocker)
Tincture of Benzoin (dermatologic preparation)
Tinidazole (amebicide)
Titanium dioxide (dermatologic preparation)
Tobramycin sulfate (antibiotic)
Tolazamide (oral antidiabetic agent)
Tolazoline HCl (vasodilator)
Tolbutamide (oral antidiabetic agent)
Tolmetin sodium (nonsteroidal antiinflammatory agent)
Tranylcypromine sulfate (MAO inhibitor, antidepressant)
Trazodone HCl (antidepressant)
Tretinoin (dermatologic preparation)
Triacetin (dermatologic preparation)
Triamcinolone preparations (corticosteroids)
Triamterene (diuretic)
Triazolam (hypnotic)
Trichlormethiazide (diuretic)
Tridihexethyl chloride (anticholinergic)
Triethanolamine polypeptide oleate-condensate (topical enzyme)
Triethanolamine salicylate (topical antiinflammatory preparation)
Triethylenethiophosphoramide (antineoplastic agent)
Trifluoperazine HCl (antipsychotic agent)
Triflupromazine HCl (antipsychotic)
Trihexyphenidyl preparations (anticholinergics, antiparkinson drugs)
Triiodothyronine (thyroid hormone)
Trimeprazine tartrate (antipsychotic agent)
Trimethadione (anticonvulsant)
Trimethaphan camsylate (antihypertensive)
Trimethobenzamide HCl (antiemetic)
Trimethoprim (antimicrobial agent)
Trimipramine maleate (antidepressant)
Tripelennamine preparations (dermatologic preparations)
Triprolidine HCl (antihistamine)
Troleandomycin (antibiotic)
Trypsin (digestive enzyme)
L-Tryptophan (amino acid)
Tuberculin test materials (biological preparations)
Tubocurarine chloride (neuromuscular blocker)
Tybamate (antianxiety agent)
Typhoid vaccine (biological preparation)

U

Undecylenic acid (antifungal preparation)
Urea preparations (dermatologic preparations)
Urokinase (enzyme)

V

Valproic acid (anticonvulsant)
Vancomycin hydrochloride (antibiotic)
Vasopressin (antidiuretic hormone)
Verapamil HCl (antianginal agent)
Versenate, calcium disodium (heavy metal antigonists)
Vidarabine (antiviral agent)
Vinblastine sulfate (antineoplastic agent)
Vincristine sulfate (antineoplastic agent)
Vitamin A preparations
Vitamin A and D preparations
Vitamin B_1 preparations
Vitamin B_2 preparations
Vitamin B_6 preparations
Vitamin B_{12} preparations
Vitamin B complex preparations

Appendix B

INDEX OF DRUGS BY TRADE NAME

Trade Name	Generic Name	Classification	Significant or Serious Reactions
A			
Abbokinase	Urokinase	Enzyme	
Accurbron	Theophylline	Bronchodilator	
Accutane	Isotretinoin	Dermatologic preparation	
Achromycin	Tetracycline	Antibiotic	
Achromycin V	Tetracycline	Antibiotic	
Achrostatin V	Tetracycline	Antibiotic	
Acthar	Corticotropin	Hormone	Cushing's syndrome
Actidil	Triprolidine	Antihistamine	
Actifed	Triprolidine	Antihistamine	
	Pseudoephedrine	Decongestant	
Actinomycin D (see Cosmegen)			
Acyclovir			
Adapin	Doxepin HCl	Antidepressant	
Adipex-P	Phentermine	Sympathomimetic	
Adriamycin	Doxorubicin HCl	Antineoplastic agent	Bone marrow depression/cardio-toxicity
Adrucil	Fluorouracil	Antineoplastic agent	Bone marrow depression
Aerodine	Povidone-iodine	Dermatologic preparation	
Aerosporin	Polymixin B sulfate	Topical antibiotic	
Afrin	Oxymetazoline	Sympathomimetic	
Afrinol	Pseudoephedrine	Sympathomimetic	
Aftate	Tolnaftate	Topical antifungal agent	
Agoral Plain	Mineral oil	Laxative	
A-hydroCort	Hydrocortisone	Corticosteroid	Cushing's syndrome
Akarpine	Pilocarpine	Topical cholinergic	
Ak-eon	Naphazoline	Sympathomimetic	
Ak-dilate	Phenylephrine	Sympathomimetic	
Akineton	Biperiden	Anticholinergic	
Ak-nefrin	Phenylephrine	Sympathomimetic	
Ak-pentolate	Cyclopentolate	Topical anticholinergic	
Akrinol	Acrisorcin	Dermatologic preparation	
Albalon	Naphazoline	Sympathomimetic	

Albay	Hymenoptera venom allergens	Biological preparation	
Albuminar	Albumin (human)	Biological preparation	
Albutein	Albumin (human)	Biological preparation	
Alcaine	Proparacaine HCl	Topical anesthetic	
Alcopar	Bephenium hydroxynaphthoate	Anthelmintic	
Aldactazide	Spironolactone	Diuretic	Hyperkalemia
	Hydrochlorothiazide	Diuretic	Hypokalemia
Aldactone	Spironolactone	Diuretic	Hyperkalemia
Aldoclor	Methyldopa	Antihypertensive	Hemolytic anemia
	Chlorothiazide	Diuretic	Hypokalemia
Aldomet	Methyldopa	Antihypertensive	Hemolytic anemia
Aldoril	Methyldopa	Antihypertensive	Hemolytic anemia
	Hydrochlorothiazide	Diuretic	Hypokalemia
Alkeran	Melphalan	Antineoplastic agent	Bone marrow depression
Alkergot (see Hydergine)			
Almocarpine	Pilocarpine HCl	Cholinergic	
Alophen	Phenolphthalein	Laxative	
Alpha Chymar	Chymotrypsin	Enzyme	
Alphaderm	Hydrocortisone	Corticosteroid	
Alphadrol	Fluprednisolone	Corticosteroid	
AlphaRedisol	Hydroxocobalamin	Vitamin B_{12}	
ALternaGEL	Aluminum hydroxide	Antacid	
Aludrox	Aluminum hydroxide	Antacid	
Alupent	Metaproterenol sulfate	Sympathomimetic	
Ambenyl Expectorant	Bromodiphenhydramine, diphenhydramine, guaiacol sulfonate, codeine sulfate	Expectorant mixture	
Amcill	Ampicillin	Antibiotic	Anaphylaxis
Amen	Medroxyprogesterone acetate	Progestin	Thromboembolism
Americaine	Benzocaine	Topical anesthetic	
Amicar	Aminocaproic acid	Plasmin and plasminogen inhibitor	
Amidate	Etomidate	General anesthetic	
Amikin	Amikacin sulfate	Antibiotic	
Aminodur	Aminophylline	Bronchodilator	

(Continued)

Trade Name	Generic Name	Classification	Significant or Serious Reactions
Amnestrogen	Estrogen, esterified	Estrogen	Thromboembolism
Amoxil	Amoxicillin trihydrate	Antibiotic	Anaphylaxis
Amphojel	Aluminum hydroxide	Antacid	
Amytal	Amobarbital	Hypnotic	Respiratory depression
Anabolin	Methandriol	Androgen	
Anacel	Tetracaine HCl	Local anesthetic	
Anadrol-50	Oxymetholone	Androgen	
Anaprox	Naproxen sodium	Antiinflammatory agent	Peptic ulcer
Anaspaz	Hyoscyamine sulfate	Anticholinergic	
Anavar	Oxandrolone	Androgen	
Ancef	Cefazolin sodium	Antibiotic	
Ancobon	Flucytosine	Antifungal agent	Leukopenia, thrombocytopenia
Andriol	Methandriol	Androgen	
Andro-cyp	Testosterone cypionate	Androgen	
Androlone	Nadrolone phenpropionate	Androgen	
Andryl	Testosterone enanthate	Androgen	
Anectine	Succinylcholine HCl	Neuromuscular blocker	
Angex	Lidoflazine	Antianginal agent	Ventricular arrhythmia
Anhydron	Cyclothiazide	Diuretic	Hypokalemia
Anspor	Cephradine	Antibiotic	Hypersensitivity
Antabuse	Disulfiram	Antialcoholic agent	Disulfiram-alcohol reaction
Antepar	Piperazine citrate	Anthelmintic	
Antilirium	Physostigmine salicylate	Topical cholinergic	
Antiminth	Pyrantel pamoate	Anthelmintic	
Antivert	Meclizine HCl	Antihistamine	
Antrenyl	Oxyphenonium bromide	Anticholinergic	
Anturane	Sulfinpyrazone	Uricosuric	
Apogen	Gentamicin sulfate	Antibiotic	Ototoxicity, nephrotoxicity
Apresoline HCl	Hydralazine HCl	Antihypertensive	Arrhythmias, "lupus syndrome"
Aptine	Alprenolol	Antihypertensive	A-V block, congestive heart failure, bronchospasm
AquaMEPHYTON	Phytonadione	Vitamin K preparation	
Aquasol A	Vitamin A		
Aquatag	Benzthiazide	Diuretic	Hypokalemia

Aquatensen	Methylclothiazide	Diuretic	Hypokalemia
Aralen Phosphate	Chloroquine phosphate	Antimalarial	
Aramine	Metaraminol bitartrate	Sympathomimetic	
Arfonad	Trimethaphan camsylate	Antihypertensive	
Argyrol	Silver protein	Disinfectant	
Aristocort	Triamcinolone	Corticosteroid	
Aristospan	Triamcinolone hexacetonide	Corticosteroid	
Arlidin	Nylidrin HCl	Vasodilator	
Arsobal	Melarsoprol	Antiprotozoal agent	Toxic encephalopathy
Artane	Trihexyphenidyl HCl	Anticholinergic	
Ascriptin	Aspirin	Nonsteroidal antiinflammatory	Peptic ulcer, GI bleeding
Asellacrin	Somatropin	Hormone	
Asendin	Amoxapine	Antidepressant	
Astiban	Stibocaptate	Anthelmintic	
Atabrine HCl	Quinacrine HCl	Antimalarial agent	Toxic psychosis
Atarax	Hydroxyzine HCl	Antihistamine	
Athrombine-K	Warfarin potassium	Anticoagulant	Bleeding diathesis
Ativan	Lorazepam	Antianxiety agent	
Atromid-S	Clofibrate	Antilipemic	
Atropisol	Atropine sulfate	Anticholinergic	
Atrovent	Ipratropium	Anticholinergic	
A/T/S	Erythromycin	Antibiotic	
Aureomycin	Chlortetracycline	Antibiotic	
Aventyl HCl	Nortriptyline HCl	Antidepressant	
Avitene	Microfibrillar collagen hemostat	Hemostatic agent	
Avlosulfon	Dapsone	Antileprosy agent	Sulfone syndrome
Aygestin	Norethindrone acetate	Progestin	
Azlin	Azlocillin sodium	Antibiotic	Anaphylaxis
Azo Gantanol	Sulfamethoxazole	Antibiotic	Nephrotoxicity, allergy
	Phenazopyridine HCl	Urinary analgesic	Blood dyscrasia
Azo Gantrisin (see Azo Gantanol)			
Azolid	Phenylbutazone	Nonsteroidal antiinflammatory	Agranulocytosis, nephrotoxicity
Azotrex	Sulfamethoxazide	Antibiotic	Blood dyscrasias, allergy, nephrotoxicity
	Phenazopyridine HCl	Urinary analgesic	
	Tetracycline phosphate	Antibiotic	
Azulfidine	Sulfasalazine	Antibiotic, antiinflammatory	Macrocytic anemia

(Continued)

Trade Name	Generic Name	Classification	Significant or Serious Reactions
B			
Bacarate	Phendimetrazine tartrate	Sympathomimetic	
Baciguent	Bacitracin	Topical antibiotic	
Bactocill	Oxacillin sodium	Antibiotic	Anaphylaxis
Bactrim	Sulfamethoxazole	Antibiotic	Nephrotoxicity, allergy
	Trimethoprim	Antibiotic	Blood dyscrasias
BAL in oil	Dimercaprol	Heavy metal antagonist	Hypertension, nephrotoxicity
Banthīne	Methantheline bromide	Anticholinergic	
Basaljel	Aluminum hydroxide	Antacid	
Because	Nonoxynol-9	Contraceptive cream	
Beclovent	Beclomethasone dipropionate	Topical steroid inhalant	Cushing's syndrome
Beconase (see Beclovent)			
Belap	Belladonna	Anticholinergic	
	Phenobarbital	Hypnotic	
Belladenal (see Belap)			
Bellergal	Belladonna	Anticholinergic	
	Ergotamine tartrate	Antimigraine drug	Peripheral vasoconstriction
	Phenobarbital	Hypnotic	
Benadryl	Diphenhydramine HCl	Antihistamine	
Bendectin	Doxylamine succinate	Antihistamine	
	Pyridoxine HCl	Vitamin B preparation	
Benemid	Probenecid	Antigout agent	
Benisone	Betamethasone benzoate	Corticosteroid	Cushing's syndrome
Benoquin	Monobenzone	Dermatologic preparation	
Benoxyl	Benzoyl peroxide	Dermatologic preparation	
Bentyl	Dicyclomine HCl	Anticholinergic	
Benylin	Diphenhydramine HCl	Antihistamine	
Benzac (see Benoxyl)			
Benzedrex	Propylhexedrine	Sympathomimetic	
Benzedrine	Amphetamine sulfate	Sympathomimetic	
Berubigen	Cyanocobalamin	Vitamin	
Betadine	Povidone-iodine	Dermatologic preparation	

Betalin S	Thiamine HCl	Vitamin B preparation	
Betalin 12	Cyanocobalamin	Vitamin B preparation	
Betapen	Penicillin VK	Antibiotic	Anaphylaxis
Beuron	Thiamine HCl	Vitamin B	
Bicillin	Penicillin G benzathine	Antibiotic	Anaphylaxis
BiCNU	Carmustine	Antineoplastic agent	Bone marrow depression, pulmonary fibrosis
Bilarcil	Metrifonate	Anthelmintic	
Biopar	Cyanocobalamin	Vitamin B_{12}	
	Intrinsic factor	Enzyme	
Biotres	Bacitracin, polymyxin B	Topical antibiotic	
Biozyme-C	Collagenase	Enzyme	
Biphetamine	Dextroamphetamine	Sympathomimetic	
	Amphetamine	Sympathomimetic	
Blanex (see Parafon Forte)			
Blenoxane	Bleomycin sulfate	Antineoplastic agent	Skin reactions, pulmonary fibrosis
Bleph-10 Liquifilm	Sulfacetamide sodium	Topical antibiotic	
Blocadren	Timolol maleate	Antianginal agent	Heart block, congestive heart failure
Bonine	Meclizine HCl	Antihistamine	
Breokinase	Streptokinase	Enzyme	
Breonesin	Guaifenesin	Expectorant	
Brethine	Terbutaline sulfate	Sympathomimetic	
Bretylol	Bretylium tosylate	Antiarrhythmic	Hypotension, arrhythmias
Brevicon	Norethindrone ethinyl estradiol	Contraceptive hormone	Thromboembolism
Brevital Sodium	Methohexital sodium	General anesthetic	
Bricanyl	Terbutaline sulfate	Sympathomimetic	
Bristagen	Gentamicin sulfate	Antibiotic	Nephrotoxicity, ototoxicity
Bristamycin	Erythromycin stearate	Antibiotic	
Brondecon	Oxytriphylline	Bronchodilator	
	Guaifenesin	Expectorant	
Bronkodyl	Theophylline	Bronchodilator	
Bronkometer	Isoetharine mesylate	Sympathomimetic	
Bronkosol	Isoetharine HCl	Sympathomimetic	
Bucladin-S	Buclizine HCl	Antihistamine	

(Continued)

Trade Name	Generic Name	Classification	Significant or Serious Reactions
Bumex	Bumetanide	Diuretic	Electrolyte disorders
Buminate	Albumin (human)	Biological preparation	
Buprenex	Buprenorphine HCl	Narcotic analgesic	
Burntame	Benzocaine	Topical anesthetic	
Butazolidin	Phenylbutazone	Nonsteroidal antiinflammatory agent	Agranulocytosis, renal failure, peptic ulcer, hepatitis
Butesin Picrate	Butamben picrate	Topical anesthetic	
Butabell	Belladonna	Anticholinergic	
	Butabarbital sodium	Hypnotic	
Buticaps	Butabarbital sodium	Hypnotic	
Butisol sodium	Butabarbital sodium	Hypnotic	
C			
Cafergot	Ergotamine tartrate	Antimigraine agent	Peripheral vasoconstriction
	Caffeine	Cerebral stimulant	
Caladryl	Diphenhydramine HCl	Antihistamine	
Calan	Verapamil HCl	Calcium channel blocker	
Calcidrine Syrup	Codeine	Narcotic analgesic	Dependency
	Calcium iodide	Expectorant	Hypersensitivity
Calcimar	Calcitonin	Hormone	Hypersensitivity
Calciparine	Heparin calcium	Anticoagulant	Bleeding diathesis
Calcium Disodium Versenate	Edetate calcium disodium	Heavy metal antagonist	Nephrotoxicity
Calderol	Calcifediol	Vitamin D preparation	
Camalox	Aluminum hydroxide	Antacid	
	Magnesium hydroxide	Antacid	
	Calcium carbonate	Antacid	
Candex	Nystatin	Antifungal agent	
Cantharone	Cantharidin	Dermatologic preparation	
Cantil	Mepenzolate bromide	Anticholinergic	
Capastat Sulfate	Capreomycin sulfate	Antimycobacterial agent	Nephrotoxicity
Capoten	Captopril	Antihypertensive	Pancytopenia, nephrotoxicity
Carafate	Sucralfate	Antiulcer drug	
Carbacel	Carbachol	Cholinergic	
Carbocaine	Mepivacaine HCl	Local anesthetic	
Cardilate	Erythrityl tetranitrate	Antianginal agent	Hypotension

Cardioquin	Quinidine polygalacturonate	Antiarrhythmic	Arrhythmias, congestive heart failure
Cardizem	Diltiazem HCl	Antianginal agent	A-V block
Catapres	Clonidine HCl	Antihypertensive	Hypotension, paradoxical hypertension
Ceclor	Cefaclor	Antibiotic	
Cedilanid-D	Deslanoside	Digitalis preparation	Arrhythmias
CeeNU	Lomustine	Antineoplastic agent	Bone marrow depression
Cefadyl	Cephapirin sodium	Antibiotic	
Celbenin	Methicillin	Antibiotic	Anaphylaxis
Celestrone	Betamethasone	Corticosteroid	Cushing's syndrome
Celontin	Methsuximide	Anticonvulsant	Pancytopenia, ataxia
Centrax	Prazepam	Antianxiety agent	
Cephulac	Lactulose	Ammonium binding agent	
Cerubidine	Daunorubicin HCl	Antineoplastic agent	Bone marrow depression, cardiomyopathy
Cerumenex	Triethanolamine polypeptide oleate	Dermatologic preparation	
Cetacort	Hydrocortisone	Corticosteroid	
Cetamide	Sulfacetamide sodium	Topical antibiotic	
Chardonna-2	Belladonna	Anticholinergic	
	Phenobarbital	Hypnotic	
Chealamide	Edetate disodium	Heavy metal antagonist	Nephrotoxicity
Chenix	Chenodeoxycholic acid	For gallstone dissolution	
Cheracol	Codeine phosphate	Antitussive agent	
	Guaifenesin	Expectorant	
Chloromycetin	Chloramphenicol	Antibiotic	Aplastic anemia
Chloroptic S.O.P.	Chloramphencol	Topical antibiotic	
Chlor-Trimeton	Chlorpheniramine maleate	Antihistamine	
Cholan HMB	Dehydrocholic acid	Bile salt	
	Phenobarbital	Hypnotic	
	Homatropine methylbromide	Anticholinergic	
Choledyl	Oxtriphylline	Bronchodilator	
Choloxin	Dextrothyroxine sodium	Antilipemic agent	
Chronulac (see Cephulac)			
Cibalith	Lithium citrate	Antidepressant	Nephrotoxicity, convulsions

(Continued)

Trade Name	Generic Name	Classification	Significant or Serious Reactions
Cidex	Glutaral	Dermatologic preparation	
Cinobac	Cinoxacin	Antimicrobial agent	
Cin-Quin	Quinidine sulfate	Antiarrhythmic	Arrhythmias, congestive heart failure
Citanest	Prilocaine HCl	Local anesthetic	
Claforan	Cefotaxime sodium	Antibiotic	
Cleocin	Clindamycin HCl	Antibiotic	Pseudomembranous colitis
Clērz	Hydroxyethylcellulose	Ophthalmic preparation	
Clinoril	Sulindac	Nonsteroidal antiinflammatory agent	Peptic ulcer, GI bleeding
Clistin	Carbinoxamine maleate	Antihistamine	
Cloderm	Clocortolone pivalate	Dermatologic preparation	
Clomid	Clomiphene citrate	Infertility agent	Ovarian cysts
Clonopin	Clonazepam	Anticonvulsant	
Cloxapen	Cloxacillin sodium	Antibiotic	Anaphylaxis
Coast	Triclocarban	Dermatologic preparation	
Cogentin	Benztropine mesylate	Anticholinergic	
Colace	Docusate sodium	Laxative	
ColBENEMID	Colchicine	Antigout agent	
	Probenecid	Uricosuric agent	
Colestid	Colestipol	Antilipemic agent	
Collyrium	Boric acid, sodium borate, thimerosal, antipyrine	Ophthalmologic preparation	
Coly-Mycin M	Colistimethate sodium	Antibiotic	Nephrotoxicity
Coly-Mycin S	Colistin sulfate	Antibiotic	Nephrotoxicity
Combid	Prochlorperazine maleate	Antipsychotic	Extrapyramidal reactions
	Isopropamide iodide	Anticholinergic	
Combipres	Clonidine HCl	Antihypertensive	Hypotension, pardoxical hypertension, hypokalemia
	Chlorthalidone	Diuretic	
Comfolax	Docusate sodium	Laxative	
Comfort Drops	Edetate disodium, benzalkonium chloride	Ophthalmologic preparation	

Comhist LA	Phenylephrine HCl	Sympathomimetic	
	Phenyltoloxamine citrate	Antihistamine	
	Chlorpheniramine maleate	Antihistamine	
	Atropine sulfate	Anticholinergic	
Compazine	Prochlorperazine	Antipsychotic agent	Extrapyramidal reaction
Comtrex	Phenylpropanolamine HCl	Sympathomimetic	
	Chlorpheniramine maleate	Antihistamine	
	Acetaminophen	Nonnarcotic analgesic	
	Dextromethorphan HBr	Antitussive	
Conar	Noscapine	Antihistamine	
	Guaifenesin	Expectorant	
	Phenylephrine HCl	Sympathomimetic	
Constant-T	Theophylline	Bronchodilator	
Contac	Phenylpropanolamine HCl	Sympathomimetic	
	Chlorpheniramine maleate	Antihistamine	
Coramine	Nikethamide	CNS stimulant	
Cordran	Flurandrenolide	Topical corticosteroid	
Corgard	Nadolol	Antihypertensive	Hypotension, A-V block
Coricidin D	Phenylpropanolamine HCl	Sympathomimetic	
	Chlorpheniramine maleate	Antihistamine	
	Aspirin	Nonsteroidal antiinflammatory agent	Peptic ulcer, GI bleeding
Cort-Dome	Hydrocortisone acetate	Topical corticosteroid	
Cortef	Hydrocortisone	Corticosteroid	Cushing's syndrome
Cortenema	Hydrocortisone	Corticosteroid	
Cortigel	Corticotropin	Corticotropic hormone	Cushing's syndrome
Cortisporin	Hydrocortisone acetate	Topical corticosteroid	
	Neomycin	Topical antibiotic	
	Polymyxin B	Topical antibiotic	
	Gramicidin	Topical antibiotic	
Cortone	Cortisone acetate	Corticosteroid	Cushing's syndrome
Cortril Acetate	Hydrocortisone	Corticosteroid	Cushing's syndrome
Cortrophin	Corticotropin	Corticosteroid	Cushing's syndrome
Cortrosyn	Cosyntropin	Corticotropic hormone	Cushing's syndrome
Cosmegen	Dactinomycin	Antineoplastic agent	Bone marrow depression
Cotazym	Pancrelipase	Enzyme	
Cotropic Gel	Corticotropin	Pituitary hormone	Cushing's syndrome
Coumadin	Warfarin sodium	Anticoagulant	Bleeding diathesis
Crescormon (see Asellacrin)			

(Continued)

Trade Name	Generic Name	Classification	Significant or Serious Reactions
Crysticillin	Penicillin G procaine	Antibiotic	Anaphylaxis
Crystodigin	Digitoxin	Digitalis preparation	Arrhythmias
Cuprimine	Penicillamine	Heavy metal antagonist	Bone marrow depression, nephrotoxicity, allergic reactions
Curretab	Medroxyprogesterone acetate	Progestin	
Cyclaine	Hexylcaine HCl	Local anesthetic	
Cyclapen-W	Cyclacillin	Antibiotic	Hypersensitivity
Cyclocort	Amcinonide	Topical corticosteroid	
Cyclogyl	Cyclopentolate HCl	Ophthalmologic preparation	
Cyclopar	Tetracycline HCl	Antibiotic	
Cyclospasmol	Cyclandelate	Vasodilator	
Cystospaz	Hyoscyamine	Anticholinergic	
Cytellin	Sitosterols	Antilipemic	
Cytomel	Liothyronine sodium	Thyroid hormone	Thyrotoxicosis
Cytosar-U	Cytarabine	Antineoplastic agent	Bone marrow depression
Cytoxan	Cyclophosphamide	Antineoplastic agent	Bone marrow depression, cardiotoxicity, hemorrhagic cystitis
D			
Dagenan	Sulfapyridine	Antibiotic	
Dalmane	Flurazepam HCl	Hypnotic	
Danocrine	Danazol	Androgen	
Dantrium	Dantrolene sodium	Skeletal muscle relaxant	
Daranide	Dichlorphenamide	Diuretic	
Daraprim	Pyrimethamine	Antiprotozoal agent	Blood dyscrasias
Darbid	Isopropamide iodide	Anticholinergic	
Daricon	Oxyphencyclimine HCl	Anticholinergic	
Darvocet-N	Propoxyphene napsylate	Narcotic analgesic	Dependency
Darvon preparations	Propoxyphene HCl	Narcotic analgesic	Dependency
Datril	Acetaminophen	Nonnarcotic analgesic	

Deaner	Deanol acetamidobenzoate	CNS stimulant	
Debrox	Carbamide peroxide	Topical otologic preparation	
Decaderm	Dexamethasone	Topical corticosteroid	
Decadron	Dexamethasone	Corticosteroid	Cushing's syndrome
Decadron Phosphate Turbinaire	Dexamethasone	Topical corticosteroid	
Deca-Durabolin	Nandrolone decanoate	Androgen	
Decaspray	Dexamethasone	Topical corticosteroids	
Declomycin	Demeclocycline HCl	Antibiotic	Nephrogenic diabetes insipidus
Dehist	Phenylephrine HCl	Sympathomimetic	
	Phenylpropanolamine HCl	Sympathomimetic	
	Chlorpheniramine	Antihistamine	
Deladumone	Estradiol valerate	Estrogen	Thromboembolism
	Testosterone enanthate	Androgen	
Delalutin	Hydroxyprogesterone caproate	Progestin	Thromboembolism
Delaxin	Methocarbamol	Skeletal muscle relaxant	
Delestrogen	Estradiol valerate	Estrogen	Thromboembolism
Delta-Cortef	Prednisolone	Corticosteroid	
Deltasone	Prednisone	Corticosteroid	
Demerol	Meperidine HCl	Narcotic analgesic	Dependency
Demser	Metyrosine	Antihypertensive	Extrapyramidal reactions, nephrolithiasis
Demulen	Ethinyl estradiol	Estrogen	Thromboembolism
	Ethynodiol diacetate	Progestin	Thromboembolism
Dendrid	Idouridine	Antiviral agent	
Depakene	Valproic acid	Anticonvulsant	Hepatotoxicity
Depen (see Cuprimine)			
Depo-Medrol	Methylprednisolone acetate	Corticosteroid	
Depo-Provera	Medroxyprogesterone acetate	Progestin	Thromboembolism
Desenex	Undecylenic acid	Antifungal agent	
Desferal mesylate	Deferoxamine mesylate	Heavy metal antagonist	
Desoxyn	Methamphetamine HCl	Sympathomimetic	
Desyrel	Trazodone HCl	Antidepressant	
Dexampex	Dextroamphetamine sulfate	Sympathomimetic	
Dexedrine	Dextroamphetamine sulfate	Sympathomimetic	
Dexone	Dexamethasone	Corticosteroid	

(Continued)

Trade Name	Generic Name	Classification	Significant or Serious Reactions
D.H.E. 45	Dihydroergotamine mesylate	Antimigraine agent	Peripheral vasoconstriction
Diabinese	Chlorpropamide	Oral antidiabetic agent	Hypoglycemia
Diafen	Diphenylpyraline HCl	Antihistamine	
Dialose	Docusate potassium	Laxative	
Diamox	Acetazolamide	Diuretic	Hypokalemia
Diaparene	Methylbenzethonium chloride	Dermatologic preparation	
Diapid	Lypressin	Pituitary hormone	
Diasone Sodium	Sulfoxone sodium	Antimicrobial agent	
Dibenzyline	Phenoxybenzamine HCl	Vasodilator	
Dicarbosil	Calcium carbonate	Antacid	
Dicodid	Hydrocodone bitartrate	Narcotic analgesic	Dependency
Didrex	Benzphetamine HCl	Sympathomimetic	Dependency
Didronel	Etidronate disodium	Estrogen	
Dilantin	Phenytoin	Anticonvulsant	
Dilatrate-SR	Isosorbide dinitrate	Antianginal agent	Hypotension
Dilaudid	Hydromorphone HCl	Narcotic analgesic	Dependency
Dilor	Dyphylline	Bronchodilator	
Dimacol	Dextromethorphan hydrobromide	Antitussive	
	Pseudoephedrine HCl	Sympathomimetic	
	Guaifenesin	Expectorant	
	Phenylpropanolamine HCl	Sympathomimetic	
Dimetane	Brompheniramine maleate	Antihistamine	
Dimetapp	Phenylephrine HCl	Sympathomimetic	
	Brompheniramine maleate	Antihistamine	
	Phenylpropanolamine HCl	Sympathomimetic	
Diothane	Diperodon monohydrate	Topical anesthetic	
Diprosone	Betamethasone dipropionate	Topical corticosteroid	
Disipal	Orphenadrine HCl	Anticholinergic	
Ditan	Phenytoin sodium	Anticonvulsant	
Ditropan	Oxybutynin chloride	Anticholinergic	
Diucardin	Hydroflumethiazide	Diuretic	Hypokalemia
Diulo	Metolazone	Diuretic	Hypokalemia
Diupres	Chlorothiazide	Diuretic	Hypokalemia
	Reserpine	Antihypertensive	Peptic ulcer, depression
Diuril	Chlorothiazide	Diuretic	Hypokalemia

Diutensen-R	Methyclothiazide	Diuretic	Hypokalemia
	Reserpine	Antihypertensive	Peptic ulcer, depression
Dobutrex	Dobutamine HCl	Sympathomimetic	
Dolene (see Darvon)			
Dolobid	Diflunisal	Nonsteroidal antiinflammatory agent	Peptic ulcer, GI bleeding
Domol	Mineral oil	Laxative	
Donnagel	Kaolin, pectin	Antidiarrheal agent	
	Hyoscyamine sulfate	Anticholinergic	
	Atropine sulfate	Anticholinergic	
	Scopolamine hydrobromide	Anticholinergic	
Donnatal	Hyoscyamine sulfate	Anticholinergic	
	Atropine sulfate	Anticholinergic	
	Scopolamine hydrobromide	Anticholinergic	
	Phenobarbital	Hypnotic	
Dopar	Levodopa	Antiparkinsonian agent	Hypotension, dyskinesias, psychosis
Dopastat	Dopamine HCl	Sympathomimetic	
Dopram	Doxapram HCl	CNS stimulant	Laryngospasm
Dorbane (see Modane)			
Dorbantyl	Danthron	Laxative	
	Docusate sodium	Laxative	
Doriden	Glutethimide	Hypnotic	Dependency
Doxidan (see Dorbantyl)			
Dralserp	Hydralazine HCl	Antihypertensive	Angina, "lupus syndrome," arrhythmia
	Reserpine	Antihypertensive	Peptic ulcer, depression
Dramamine	Dimenhydrinate	Antihistamine	
Dristan	Phenylephrine HCl	Sympathomimetic	
	Pheniramine maleate	Antihistamine	
Drixoral	Pseudoephedrine sulfate	Sympathomimetic	
	Dexbrompheniramine maleate	Antihistamine	
Drolban	Dromostanolone	Antineoplastic agent	Virilism
Drysol	Ammonium chloride	Dermatologic preparation	

(Continued)

Trade Name	Generic Name	Classification	Significant or Serious Reactions
DTIC-Dome	Dacarbazine	Antineoplastic agent	Blood dyscrasias
Dulcolax	Bisacodyl	Laxative	
Duotrate	Pentaerythritrol	Antianginal agent	Hypotension
Durabolic	Methandriol diproprionate	Androgen	
Durabolin	Nandrolone phenpropionate	Androgen	
Duracillin A.S.	Penicillin G procaine	Antibiotic	Anaphylaxis
Duranest	Etidocaine HCl	Local anesthetic	
Duraquin	Quinidine gluconate	Antiarrhythmic	Arrhythmia, congestive heart failure
Duration	Oxymetazoline HCl	Sympathomimetic	
Duricef	Cefadroxil	Antibiotic	
Duvoid	Bethanechol chloride	Cholinergic	
Dyazide	Hydrochlorothiazide	Diuretic	Hypokalemia
	Triamterene	Diuretic	Hyperkalemia
Dycill	Dicloxacillin sodium	Antibiotic	Hypersensitivity
Dyclone	Dyclonine HCl	Topical anesthetic	
Dymelor	Acetohexamide	Oral antidiabetic agent	Hypoglycemia
Dynapen	Dicloxacillin sodium	Antibiotic	Hypersensitivity
Dyrenium	Triamterene	Diuretic	Hyperkalemia
E			
Econochlor (see Chloromycetin)			
Edecrin	Ethacrynic acid	Diuretic	
E.E.S.	Erythromycin ethylsuccinate	Antibiotic	Hepatitis
Effersyllium (see Metamucil)			
Efodine	Povidone-iodine	Dermatologic preparation	
Efricel (see Neo-Synephrine HCl)			
Efudex	Fluorouracil	Dermatologic preparation	
Elase	Fibrinolysin	Enzyme	
	Desoxyribonuclease	Enzyme	
Elavil	Amitriptyline HCl	Antidepressant	
Elixicon	Theophylline	Bronchodilator	

Elspar	Asparaginase	Antineoplastic agent	Anaphylaxis, coma
Emcyt	Estramustine phosphate sodium	Antineoplastic agent	Gynecomastia, hypercalcemia
Emete-con	Benzquinamide HCl	Antiemetic	
E-Mycin	Erythromycin	Antibiotic	
Enarax	Oxyphencyclimine HCl	Anticholinergic	
	Hydroxyzine HCl	Antihistamine	
Endep (see Elavil)			
Endrate (see Sodium Versenate)			
Enduron	Methyclothiazide	Diuretic	Hypokalemia
Enduronyl	Methyclothiazide	Diuretic	Hypokalemia
	Deserpidine	Antihypertensive	Peptic ulcer, depression
Enovid-E	Norethindrone	Androgen	
	Metranol	Estrogen	Thromboembolism
Enovil (see Elavil)			
Entex	Phenylephrine HCl	Sympathomimetic	
	Phenylpropanolamine HCl	Sympathomimetic	
	Guaifenesin	Expectorant	
Entozyme	Pancreatin	Digestive enzyme	
	Bile salts	Digestive enzyme	
Epifrin	Epinephrine HCl	Sympathomimetic	
Epitrate	Epinephrine bitartrate	Ophthalmic preparation	
Equagesic	Ethoheptazine citrate	Nonnarcotic analgesic	
	Aspirin	Nonsteroidal antiinflammatory agent	Peptic ulcer, GI bleeding
	Meprobamate	Skeletal muscle relaxant	
Equanil	Meprobamate	Skeletal muscle relaxant	
Ergomar	Ergotamine tartrate	Antimigraine agent	Peripheral vasoconstriction
Ergostat (see Ergomar)			
Erythrocin Lactobionate-I.V.	Erythromycin lactobionate	Antibiotic	
Erythrocin Stearate Filmtabs	Erythromycin stearate	Antibiotic	
Eserine	Physostigmine	Cholinergic ophthalmic preparation	

(Continued)

Trade Name	Generic Name	Classification	Significant or Serious Reactions
Esidrix	Hydrochlorothiazide	Diuretic	Hypokalemia
Esimil	Hydrochlorothiazide	Diuretic	
	Guanethidine monosulfate	Antihypertensive	Hypotension, impotence
Eskalith	Lithium carbonate	Antidepressant	Nephrotoxicity, convulsions
Estate	Estradiol valerate	Estrogen	Thromboembolism
Estinyl	Ethinyl estradiol	Estrogen	Thromboembolism
Estrace	Estradiol	Estrogen	Thromboembolism
Estratabs	Estrogens, esterified	Estrogen	Thromboembolism
Estrovis	Quinestrol	Estrogen	Thromboembolism
Ethaquin	Ethaverine	Vasodilator	
Ethrane	Enflurane	General anesthetic	
Ethril	Erythromycin stearate	Antibiotic	
Etrafon (see Triavil)			
Etrenol	Hycanthone mesylate	Anthelmintic	Postnecrotic cirrhosis
Euthroid	Levothyroxine sodium	Thyroid hormone	Thyrotoxicosis
	Liothyronine sodium	Thyroid hormone	Thyrotoxicosis
Eutonyl	Pargyline HCl	Antihypertensive	Hypertensive crisis
Eutron	Pargyline HCl	Antihypertensive	Hypertensive crisis
	Methylclothiazide	Diuretic	Hypokalemia
Evex (see Estratabs)			
Exna	Benzthiazide	Diuretic	Hypokalemia
Exsel	Selenium sulfide	Mineral	
F			
Factorate	Antihemophilic factor	Biological preparation	
Fastin	Phentermine HCl	Sympathomimetic	
Feen-a-mint	Phenolphthalein	Laxative	
Feldene	Piroxicam	Nonsteroidal antiinflammatory agent	Peptic ulcer, GI bleeding
Feminone (see Estinyl)			
Feosol	Ferrous sulfate	Mineral, hematinic	

Fergon	Ferrous gluconate	Mineral, hematinic	
Fer-In-Sol (see Feosol)			
Fermalox	Ferrous sulfate	Mineral, hematinic	
	Magnesium hydroxide	Antacid	
	Aluminum hydroxide	Antacid	
Fero-Gradumet	Ferrous sulfate	Mineral, hematinic	
Festal	Lipase	Digestive enzyme	
	Amylase	Digestive enzyme	
	Protease	Digestive enzyme	
	Hemicellulase	Digestive enzyme	
	Bile acids	Digestive enzyme	
Filibon	Multivitamin	Multivitamin	
Fiogesic	Phenylpropanolamine HCl	Sympathomimetic	
	Pheniramine maleate	Antihistamine	
	Pyrilamine maleate	Antihistamine	
	Calcium carbaspirin	Nonsteroidal antiinflammatory agent	Peptic ulcer, GI bleeding
Fiorinal	Butabarbital	Hypnotic	
	Aspirin	Nonsteroidal antiinflammatory agent	Peptic ulcer, GI bleeding
	Phenacetin	Nonnarcotic analgesic	Nephrotoxicity
	Caffeine	CNS stimulant	
Flagyl	Metronidazole	Antiprotozoal agent	Convulsions, neuropathy
Flaxedil	Gallamine triethiodide	Skeletal muscle relaxant	
Flexeril	Cyclobenzaprine HCl	Skeletal muscle relaxant	
Florinef Acetate	Fludrocortisone acetate	Topical corticosteroid	
Florone	Diflorasone diacetate	Topical corticosteroid	
Fluonid	Fluocinolone acetonide	Topical corticosteroid	
Fluoroplex	Fluorouracil	Dermatologic preparation	
Fluothane	Halothane	General anesthetic	
Forane	Isoflurane	General anesthetic	
Fostex	Sulfur salicylic acid	Dermatologic preparation	
FUDR	Floxuridine	Antineoplastic agent	Bone marrow depression
Fungizone	Amphotericin B	Antifungal agent	Nephrotoxicity
Furacin	Nitrofurazone	Topical antimicrobial agent	

(Continued)

Trade Name	Generic Name	Classification	Significant or Serious Reactions
Furadantin	Nitrofurantoin	Antimicrobial	Neuropathy, hemolytic anemia, pulmonary toxicity
Furoxone	Furazolidone	Antimicrobial	Agranulocytosis
G			
Gamastan	Immune globulin	Biological preparation	
Gammar	Immune globulin	Biological preparation	
Gantanol	Sulfamethoxazole	Antimicrobial agent	Nephrotoxicity, hypersensitivity
Gantrisin	Sulfisoxazole base	Antimicrobial agent	Nephrotoxicity, hypersensitivity
Garamycin	Gentamicin sulfate	Antimicrobial agent	Ototoxicity, nephrotoxicity
Gaviscon	Sodium alginate	Antacid	
	Alginic acid	Antacid	
	Magnesium trisilicate	Antacid	
	Aluminum hydroxide	Antacid	
Gelusil	Aluminum hydroxide	Antacid	
	Magnesium hydroxide	Antacid	
	Simethicone	Antacid	
Genoptic	Gentamicin sulfate	Antibiotic ophthalmic preparation	
Gentran 40	Dextran	Biological preparation	
Geocillin	Carbenicillin indanyl sodium	Antibiotic	Hypersensitivity, blood dyscrasias
Gitaligin	Gitalin	Digitalis preparation	Arrhythmias
Glaucon (see Epifrin)			
Glucantime	Meglumine antimoniate	Antiprotozoal agent	Antimony poisoning
Glyrol	Glycerin	Laxative	
Grifulvin V	Griseofulvin	Antifungal agent	Agranulocytosis
Grisactin (see Grifulvin)			
Gyne-Lotrimin	Clotrimazole	Topical antifungal agent	
Gynergen	Ergotamine tartrate	Antimigraine agent	Peripheral vasoconstriction

H			
Halciderm	Halcinonide	Topical corticosteroid	
Halcion	Triazolam	Hypnotic	
Haldol	Haloperidol	Antipsychotic agent	Extrapyramidal reactions
Haley's M-O	Magnesium hydroxide, mineral oil	Laxative	
Halodrin	Fluoxymesterone	Androgen	
	Ethinyl estradiol	Estrogen	Thromboembolism
Halotex	Haloprogin	Topical antifungal agent	
Harmonyl	Deserpidine	Antihypertensive	Peptic ulcer, depression
Healon	Hyaluronate sodium	Ophthalmic preparation	
Hedulin	Phenindione	Anticoagulant	Agranulocytosis, hepatitis, nephritis
Heptavax-B	Hepatitis B vaccine	Biological preparation	
Herplex Liquifilm	Idoxuridine	Antiviral ophthalmic preparation	
Hexadrol (see Decadron)			
Hiprex	Methenamine hippurate	Urinary antiseptic	
Histalog	Betazole HCl	Gastric acid stimulant	
HMS	Medrysone	Steroid ophthalmic preparation	
Homatrocel	Homatropine hydrobromide	Anticholinergic opthalmic preparation	
Humorsol	Demecarium bromide	Cholinergic ophthalmic preparation	
Humulin N	Human NPH insulin	Insulin hormone	Hypoglycemia
Hycodan	Hydrocodone bitartrate	Antitussive agent	
	Homatropine methylbromide	Anticholinergic	
Hydeltra-T.B.A.	Prednisolone tebutate	Corticosteroid	Cushing's syndrome
Hydergine	Ergoloid mesylates	CNS stimulant	
Hydrea	Hydroxyurea	Antineoplastic agent	Bone marrow depression
HydroDIURIL	Hydrochlorothiazide	Diuretic	Hypokalemia
Hydromox	Quinethazone	Diuretic	Hypokalemia
Hydropres	Hydrochlorothiazide	Diuretic	Hypokalemia
	Reserpine	Antihypertensive	Peptic ulcer, depression
Hygroton	Chlorthalidone	Diuretic	Hypokalemia
Hylorel	Guanadrel	Antihypertensive	Orthostatic hypotension

(Continued)

Trade Name	Generic Name	Classification	Significant or Serious Reactions
Hyperstat	Diazoxide	Antihypertensive	Hypotension
Hypnomidate	Etomidate	General anesthetic	Apnea, laryngospasm
Hytakerol	Dihydrotachysterol	Vitamin D analog	Hypercalcemia
Hytinic	Iron-polysaccharide complex	Iron hematinic	
Hytone	Hydrocortisone	Topical corticosteroid	
I			
Iletin I, Lente	Insulin zinc suspension	Insulin hormone	Hypoglycemia
Ilosone	Erythromycin estolate	Antibiotic	Hepatitis
Ilotycin	Erythromycin	Antibiotic	
Ilozyme	Pancrelipase	Digestive enzyme	
Imavate (see Tofranil)			
Imferon	Iron dextran	Iron hematinic	
Imodium	Loperamide HCl	Antidiarrheal agent	
Imuran	Azathioprine	Immunosuppressant	Aplastic anemia, hepatitis
Inapsine	Droperidol	Antiemetic	Extrapyramidal reactions
Inderal	Propranolol HCl	Antiarrhythmic, antihypertensive	A-V block, congestive heart failure, bronchospasm
Indocin	Indomethacin	Nonsteroidal antiinflammatory agent	Peptic ulcer, GI bleeding
Innovar	Droperidol	Antiemetic	Extrapyramidal reactions
	Fentanyl citrate	Narcotic analgesic	Apnea
Insulatard	Insulin injection isophane	Insulin hormone	Hypoglycemia
Intal	Cromolyn sodium	Antiasthmatic	
Intropin	Dopamine HCl	Sympathomimetic	
Inversine	Mecamylamine	Antihypertensive	Hypotension
Iodotope I-131	Sodium iodide I 131	Antithyroid	Hypothyroidism
Ionamin	Phentermine resin	Sympathomimetic	Dependency
Ionax	Benzalkonium chloride	Dermatologic preparation	
Iosel	Selenium sulfide	Dermatologic preparation	
Ipecac	Ipecac alkaloids	Emetic	
Ircon	Ferrous fumarate	Iron hematinic	
Ismelin	Guanethidine monosulfate	Antihypertensive	Hypotension, impotence
Ismotic	Isorbide	Ophthalmic preparation	
INH	Isoniazid	Antibiotic	Hepatitis

Isoclor	Pseudoephedrine HCl Chlorpheniramine maleate	Sympathomimetic Antihistamine	
Isodine (see Betadine)			
Isoptin	Verapamil HCl	Antianginal agent	Heart block, congestive heart failure
Isopto Carpine	Pilocarpine HCl	Cholinergic ophthalmic preparation	
Isopto Hyoscine	Scopolamine hydrobromide	Anticholinergic ophthalmic preparation	
Isordil	Isosorbide dinitrate	Antianginal agent	Hypotension
Isuprel	Isoproterenol HCl	Sympathomimetic	
K			
Kabikinase	Streptokinase	Enzyme	
Kantrex	Kanamycin sulfate	Antibiotic	Nephrotoxicity, ototoxicity
Kaochlor	Potassium chloride	Mineral	
Kaon	Potassium gluconate	Mineral	
Kaopectate	Kaolin, pectin	Antidiarrheal agent	
Kappadione	Menadiol sodium diphosphate	Vitamin K analog	
Kasof	Docusate potassium	Laxative	
Kay Ciel (see Kaochlor)			
Kayexalate	Sodium polystyrene sulfonate	Potassium binding agent	
Keflex	Cephalexin	Antibiotic	
Keflin	Cephalothin sodium	Antibiotic	
Kefzol	Cefazolin sodium	Antibiotic	
Kemadrin	Procyclidine HCl	Anticholinergic	
Kenacort	Triamcinolone	Corticosteroid	Cushing's syndrome
Kenalog	Triamcinolone acetonide	Corticosteroid	
Ketaject	Ketamine HCl	General anesthetic	
Kinesed (see Donnatal)			
Klebcil (see Kantrex)			
K-Lor (see Kaochlor)			
Klotrix (see Kaochlor)			

(Continued)

Trade Name	Generic Name	Classification	Significant or Serious Reactions
Koāte	Antihemophilic factor	Biological preparation	
Kondremul	Mineral oil	Laxative	
Konsyl (see Metamucil)			
Koromex Cream	Nonoxynol-9	Contraceptive agent	
K-Tab (see Kaochlor)			
Ku-Zyme HP	Pancrelipase	Digestive enzyme	
Kwell	Lindane	Topical scabicide	
L			
LāBID (see Elixicon)			
Lampit (see Furadantin)			
Lamprene	Clofazimine	Antimycobacterial agent	Red skin
Lanoxicaps (see Lanoxin)			
Lanoxin	Digoxin	Antiarrhythmic	Arrhythmias, heart block
Larodopa	Levodopa	Antiparkinsonian agent	Hypotension, dyskinesias, psychosis
Lasix	Furosemide	Diuretic	Hyponatremia, hypokalemia
Lavatar	Coal tar	Dermatologic preparation	
Ledercillin VK	Penicillin V potassium	Antibiotic	Anaphylaxis
Lentard	Insulin zinc suspension	Insulin hormone	Hypoglycemia
Lente Iletin (see Iletin I, Lente)			
Leukeran	Chlorambucil	Antineoplastic agent	Bone marrow depression
Levo-Dromoran	Levorphanol tartrate	Narcotic analgesic	Dependency
Levophed Bitartrate	Norepinephrine bitartrate	Sympathomimetic	
Levothroid	Levothyroxine sodium	Thyroid hormone	Thyrotoxicosis
Levsin	Hyoscyamine sulfate	Anticholinergic	
Libritabs (see Librium)			
Librium	Chlordiazepoxide	Antianxiety agent	
Lida-Mantle (see Xylocaine)			
Lidex	Fluocinonide	Topical corticosteroid	

Lidosporin Otic	Polymyxin B sulfate	Topical antibiotic	
Limbitrol	Chlordiazepoxide	Antianxiety agent	
	Amitriptyline HCl	Antidepressant	
Lincocin	Lincomycin HCl monohydrate	Antibiotic	Pseudomembranous colitis
Lioresal	Baclofen	Skeletal muscle relaxant	
Liotrix (see Euthroid)			
Lipo-Hepin	Heparin sodium	Anticoagulant	Bleeding diathesis
Liquaemin Sodium (see Lipo-Hepin)			
Liquamar	Phenprocoumon	Anticoagulant	Bleeding diathesis
Liquiprin Acetaminophen	Acetaminophen	Nonnarcotic analgesic	
Lithane	Lithium carbonate	Antidepressant	Nephrotoxicity, convulsions
Lithobid (see Lithane)			
Locorten	Flumethasone pivalate	Topical corticosteroid	
Loestrin	Ethinyl estradiol	Oral contraceptive hormone	Thromboembolism
	Norethindrone acetate		
Lomidine	Pentamidine isethionate	Antiprotozoal agent	Hepatoxicity, nephrotoxicity
Lomotil	Diphenoxylate HCL	Antidiarrheal agent	
	Atropine sulfate	Anticholinergic	
Loniten	Minoxidil	Antihypertensive	Edema, pericardial effusion, angina, hypertrichosis
Lo/Ovral	Ethinyl estradiol	Estrogen	Thromboembolism
	Norgestrel	Progestin	Thromboembolism
Lopid	Gemfibrozil	Antilipemic agent	
Lopressor	Metoprolol tartrate	Antihypertensive	Heart block, congestive heart failure
Lopurin (see Zyloprim)			
Lorelco	Probucol	Antilipemic agent	
Loroxide	Benzoyl peroxide	Dermatologic preparation	
Lotrimin	Clotrimazole	Topical antifungal agent	
Loxitane (see Asendin)			

(Continued)

Trade Name	Generic Name	Classification	Significant or Serious Reactions
Ludiomil	Maprotiline HCl	Antidepressant	
Lufyllin	Dyphylline	Bronchodilator	
Lysodren	Mitotane	Antineoplastic agent	GI reactions, CNS reactions
M			
Maalox	Aluminum hydroxide Magnesium hydroxide	Antacid	
Macrodantin (see Furadantin)			
Mallisol (see Betadine)			
Maltsupex	Potassium carbonate Malt soup extract	Laxative	
Mandelamine	Methenamine mandelate	Antimicrobial agent	
Mandol	Cefamandole nafate	Antibiotic	
Maolate	Chlorphenesin carbamate	Skeletal muscle relaxant	
Marax	Theophylline Ephedrine sulfate Hydroxyzine HCl	Bronchodilator Sympathomimetic Antihistamine	
Marcaine	Bupivacaine HCl	Local anesthetic	
Marezine	Cyclizine lactate	Antihistamine	
Marplan	Isocarboxazid	Antidepressant	Hypertensive crisis
Matulane	Procarbazine HCl	Antineoplastic agent	Bone marrow depression, neurologic reactions
Mazanor	Mazindol	Sympathomimetic	
Measurin	Aspirin	Nonsteroidal antiinflammatory agent	Peptic ulcer, GI bleeding
Mebaral	Mephobarbital	Anticonvulsant	
Meclan	Meclocycline Sulfosalicylate	Antimicrobial Dermatologic preparation	
Meclomen	Meclofenamate sodium	Nonsteroidal antiinflammatory agent	Peptic ulcer, GI bleeding
Medihaler Ergotamine	Ergotamine tartrate	Antimigraine agent	Peripheral vasoconstriction
Medihaler-Iso	Isoproterenol sulfate	Sympathomimetic	
Medrol	Methylprednisolone	Corticosteroid	Cushing's syndrome

Mefoxin	Cefoxitin sodium	Antibiotic	
Megace	Megestrol acetate	Progestin	Thromboembolism
Mellaril	Thioridazine HCl	Antipsychotic agent	Extrapyramidal reactions
Menest	Estrogen, esterified	Estrogen	Thromboembolism
Menrium	Estrogen, esterified	Estrogen	Thromboembolism
	Chlordiazepoxide	Antianxiety agent	
Mepergan	Meperidine HCl	Narcotic analgesic	Dependency
	Promethazine HCl	Antipsychotic agent	Extrapyramidal reactions
Mephyton	Phytonadione	Vitamin K analog	
Meprospan	Meprobamate	Skeletal muscle relaxant	
Mequin (see Quāālude)			
Mersol	Thimerosal	Dermatologic preparation	
Mestinon	Pyridostigmine bromide	Cholinergic	Cholinergic crisis
Metahydrin	Trichlormethiazide	Diuretic	Hypokalemia
Metamucil	Psyllium hydrophilic colloid	Laxative	
Metandren (see Oreton)			
Metaprel	Metaproterenol sulfate	Sympathomimetic	Hypokalemia
Metatensin	Trichlormethiazide	Diuretic	Depression, peptic ulcer
	Reserpine	Antihypertensive	
Methabolic	Methandriol dipropionate	Androgen hormone	
Methergine	Methylergonovine maleate	Uterine stimulant	Peripheral vasoconstriction
Meticorten	Prednisone	Corticosteroid hormone	Cushing's syndrome
Meti-Derm	Prednisolone	Topical corticosteroid	
Metimyd	Sulfacetamide	Antimicrobial agent	
	Prednisolone acetate	Corticosteroid hormone	
Metopirone	Metyrapone	Blocker of cortisol production for diagnostic use	
Metrazol	Pentylenetetrazol	Cerebral stimulant	Convulsions
Metreton	Prednisolone	Corticosteroid hormone	Cushing's syndrome
Metryl (see Flagyl)			
Metycaine HCl	Piperocaine HCl	Local anesthesic	
Mexate	Methotrexate sodium	Antineoplastic agent	Bone marrow depression, hepatoxicity

(Continued)

Trade Name	Generic Name	Classification	Significant or Serious Reactions
Mezlin	Mezlocillin sodium	Antibiotic	Anaphylaxis
Micrainin	Meprobamate	Skeletal muscle relaxant	
	Aspirin	Nonsteroidal antiinflammatory agent	Peptic ulcer, GI bleeding
Micro-K (see Kaochlor)			
Midrin	Isometheptene mucate	Sympathomimetic	
	Dichloralphenazone	Hypnotic	
	Acetaminophen	Nonnarcotic analgesic	
Migral	Ergotamine tartrate	Antimigraine agent	Peripheral vasoconstriction
	Caffeine	CNS stimulant	
	Cyclizine HCl	Antihistamine	
Milk of Magnesia	Magnesium hydroxide	Antacid	
Milontin	Phensuximide	Anticonvulsant	Bone marrow depression, nephrotoxicity
Milpath	Meprobamate	Skeletal muscle relaxant	
	Tridihexethyl chloride	Anticholinergic	
Miltown	Meprobamate	Skeletal muscle relaxant	
Minipress	Prazosin HCl	Antihypertensive	Syncope
Minizide	Prazosin HCl	Antihypertensive	
	Polythiazide	Diuretic	Hypokalemia
Minocin	Minocycline HCl	Antibiotic	Ototoxicity
Mintezol	Thiabendazole	Anthelmintic	
Miochol	Acetylcholine chloride	Cholinergic ophthalmic preparation	
Miostat	Carbachol	Cholinergic ophthalmic preparation	
Mithracin	Plicamycin	Antineoplastic agent	Bleeding diathesis, bone marrow depression
Mitrolan	Calcium polycarbophil	Laxative	
Mixtard	Insulin injection	Hormone	Hypoglycemia
Moban	Molindone HCl	Antipsychotic agent	Extrapyramidal reactions
Modane	Danthron	Laxative	
Moderil	Rescinnamine	Antihypertensive	Arrhythmias
Modicon	Ethinyl estradiol	Estrogen hormone	Thromboembolism
	Norethindrone	Progestin hormone	Thromboembolism

Moduretic	Amiloride HCl	Antihypertensive	Hyperkalemia, arrhythmias
	Hydrochlorothiazide	Diuretic	Hypokalemia
Monistat	Miconazol nitrate	Topical antifungal agent	
Monotard	Insulin zinc suspension	Hormone	Hypoglycemia
Motrin	Ibuprofen	Nonsteroidal antiinflammatory agent	Peptic ulcer, GI bleeding
Moxam	Moxalactam disodium	Antibiotic	Hypersensitivity, coagulopathy
Mucomyst	Acetylcysteine	Expectorant	
Mustargen	Mechlorethamine HCl	Antineoplastic agent	Bone marrow depression
Mutamycin	Mitomycin	Antineoplastic agent	Bone marrow depression, nephrotoxicity
Myambutol	Ethambutol HCl	Antimycobacterial agent	Optic neuritis
Mycelex (see Lotrimin)			
Mycifradin	Neomycin sulfate	Topical antibiotic	
Mycitracin	Bacitracin	Topical antibiotic	
	Polymyxin B	Topical antibiotic	
	Neomycin	Topical antibiotic	
Mycolog	Triamcinolone acetonide	Topical corticosteroid	
	Neomycin sulfate	Topical antibiotic	
	Gramicidin	Antibiotic	
	Mystatin	Antifungal agent	
Mycostatin	Mystatin	Antifungal agent	
Mylanta	Aluminum hydroxide	Antacid	
	Magnesium hydroxide	Antacid	
	Simethicone	Antacid	
Myleran	Busulfan	Antineoplastic agent	Bone marrow depression
Mylicon	Simethicone	Antacid	
Myochrysine	Gold sodium thiomalate	Antiinflammatory metal	Dermatitis, nephrotoxicity, bone marrow depression
Myotonachol (see Urecholine)			
Mysoline	Primidone	Anticonvulsant	Megaloblastic anemia
Mysteclin-F	Tetracycline HCl	Antibiotic	
	Amphotericin B	Antifungal agent	Nephrotoxicity

(Continued)

Trade Name	Generic Name	Classification	Significant or Serious Reactions
Mytelase	Ambenonium chloride	Cholinergic	Cholinergic crisis
Mytrate	Epinephrine bitartrate	Sympathomimetic	
Mytrex (see Mycolog)			
N			
Naldecon	Phenylpropanolamine HCl	Sympathomimetic	
	Phenylephrine HCl	Sympathomimetic	
	Phenyltoloxamine citrate	Antihistamine	
	Chlorpheniramine maleate	Antihistamine	
Nalfon	Fenoprofen calcium	Nonsteroidal antiinflammatory agent	Peptic ulcer, GI bleeding
Nandrolin	Nandrolone phenpropionate	Androgen hormone	
Naphcon	Naphazoline HCl	Ophthalmic preparation	
Naprosyn	Naproxen	Nonsteroidal antiinflammatory agent	Peptic ulcer, GI bleeding
Naqua	Trichlormethiazide	Diuretic	Hypokalemia
Narcan	Naloxone HCl	Narcotic antagonist	
Nardil	Phenelzine sulfate	Antidepressant	Hypertensive crisis
Nasalide	Flunisolide	Topical corticosteroid	
Natabec	Multivitamin	Multivitamin	
Natalins	Multivitamin	Multivitamin	
Naturetin	Bendroflumethiazide	Diuretic	Hypokalemia
Navane	Thiothixene	Antipsychotic agent	
Naxamide	Ifosfamide	Antineoplastic agent	
Nebcin	Tobramycin sulfate	Antibiotic	
NegGram	Nalidixic acid	Antimicrobial agent	
Nema Worm Capsules	Tetrachloroethylene	Anthelmintic	
Neobiotic	Neomycin sulfate	Antibiotic	Insignificant unless given parenterally
Neo-Cortef	Neomycin sulfate	Topical antibiotic	
	Hydrocortisone acetate	Corticosteroid	
Neodecadron	Neomycin sulfate	Topical antibiotic	
	Dexamethasone	Corticosteroid	

Neo-Hydeltrasol	Neomycin sulfate	Ophthalmic antibiotic	
	Prednisolone sodium phosphate	Corticosteroid preparation	
Neoloid	Castor oil	Laxative	
Neo-Medrol Acetate	Neomycin sulfate	Topical antibiotic	
	Methylprednisolone	Corticosteroid	
Neo-Polycin	Polymyxin B sulfate	Topical antibiotic	
	Bacitracin zinc	Topical antibiotic	
	Neomycin sulfate	Topical antibiotic	
Neosporin (see Neo-Polycin)			
Neo-Synephrine HCl	Phenylephrine HCl	Sympathomimetic	
Neothylline	Dyphylline	Sympathomimetic	
Nervine	Phyllamine	Antihistamine	
Netromycin	Netilmicin	Antibiotic	
Niclocide	Niclosamide	Anthelmintic	
Nicobid	Niacin	Vitamin	
Nicotinex	Niacin	Vitamin	
Niferex	Iron-polysaccharide complex	Mineral, hematinic	
Nilstat	Nystatin	Antifungal agent	
Nipride	Sodium nitroprusside	Antihypertensive agent	Hypotension
Nisentil	Alphaprodine HCl	Narcotic analgesic	Dependency
Nitro-Bid	Nitroglycerin	Antianginal agent	Hypotension
Nitro-Dur	Nitroglycerin	Antianginal agent	Hypotension
Nitroglyn	Nitroglycerin	Antianginal agent	Hypotension
Nitrol	Nitroglycerin	Antianginal agent	Hypotension
Nitropress (see Nipride)			
Nitrospan	Nitroglycerin	Antianginal agent	Hypotension
Nitrostat	Nitroglycerin	Antianginal agent	Hypotension
Nizoral	Ketoconazole	Antifungal agent	
Noctec	Chloral hydrate	Hypnotic	Dependency
Nolamine	Phenylpropanolamine HCl	Sympathomimetic	
	Chlorpheniramine maleate	Antihistamine	
	Phenindamine	Antihistamine	
	Phenindamine tartrate	Antihistamine	

(Continued)

Trade Name	Generic Name	Classification	Significant or Serious Reactions
Noludar	Methyprylon	Hypnotic	Dependency
Nolvadex	Tamoxifen citrate	Antineoplastic agent	
Norflex	Orphenadrine citrate	Skeletal muscle relaxant	
Norgesic	Orphenadrine citrate	Skeletal muscle relaxant	
	Aspirin	Nonsteroidal antiinflammatory agent	Peptic ulcer, GI bleeding
	Caffeine	Cerebral stimulant	
Norinyl	Norethindrone	Progestin hormone	Thromboembolism
	Mestranol	Estrogen hormone	
Norisodrine Sulfate	Isoproterenol HCl	Sympathomimetic	
Norlestrin	Norethindrone acetate	Progestin hormone	Thromboembolism
	Ethinyl estradiol	Estrogen hormone	
Norlutate	Norethindrone acetate	Progestin hormone	Thromboembolism
Norpace	Disopyramide phosphate	Antiarrhythmic agent	Hypotension, congestive heart failure
Norpramin	Desipramine HCl	Antidepressant	
Novafed	Pseudoephedrine HCl	Sympathomimetic	
Novahistine-DH	Codeine phosphate	Antitussive agent	
	Chlorpheniramine maleate	Antihistamine	
	Phenylpropanolamine HCl	Sympathomimetic	
Novocain	Procaine HCl	Local anesthetic	
Novrad	Levopropoxyphene	Antitussive agent	
NPH Iletin I	Insulin injection isophane	Hormone	
NTZ Nasal	Phenylephrine HCl	Sympathomimetic	
	Phenyldiamine HCl	Sympathomimetic	
Nubain	Nalbuphine HCl	Narcotic analgesic	Dependency
Numorphan	Oxymorphone HCl	Narcotic analgesic	Dependency
Nupercaine	Dibucaine HCl	Topical anesthetic	
Nutraplus	Urea	Dermatologic preparation	
Nydrazid	Isoniazid	Antimycobacterial agent	Hepatotoxicity
Nytol	Pyrilamine	Antihistamine	

O			
Omnipen	Ampicillin	Antibiotic	Anaphylaxis
Oncovin	Vincristine sulfate	Antineoplastic agent	Leukopenia, neuropathy
Onset	Isosorbid dinitrate	Antianginal agent	Hypotension
Ophthochlor	Chloramphenicol	Ophthalmic antibiotic preparation	
Opticrom	Cromolyn	Ophthalmic preparation	
Optimine	Azatadine maleate	Antihistamine	
Orasone	Prednisone	Corticosteroid	Cushing's syndrome
Oratrol	Dichlorphenamide	Carbonic anhydrase inhibitor	
Oretic (see Hydro-DIURIL)			
Oreton	Methyltestosterone	Androgen	
Orgatrax (see Vistaril)			
Orinase	Tolbutamide	Oral antidiabetic agent	Hypoglycemia
Ornade	Phenylpropanolamine HCl	Sympathomimetic	
	Chlorpheninamine maleate	Antihistamine	
Ortho-Novum preparations	Norethindrone	Progestin	Thromboembolism
	Ethinyl estradiol	Estrogen	
Os-Cal	Calcium carbonate	Mineral	
Otobione	Neomycin sulfate	Topical preparation	
	Polymyxin B sulfate	Topical preparation	
	Hydrocortisone	Topical preparation	
Otobiotic	Neomycin sulfate	Topical otic antibiotic	
Otrivin	Xylometazoline HCl	Topical nasal sympathomimetic	
Ovcon	Norethindrone	Progestin	Thromboembolism
Ovral	Ethinyl estradiol	Estrogen	Thromboembolism
	Norgestrel	Progestin	Thromboembolism
Ovrette	Norgestrel	Progestin	Thromboembolism
Ovulen	Ethynodiol diacetate	Progestin	Thromboembolism
	Mestranol	Estrogen	
Oxalid	Oxyphenbutazone	Nonsteroidal antiinflammatory agent	Bone marrow depression, hepatitis, nephrotoxicity, peptic ulcer
Oxsoralen	Methoxsalen	Dermatologic preparation	
Oxylone	Fluorometholone	Topical corticosteroid	

(Continued)

Trade Name	Generic Name	Classification	Significant or Serious Reactions
P			
P-200 (see Pavabid)			
Pagitane HCl	Cycrimine HCl	Anticholinergic	
Pallace	Megestrol acetate	Estrogen	Thromboembolism
Pamelor	Nortriptyline HCl	Antidepressant	
Pamine	Methscopolamine bromide	Anticholinergic	
Pancrease	Pancrelipase	Digestive enzyme	
Panheprin	Heparin sodium	Anticoagulant	Bleeding diathesis
Panmycin	Tetracycline	Antibiotic	
Panwarfin	Warfarin sodium	Anticoagulant	Bleeding diathesis
Paradione	Paramethadione	Vitamin K analog	
Paraflex	Chlorzoxazone	Skeletal muscle relaxant	
Parafon Forte	Chlorzoxazone	Skeletal muscle relaxant	
	Acetaminophen	Nonnarcotic analgesic	
Paral	Paraldehyde	Hypnotic	Pulmonary edema on IV use
Parasal Sodium	Aminosalicylate sodium	Antimycobacterial agent	Peptic ulcer, GI bleeding
Paredrine	Hydroxyamphetamine hydrobromide	Sympathomimetic	
Parepectolin	Pectin	Antidiarrheal	
	Kaolin	Antidiarrheal	
	Opium tincture	Narcotic antidiarrheal	Dependency
Parest	Methaqualone HCl	Hypnotic	Dependency
Parlodel	Bromocriptine mesylate	Antiparkinsonian agent	Psychosis, extrapyramidal reactions
Pathibamate (see Milpath)			
Pathilon	Tridihexethyl chloride	Anticholinergic	
	Phenobarbital	Hypnotic	Dependency
Pathocil	Dicloxacillin sodium	Antibiotic	Anaphylaxis
Pavabid	Papaverine HCl	Vasodilator	
Paveril	Dioxyline	Vasodilator	
Pavulon	Pancuronium bromide	Neuromuscular blocker	Respiratory paralysis
Paxipam	Halazepam	Antianxiety agent	
PBZ	Tripelennamine citrate	Antihistamine	

Pediamycin	Erythromycin ethylsuccinate	Antibiotic	
Pediazole	Erythromycin ethylsuccinate	Antibiotic	
	Sulfisoxazole acetyl	Antimicrobial agent	Nephrotoxicity, hypersensitivity
Peganone	Ethotoin	Anticonvulsant	
Penthrane	Methoxyflurane	General anesthetic	Hepatotoxicity, nephrotoxicity
Pentids	Penicillin G potassium	Antibiotic	Anaphylaxis
Pentostam	Sodium stibogluconate	Antiprotozoal agent	
Pentothal	Thiopental sodium	General anesthetic	Respiratory depression
Pentritol (see Peritrate)			
Pen-Vee K	Penicillin V potassium	Antibiotic	Anaphylaxis
Pepto-Bismol	Bismuth subsalicylate	Antidiarrheal agent	
Percocet-5	Oxycodone HCl	Narcotic analgesic	Dependency
	Acetaminophen	Nonnarcotic analgesic	
Percodan	Oxycodone HCl	Narcotic analgesic	Dependency
	Oxycodone terephthalate	Narcotic analgesic	
	Aspirin	Nonsteroidal antiinflammatory agent	
Percogesic	Acetaminophen	Nonnarcotic analgesic	
	Phenyltoloxamine citrate	Nonnarcotic analgesic	
Percorten Pivalate	Desoxycorticosterone pivalate	Corticosteroid	Cushing's syndrome
Pergonal	Menotropins	Pituitary hormone	
Periactin	Cyproheptadine HCl	Antihistamine	
Peri-Colace	Casanthranol, docusate sodium	Laxatives	
Peritrate	Pentaerythritol tetranitrate	Antianginal agent	Hypotension
Permitil	Fluphenazine HCl	Antipsychotic agent	Extrapyramidal reactions
Persantine	Dipyridamole	Antianginal agent	
Pertofrane (see Norpramin)			
Petrogalar Plain	Mineral oil	Laxative	
Pharmalgen	Hymenoptera venom allergens	Biological preparations	
Phase III	Triclosan	Dermatologic preparations	
Phazyme	Simethicone	Digestive enzyme	
	Pancreatin	Digestive enzyme	
Phenergan	Promethazine HCl	Antihistamine (antiemetic)	

(Continued)

Trade Name	Generic Name	Classification	Significant or Serious Reactions
Phenergan Expectorant	Promethazine HCl	Antihistamine	
	Guaiacolsulfonate potassium, citric acid, sodium citrate	Expectorants	
Phenolax	Phenolphthalein	Laxative	
Phentrol (see Fastin)			
Phenurone	Phenacemide	Anticonvulsant	Bone marrow depression, hepatotoxicity
pHisoHex	Hexachlorophene	Detergent dermatologic preparation	
Phyllocontin	Aminophylline	Bronchodilator	
Pilocar	Pilocarpine HCl	Cholinergic ophthalmic preparation	
Pilocel (see Pilocar)			
Pipracil	Piperacillin sodium	Antibiotic	Hypersensitivity
Pitocin	Oxytocin	Pituitary hormone	Anaphylaxis
Pitressin Synthetic Tannate	Vasopressin	Pituitary hormone	Anaphylaxis
Placidyl	Ethchlorvynol	Hypnotic	Dependency
Plaquenil Sulfate	Hydroxychloroquine	Antimalarial agent	Retinopathy
Plasmanate	Plasma protein fraction	Volume expander	Hypersensitivity
Platinol	Cisplatin	Antineoplastic agent	Bone marrow depression, ototoxicity, nephrotoxicity
Plegine	Phendimetrazine tartrate	Sympathomimetic	
Podoben	Podophyllin	Dermatologic preparation	
Polaramine	Dexchlorpheniramine maleate	Antihistamine	
Polycillin	Ampicillin	Antibiotic	Anaphylaxis
Polydine (see Betadine)			
Polymox (see Amoxil)			
Polysporin	Bacitracin Polymyxin B	Topical antibiotic	

Pondimin	Fenfluramine HCl	Sympathomimetic	
Ponstel	Mefenamic acid	Nonnarcotic analgesic	
Pontocaine HCl	Tetracaine HCl	Topical anesthetic	
Potassium Triplex	Potassium bicarbonate Potassium gluconate Potassium citrate Ammonium chloride	Oral potassium solution	
Povan	Pyrvinium pamoate	Anthelmintic	
Pragmatar	Coal tar, sulfur, salicylic acid	Dermatologic preparation	
Predalone RP	Prednisolone acetate	Corticosteroid	Cushing's syndrome
Pregnyl	Gonadotropin, chorionic	Hormone	
Preludin	Phenmetrazine HCl	Sympathomimetic	
Premarin	Estrogens, conjugated	Estrogen	Thromboembolism
Pre-Pen	Benzylpenicilloyl-poly-L-lysine	Skin test for penicillin allergy	
Pre-Sate	Chlorphentermine HCl	Sympathomimetic	
Principen (see Polycillin)			
Prioderm	Malathion	Topical pediculicidal agent	
Privine HCl	Naphazoline HCl	Sympathomimetic nasal preparation	
Pro-Banthine	Propantheline bromide	Anticholinergic	
Procan	Procainamide HCl	Antiarrhythmic	Agranulocytosis, "lupus syndrome"
Procardia	Nifedipine	Antianginal agent	Hypotension, edema
Proctofoam-HC	Hydrocortisone Pramoxine HCl	Topical rectal corticosteroid Topical anesthetic	
Profasi HP (see Pregnyl)			
Proglycem (see Hyperstat)			
Proketazine	Carphenazine maleate	Antipsychotic agent	Extrapyramidal reactions
Prolixin	Fluphenazine	Antipsychotic agent	Extrapyramidal reactions

(Continued)

Trade Name	Generic Name	Classification	Significant or Serious Reactions
Proloid	Thyroglobulin	Thyroid hormone	Thyrotoxicosis
Proloprim	Trimethoprim	Antimicrobial agent	
Pronestyl	Procainamide HCl	Antiarrhythmic	Agranulocytosis, "lupus syndrome"
Propadrine	Phenylpropanolamine HCl	Sympathomimetic	
Prostigmin	Neostigmine bromide	Cholinergic	
Prostin E_2	Dinoprostone	Prostaglandin hormone	
Prostin F_2 Alpha	Dinoprost tromethethamine	Prostaglandin hormone	
Protaphane	Insulin injection isophane	Insulin	Hypoglycemia
Proventil	Albuterol sulfate	Sympathomimetic	
Provera	Medroxyprogesterone acetate	Progestin	Thromboembolism
Purified Lente	Insulin zinc suspension	Insulin	Hypoglycemia
Purified NPH	Insulin injection isophane	Insulin	Hypoglycemia
Purinethol	Mercaptopurine		
Purodigin	Digitoxin	Digitalis preparation	Cardiac arrhythmias
Pyopen	Carbenicillin disodium	Antibiotic	Anaphylaxis
Pyridium	Phenazopyridine HCl		
Q			
Quāālude	Methaqualone	Hypnotic	Dependency
Quadrinal	Theophylline	Bronchodilator	Arrhythmias
	Ephedrine HCl	Sympathomimetic	Arrhythmias
	Butabarbital	Hypnotic	Dependency
	Guaifenesin	Expectorant	
Quarzan	Clidinium bromide	Anticholinergic	
Quelicin	Succinylcholine chloride	Neuromuscular blocker	Respiratory paralysis
Questran	Cholestyramine resin	Antilipemic agent	
Quibron	Theophylline	Bronchodilator	Arrhythmias
	Guaifenesin	Expectorant	
Quide	Piperacetazine	Antipsychotic agent	Extrapyramidal reactions
Quinaglute	Quinidine gluconate	Antiarrhythmic agent	Arrhythmias, heart block
Quinidex	Quinidine sulfate	Antiarrhythmic agent	Arrhythmias, heart block
R			
Raudixin	Rauwolfia serpentina	Antihypertensive	Ulcers, depression
Rauwiloid	Alseroxylon	Antihypertensive	Ulcers, depression

Rauzide	Rauwolfia serpentina	Antihypertensive	Ulcers, depression
	Bendroflumethiazide	Diuretic	Hypokalemia
Redisol	Cyanocobalamin	Vitamin B_{12}	
Regitine	Phentolamine	Vasodilator	Hypotension
Reglan	Metoclopramide	Miscellaneous gastrointestinal drug	Extrapyramidal reactions
Regonol (see Mestinon)			
Regroton	Reserpine	Antihypertensive	Ulcers, depression
	Chlorthalidone	Diuretic	Hypokalemia
Rela	Carisoprodol	Skeletal muscle relaxant	
Relafact	Protirelin	Thyrotropin releasing hormone	Thyrotoxicosis
Remsed	Promethazine HCl	Antipsychotic agent	Extrapyramidal reactions
Renalgin (see Hiprex)			
Renese	Polythiazide	Diuretic	Hypokalemia
Renoquid	Sulfacytine	Antimicrobial agent	Allergic reactions, blood dyscrasias
Repen-VK	Penicillin V potassium	Antibiotic	Anaphylaxis
Reserpoid (see Serpasil)			
Resolve	Dyclonine HCl	Topical anesthetic	
Restoril	Temazepam	Hypnotic	Dependency
Retin-A	Tretinoin	Dermatologic preparation	
Rhinex	Phenylephrine HCl	Sympathomimetic	
	Chlorpheniramine maleate	Antihistamine	
	Aspirin	Nonsteroidal antiinflammatory agent	
RhoGAM	Rh_0 (D) immune globulin	Biological preparation	Anaphylaxis, serum sickness
Ridaura (see Myochrysine)			
Rifadin	Rifampin	Antimycobacterial agent	Hepatitis
Rifamate	Rifampin isoniazid	Antimycobacterial agent	Hepatitis

(Continued)

Trade Name	Generic Name	Classification	Significant or Serious Reactions
Rimactane (see Rifadin)			
Riopan	Aluminum hydroxide	Antacid	Constipation
Ritalin	Methylphenidate HCl	Cerebral stimulant	Dependency
Ro Trim (see Fastin)			
Robamox	Amoxicillin trihydrate	Antibiotic	Anaphylaxis
Robaxin	Methocarbamol	Skeletal muscle relaxant	
Robaxisal	Methocarbamol	Skeletal muscle relaxant	
	Aspirin	Nonsteroidal antiinflammatory agent	Ulcers, GI bleeding
Robicillin VK (see Pen-Vee K)			
Robimycin (see Erythrocin)			
Robinul	Glycopyrrolate	Anticholinergic	
Robitet	Tetracycline HCl	Antibiotic	
Robitussin	Guaifenesin	Expectorant	
Rocaltrol	Calcitrol	Vitamin D derivative	
Rolaids	Dihydroxyaluminum sodium carbonate	Antacid	
Rondec	Pseudoephedrine HCl	Sympathomimetic	
	Carbinoxamine maleate	Antihistamine	
Rondomycin	Methacycline HCl	Antibiotic	
Roniacol	Nicotinyl alcohol	Vasodilator	
Rubramin PC	Cyanocobalamin	Vitamin B_{12}	
Rufen (see Motrin)			
Rynatan	Phenylephrine tannate	Sympathomimetic	
	Chlorpheniramine tannate	Antihistamine	
Rynatuss	Carbetapentane tannate	Antitussive agent	
	Chlorpheniramine tannate	Antihistamine	
	Ephedrine tannate	Sympathomimetic	
	Phenylephrine tannate	Sympathomimetic	

S			
Saluron	Hydroflumethiazide	Diuretic	Hypokalemia
Salutensin	Hydroflumethiazide	Diuretic	
	Reserpine	Antihypertensive	Ulcers, depression
Sandril (see Serpasil)			
Sanorex	Mazindol	Sympathomimetic	
Sansert	Methysergide maleate	Antimigraine agent	Retroperitoneal fibrosis
Sarenin	Saralasin acetate	Antihypertensive	Hypertension
S.A.S. - 500 (see Azulfidine)			
Sātric (see Flagyl)			
Savacort	Prednisolone acetate	Corticosteroid	Cushing's syndrome
Scabene	Lindane	Topical scabicidal agent	
Seconal	Secobarbital	Hypnotic	Dependency
Sectral	Acebutolol	Antihypertensive	A-V block
Sed-Tens-Se	Homatropine methylbromide	Anticholinergic	
Senokot	Senna pod preparation	Laxative	
Sensorcaine	Bupivacaine HCl	Local anesthetic	
Septisol	Hexachlorophen	Detergent	
Septra (see Bactrim)			
Ser-Ap-Es	Reserpine	Antihypertensive	Ulcers, depression
	Apresoline	Antihypertensive	
	Hydrochlorothiazide	Diuretic	Hypokalemia
Serax	Oxazepam	Antianxiety agent	
Serentil	Mesoridazine besylate	Antipsychotic agent	Extrapyramidal reactions
Seromycin	Cycloserine	Antimycobacterial agent	
Serophene	Clomiphene citrate	Miscellaneous infertility agent	
Serpasil	Reserpine	Antihypertensive	Ulcers, depression
Servin	Carbaryl	Pediculicidal agent	
Silain (see Mylicon)			
Silvadene	Silver sulfadiazine	Antimicrobial agent	

(Continued)

Trade Name	Generic Name	Classification	Significant or Serious Reactions
Sinemet	Levodopa	Antiparkinson agent	Dyskinesia
	Carbidopa	Antiparkinson agent	
Sinequan	Doxepin HCl	Antidepressant	
Sinutab	Phenylpropanolamine HCl	Sympathomimetic	
	Phenyltoloxamine citrate	Antihistamine	
Slo-Phyllin	Theophylline	Bronchodilator	Cardiac arrhythmias
Slow-K	Potassium chloride	Electrolyte	Jejunal ulcers
Sodium Edecrin (see Edecrin)			
Sodium Versenate	Edetate disodium	Used to treat hypercalcemia	
Solarcaine	Benzocaine	Topical anesthetic	
Solfoton	Phenobarbital	Anticonvulsant	
Solganal (see Myochrysine)			
Solu-Cortef	Hydrocortisone sodium succinate	Corticosteroid	Cushing's syndrome
Solu-Medrol	Methylprednisolone	Corticosteroid	Cushing's syndrome
	Sodium succinate	Corticosteroid	
Soma	Carisoprodol	Skeletal muscle relaxant	
Soma Compound	Carisoprodol	Skeletal muscle relaxant	
	Phenacetin	Analgesic	
	Caffeine	Cerebral stimulant	
Sominex	Pyrilamine	Antihistamine	
Somophyllin	Theophylline	Bronchodilator	
Sorbitrate	Isosorbide dinitrate	Antianginal agent	Hypotension
Sotalex	Sotalol	Antihypertensive	A-V block
Sparine	Promazine HCl	Antipsychotic agent	Extrapyramidal reactions
Spectrobid	Bacampicillin HCl	Antibiotic	Anaphylaxis
SPRX - 105	Phendimetrazine tartrate	Sympathomimetic	Dependency
Stadol	Butorphanol tartrate	Narcotic analgesic	
Staphcillin	Methicillin sodium	Antibiotic	Anaphylaxis, nephrotoxicity
Staticin (see Erythrocin)			
Statobex	Phendimetrazine tartrate	Sympathomimetic	Dependency
Stelazine	Trifluoperazine HCl	Antipsychotic agent	Extrapyramidal reactions

Sterane	Prednisolone	Corticosteroid	Cushing's syndrome
Steribolic	Methandriol dipropionate	Androgen	
Stilphostrol	Diethylstilbestrol diphosphate	Estrogen	Neoplasm, thromboembolism
Stoxil	Idoxuridine	Antiviral agent	
Streptase	Streptokinase	Enzyme	
Sublimaze	Fentanyl citrate	General anesthetic	Rigidity
Sucostrin	Succinylcholine chloride	Neuromuscular blocker	Respiratory paralysis
Sudafed	Pseudoephedrine HCl	Sympathomimetic	
Sulamyd	Sulfacetamide sodium	Topical antimicrobial agent	
Sulfacet-15 (see Sulamyd)			
Sulfamylon	Mafenide acetate	Topical antimicrobial agent	
Sulfose	Trisulfapyrimidine	Antimicrobial agent	
Sultrin	Sulfathiazole	Antimicrobial agent	
	Sulfacetamide, sulfabenzamide	Vaginal cream	
Sumox	Amoxicillin trihydrate	Antibiotic	Anaphylaxis
Sumycin	Tetracycline	Antibiotic	
Supen	Ampicillin	Antibiotic	
Surfak	Docusate calcium	Laxative	
Surfol	Mineral oil	Laxative	
Surgicel	Cellulose, oxidized regenerated	Topical coagulant	
Surital	Thiamylal sodium	General anesthetic	Laryngospasm, respiratory depression
Surmontil	Trimipramine maleate	Antidepressant	
Susadrin	Nitroglycerin	Antianginal agent	Hypotension
Sus-Phrine	Epinephrine	Sympathomimetic	
Sustaire	Theophylline	Bronchodilator	
Sux-cert (see Anectine)			
Symmetrel	Amantadine HCl	Antiparkinsonian agent	
Synacort	Hydrocortisone	Topical corticosteroid	
Synalar	Fluocinolone acetonide	Topical corticosteroid	
Synalgos	Aspirin	Analgesic	
	Caffeine	CNS stimulant	
	Promethazine HCl	Antihistamine	

(Continued)

Trade Name	Generic Name	Classification	Significant or Serious Reactions
Synemol (see Synalar)			
Synkayvite	Menadiol sodium diphosphate	Vitamin K preparation	
Syntocinon	Oxytocin	Pituitary hormone	
T			
Tacaryl	Methdilazine	Antihistamine	
TACE	Chlorotrianisene	Estrogen	
Tagamet	Cimetidine	Miscellaneous gastrointestinal agent	
Talwin	Pentazocine lactate	Analgesic	Hallucinations, dependency
Tandearil	Oxyphenbutazone	Nonsteroidal antiinflammatory agent	Agranulocytosis
Tao	Troleandomycin	Antibiotic	
Tapazole	Methimazole	Antithyroid drug	Agranulocytosis
Taractan	Chlorprothixene	Antipsychotic agent	Extrapyramidal reactions, cholestatic jaundice
Tavist	Clemastine fumarate	Antihistamine	
Tegopen	Cloxacillin sodium	Antibiotic	Anaphylaxis
Tegretol	Carbamazepine	Anticonvulsant	Agranulocytosis
Teldrin	Pseudoephedrine	Sympathomimetic	
Teldrin Multi-Symptom	Chlorpheniramine maleate	Antihistamine	
	Acetaminophen	Nonnarcotic analgesic	
Temaril	Trimeprazine tartrate	Antihistamine	Extrapyramidal reactions, hepatitis
Tempra (see Tylenol)			
Tenormin	Atenolol	Antihypertensive	Heart block
Tensilon	Edrophonium chloride	Cholinergic drug	Cholinergic crisis
Tenuate	Diethylpropion HCl	Sympathomimetic	Dependency
Tepanil (see Tenuate)			
Terfonyl (see Sulfose)			
Terramycin	Oxytetracycline base	Antibiotic	

Teslac	Testolactone	Androgen	Cholestatic jaundice
Tessalon	Benzonatate	Antitussive agent	
Testred (see Oreton)			
Tetracyn	Tetracycline	Antibiotic	
Tetrastatin	Tetracycline	Antibiotic	
	Nystatin	Antifungal agent	
Tetrex	Tetracycline phosphate	Antibiotic	
Theoclear	Theophylline	Bronchodilator	
Theolair	Theophylline	Bronchodilator	
Theophyl	Theophylline	Bronchodilator	
Theostat	Theophylline	Bronchodilator	
Theragran	Multivitamins and minerals		
Thiosulfil	Sulfamethizole	Antimicrobial agent	Hypersensitivity
Thorazine	Chlorpromazine	Antipsychotic agent	Cholestatic jaundice, extrapyramidal reactions
Thyrar	Thyroid USP	Thyroid hormone	Thyrotoxicosis
Thyrolar (see Euthroid)			
Thytropar	Thyrotropin	Thyroid stimulating hormone	Thyrotoxicosis
Ticar	Ticarcillin disodium	Antibiotic	Anaphylaxis
Tigan	Trimethobenzamide HCl	Antiemetic agent	Convulsions, extrapyramidal reactions
Tinactin	Tolnaftate	Topical antifungal agent	
Tindal	Acetophenazine maleate	Antipsychotic agent	Extrapyramidal reactions
T-Ionate-P.A.	Testosterone cypionate	Androgen	Jaundice
Titralac	Calcium carbonate	Antacid	
Tobrex	Tobramycin	Antibiotic	Nephrotoxicity, ototoxicity
Tofranil	Imipramine HCl	Antidepressant	
Tolectin	Tolmetin sodium	Nonsteroidal antiinflammatory agent	Ulcers, GI bleeding
Tolinase	Tolazamide	Oral antidiabetic agent	Hypoglycemia
Topex	Benzoyl peroxide	Dermatologic preparation	
Topicort	Desoximetasone	Topical corticosteroid	
Topsyn (see Lidex)			
Torecan	Thiethylperazine maleate	Antiemetic agent	Extrapyramidal reactions

(Continued)

Trade Name	Generic Name	Classification	Significant or Serious Reactions
Totacillin (see Polycillin)			
Tral	Hexocycilium methylsulfate	Anticholinergic	
Transderm-Nitro	Nitroglycerin	Antianginal agent	
Transderm-Scōp	Scopolamine	Anticholinergic	
Tranxene	Chlorazepate dipotassium	Antianxiety agent	
Trasicor	Oxprenolol	Antihypertensive agent	Heart block
Trecator-SC	Ethionamide	Antimycobacterial agent	Hepatotoxicity, peripheral neuritis
Tremin (see Artane)			
Trest	Methixene HCl	Anticholinergic	
Triacet (see Aristocort)			
Triaminic	Phenylpropanolamine HCl	Sympathomimetic	
	Pheniramine maleate	Antihistamine	
Triaprin	Acetaminophen	Analgesic	
	Salicylamide	Analgesic	
	Pentobarbital	Hypnotic	Dependency
Triavil	Perphenazine	Antipsychotic agent	Extrapyramidal reactions
	Amitriptyline HCl	Antidepressant	
Tridesilon	Desonide	Topical corticosteroid	
Tridil	Nitroglycerin	Antianginal agent	Hypotension
Tridione	Trimethadione	Anticonvulsant	Dermatitis, aplastic anemia, nephrotoxicity, hepatotoxicity
Trigot (see Hydergine)			
Trilafon	Perphenazine	Antipsychotic agent	Extrapyramidal reactions
Trimox	Amoxicillin trihydrate	Antibiotic	Anaphylaxis
Trimpex (see Proloprim)			
Trinsicon	Ferrous fumarate	Vitamin preparation	
	Cyanocobalamin		
	Intrinsic factor		
	Folic acid		
	Ascorbic acid		

Trisoralen	Trioxsalen	Dermatologic preparation	
Triten	Dimethindene maleate	Antihistamine	
Tri-Vi-Sol	Multivitamin	Multivitamin	
Trobicin	Spectinomycin HCl	Antibiotic	
Trocinate	Thiphenamil HCl	Anticholinergic	
Tronolane	Pramoxine HCl	Topical anesthetic	
Tums	Calcium carbonate	Antacid	
Tusscapine	Noscapine	Antitussive agent	
Tussionex	Hydrocodone	Antitussive agent	
	Phenyltoloxamine	Cation exchange resin	
Tuss-Ornade	Carmiphen edisylate	Antitussive agent	
	Phenylpropanolamine	Sympathomimetic	
Tylenol	Acetaminophen	Nonnarcotic analgesic	
Tylox	Oxycodone HCl	Narcotic analgesic	
	Oxycodone terephthalate	Narcotic analgesic	
	Acetaminophen	Nonnarcotic analgesic	
Tyzine	Tetrahydrozoline HCl	Topical sympathomimetic agent	
U			
Ultracef	Cefadroxil	Antibiotic	Hypersensitivity
Ultralente Iletin I	Insulin zinc suspension	Insulin	Hypoglycemia
Unipen	Nafcillin sodium	Antibiotic	Hypersensitivity
Unipres	Hydralazine HCl	Antihypertensive	"Lupus syndrome"
	Hydrochlorothiazide	Diuretic	Hypokalemia
Unisom	Doxylamine	Antihistamine hypnotic	
Urecholine	Bethanechol chloride	Cholinergic	
Urex (see Hiprex)			
Urispas	Flavoxate HCl	Anticholinergic	
Urobiotic	Oxytetracycline HCl	Antibiotic	
	Sulfamethizole	Antimicrobial agent	Hypersensitivity
	Phenazopyridine HCl	Urinary analgesic	
Uticillin VK (see Pen-Vee K)			
Uticort	Betamethasone benzoate	Topical corticosteroid	

(Continued)

Trade Name	Generic Name	Classification	Significant or Serious Reactions
V			
Vagisec	Nonoxynol-9, edetate sodium, docusate sodium	Topical vaginal preparation	
Valisone	Betamethasone valerate	Topical corticosteroid	
Valium	Diazepam	Antianxiety agent	
Valmid	Ethinamate	Hypnotic	
Valpin 50	Anisotropine methylbromide	Anticholinergic	
Valrelease	Diazepam	Antianxiety agent	
Vancenase	Beclomethasone dipropionate	Topical corticosteroid inhalant	
Vanceril (see Vancenase)			
Vancocin HCl	Vancomycin HCl	Antibiotic	Ototoxicity, nephrotoxicity
Vanobid	Candicidin	Antifungal agent	
Vansil	Oxamniquine	Anthelmintic	Seizures
Vaponefrin	Epinephrine HCl	Sympathomimetic	Arrhythmias, hypertension
Vasodilan	Isoxsuprine HCl	Vasodilator	
Vasosulf	Sulfacetamide sodium	Topical antimicrobial agent	
V-Cillin K (see Pen-Vee K)			
Veetids (see Pen-Vee K)			
Velban	Vinblastine sulfate	Antineoplastic agent	Peripheral neuropathy
Velosef	Cephradine	Antibiotic	Hypersensitivity
Ventolin (see Proventil)			
Vermox	Mebendazole	Anthelmintic	
Versapen	Hetacillin	Antibiotic	Anaphylaxis
Vescol	Labetalol HCl	Antihypertensive	Heart block, bronchospasm
Vesprin	Triflupromazine HCl	Antipsychotic agent, antiemetic agent	Extrapyramidal reactions
Vibramycin	Doxycycline	Antibiotic	

Vioform	Iodochlorhydroxyquin	Topical antimicrobial agent	
Viokase	Pancreatin	Digestive enzyme	
Vira-A	Vidarabine	Antiviral agent	
Viroptic	Trifluridine	Topical antiviral agent	
Visine	Tetrahydrozoline HCl	Topical sympathomimetic	
Visken	Pindolol	Antihypertensive	Heart block, paradoxical hypertension
Vistaril	Hydroxyzine HCl	Antihistamine	
		Antianxiety agent	
Vitron-C	Multivitamin and mineral preparation	Multivitamin hematinic	
Vivactil	Protriptyline HCl	Antidepressant	
Vivonex	Nutritional preparation		
Vontrol	Diphenidol HCl	Antiemetic, antivertigo agent	Hallucinations, psychosis
Voranil	Clortermine HCl	Sympathomimetic	Dependency
W			
Wehless-35	Phendimetrazine tartrate	Sympathomimetic	Dependency
Wescohex (see pHisoHex)			
Westcort	Hydrocortisone valerate	Topical corticosteroid	
Wigraine	Ergotamine tartrate	Antimigraine agent	
	Caffeine	Cerebral stimulant	
	Belladonna alkaloids	Anticholinergic	
WinGel	Aluminum hydroxide	Antacid	
	Magnesium hydroxide	Antacid	
Winstrol	Stanozolol	Androgen	Masculinization
Wyamycin E	Erythromycin ethylsuccinate	Antibiotic	Hepatotoxicity
Wyanoids HC		Topical rectal preparation	
Wycillin	Penicillin G procaine	Antibiotic	Anaphylaxis
Wydase	Hyaluronidase	Enzyme	
Wymox	Amoxicillin trihydrate	Antibiotic	Anaphylaxis
Wytensin	Guanabenz acetate	Antihypertensive	Hypotension arrhythmias

(Continued)

Trade Name	Generic Name	Classification	Significant or Serious Reactions
X			
Xanax	Alprazolam	Antianxiety agent	
Xylocaine	Lidocaine	Antiarrhythmic agent Local anesthetic	Convulsions, heart block
Y			
Yodoxin	Iodoquinol	Amebicidal agent	Myelo-optic neuropathy
Yutopar	Ritodrine HCl	Uterine stimulant	Hypertension, tachycardia
Z			
Zanosar	Streptozocin	Antineoplastic agent	Nephrotoxicity
Zantac	Ranitidine HCl	Miscellaneous gastrointestinal agent	
Zarontin	Ethosuximide	Anticonvulsant	
Zaroxolyn	Metolazone	Diuretic	Hypokalemia
Zephiran	Benzalkonium chloride	Topical antimicrobial agent	
Zide (see Hydro-DIURIL)			
Zovirax	Acyclovir	Topical antiviral agent	Hypersensitivity
Zyloprim	Allopurinol	Antigout agent	Hepatotoxicity

INDEX

Page numbers followed by f represent figures; those followed by t represent tables.